A Clinical Guide to
ADVANCED MINIMUM
INTERVENTION RESTORATIVE
DENTISTRY

A Clinical Guide to ADVANCED MINIMUM INTERVENTION RESTORATIVE DENTISTRY

Professor Avijit Banerjee

BDS MSc PhD (Univ. of Lond) LDS FDS (Rest Dent) FDS RCS
(Eng) FCGDent FICD FHEA

Chair in Cariology & Operative Dentistry; Programme Director,
Masters in Advanced Minimum Intervention Restorative Dentistry,
Faculty of Dentistry, Oral & Craniofacial Sciences,
King's College London

Honorary Consultant, Restorative Dentistry, Guy's & St. Thomas'
Hospitals Trust
London, UK

ELSEVIER

ISBN: 978-0-443-10971-3

Content Strategist: Alexandra Mortimer
Content Project Manager: Ayan Dhar
Design: Miles Hitchen
Marketing Manager: Deborah Watkins

Printed in India by Replika Press Pvt Ltd.

Last digit is the print number: 9 8 7 6 5 4 3 2 1

Working together to grow libraries in developing countries

www.elsevier.com • www.bookaid.org

FOREWORD

Conserving teeth continues to dominate the clinical practice of dentistry. As such, this clinical guide—a most welcome addition to the dental literature—is central to adopting and applying a person-focused, minimum intervention oral healthcare framework, including minimally invasive operative dentistry, in the best interests of patients and, amongst other things, using state-of-the-art, sustainable dental biomaterials and technologies to best possible advantage.

Professor H.M. Pickard, the original author of *Pickard's Guide to Minimally Invasive Operative Dentistry*, would be amazed but delighted to read this contemporary clinical guide. How operative dentistry has moved on and evolved, with Avijit Banerjee being the third-generation proponent of Professor Pickard's quest to promote the application of best available evidence in the management of diseased and damaged teeth. Mechanistic, extensively interventive approaches based on cavity preparations of prescribed design are well and truly assigned to history, having been replaced by non-, micro- and minimally invasive approaches as part of minimum intervention oral care (MIOC), which in turn is part of sustainable holistic, whole-patient healthcare. Also, the time has come where patients are cared for by a dentist-led team of oral healthcare professionals, rather than being treated by a dentist variously supported by different dental personnel.

This clinical guide champions the adoption and practice of MIOC, specifically in the prevention and management of dental caries and toothwear. Importantly, this guide promotes the integration of prevention; minimally invasive operative dentistry; and phased, personalised patient care pathways—a powerful triad of

sustainable measures to combat and control dental caries and toothwear, let alone related oral disease.

Notwithstanding the above, this carefully crafted guide is a pleasure to read. It makes full use of bullet points, tables, diagrams and flowcharts and includes a large number of high-quality clinical images to enhance the clear, concise, easy-to-read text. Professor Banerjee is to be congratulated on his meticulous, well-planned, thought-provoking work, providing dental students and graduate dentists, dental therapists, dental hygienists and others seeking to update their knowledge and understanding of the conservation of teeth with a superb guide to advanced minimum intervention restorative dentistry.

It is hoped that the guide realises its goals of enhanced understanding and ever-increasing adoption and widespread practice of MIOC, resulting in more high-quality clinical outcomes, increased longevity of restorations, and many more patients valuing and taking responsibility for their oral health.

This clinical guide supersedes existing textbooks on operative and conservative dentistry. It's time to get up to date on the core element of the clinical practice of dentistry!

Professor Sir Nairn Wilson CBE DSc(*h.c.*) DDent(*h.c.*) PhD MSc BDS FCGDent FDS *RCS Edin, Eng (Hon) & RCPS Glasg(Hon)* FFD*(Hon)* FCDSHK*(Hon)* DRD FHEA FICD FACD FADM FPFA FKC

Emeritus Professor of Dentistry, King's College London, President Emeritus, College of General Dentistry

PREFACE

With the ongoing advances in the clinical practice of conservative dentistry, and after having the honour of co-authoring the last two editions of *Pickard's Guide to Minimally Invasive Operative Dentistry*, published over the last 15 years, I felt in 2021 that it was high time to revisit the discipline of advanced minimum intervention restorative dentistry.

It is my privilege to author this work, building on the legacy of Professor H.M. Pickard and past authors of his eponymous textbook, the late Professor Bernard Smith, Professor Edwina Kidd and more recently, Professor Timothy Watson, all titans in the fields of restorative dentistry, cariology and dental biomaterials science as well as being my teachers, gurus, colleagues and friends over the years.

A Clinical Guide to Advanced Minimum Intervention Restorative Dentistry aims to describe the clinical implementation of the *minimum intervention oral care (MIOC)* delivery framework in primary care, specifically to manage dental caries and toothwear. This is the modern oral healthcare team–delivered, person-focused, prevention-based and risks/needs-related approach to managing patients with oral and dental disease. The beauty of MIOC lies in its pragmatic simplicity, utilising the oral healthcare workforce, resources and technology available in general dental practice to develop phased, personalised care pathways based on the four interlinking clinical domains of (1) *identifying/determining* the problem, (2) *preventing* lesions/*controlling* disease processes, (3) *minimally invasive* operative interventions (often known as minimally invasive dentistry; MID) and (4) person-focused *recall/reassessment/active surveillance*.

This book is ideal for student and graduate dentists, dental hygienists, dental therapists and those taking further professional education courses worldwide (including dental nursing, dental hygiene and therapy as well as specialist training programmes). It will take the reader on a journey, from appreciating the latest concepts in the aetiology and histopathological development of dental disease, through the clinical management pathway following the four clinical domains of MIOC highlighted above, with the goal of delivering better long-term oral health to patients and populations as a whole.

Using bullet points, tables, diagrams, flowcharts and high-quality clinical images throughout, this easy-to-read book will enable the reader to learn how to detect, diagnose and risk/susceptibility assess patients with dental disease and conditions affecting the teeth, implementing prevention-based clinical management protocols based upon behaviour modelling. It makes the most of the latest minimally invasive operative technologies, techniques and dental bioactive/bio-interactive materials to conserve, protect and maintain viable dental tissues and the tooth restoration complex for life.

This new book has been enhanced significantly by the reproduction of many high-quality clinical images to help illustrate scientific concepts and clinical protocols. I must personally thank Drs. Michael Thomas, Bhupinder Dawett and Petros Mylonas individually for their unerring assistance in helping me to coordinate and providing a number of these valuable additions. Additionally, I wish to thank my many colleagues and friends from around the world who have permitted me to use their excellent images. They are all duly acknowledged in the captions to the relevant figures together with a source of the original publication where applicable. Dr. Len D'Cruz is acknowledged for his wonderful artwork used on the front cover of the book.

I hope I have reinforced the link between prevention, minimally invasive operative dentistry and phased personalised patient care. This *minimum intervention oral care* philosophy must underpin the sustainable holistic approach to delivering better oral health in the long term in primary care, with an increasing emphasis placed upon the differing important roles of the oral healthcare team. The operative skill set of a new graduate has evolved to encompass not only the techniques, materials and science of minimally invasive dentistry but also the behaviour and expectation management of their patients. Without patients taking responsibility for and valuing their own oral health, even the best operative dentistry will fail, regardless of the materials used and the skills of the operator. As a result of the United Nations Environment Programme Minamata Treaty in 2013, the global environmental impact of the production, use and disposal of dental amalgam has led to recommendations for a phase-out of its clinical use, starting as early as 2025 in some countries, possibly including the United Kingdom soon after. The treaty highlighted the need for increased dental research into caries prevention and alternative, sustainable restorative materials/procedures in conjunction with better professional (and patient) education in their application and maintenance. I sincerely hope that this book goes some way towards achieving the latter.

A.B.
October 2023

CONTENTS

Dental Hard Tissue Pathologies

CHAPTER OUTLINE

1.1 DENTAL CARIES

1.1.1 What Is It?

'It is, in its earliest stages, a reversible but potentially progressive non-communicable disease of the dental hard tissues, instigated histo-pathologically by the action of oral bacteria upon fermentable carbohydrates in the dental plaque biofilm stagnating on susceptible tooth surfaces (the caries process), ultimately leading to tissue damage caused by bacterially-generated acid mineral dissolution (demineralisation) and proteolytic destruction of the organic component of the dental tissues (the carious lesion).'

Dental caries has been classified as one of the most prevalent untreated, non-communicable diseases affecting adults and children globally, by the Global Burden of Disease study carried out by the World Health Organization from 1990 to 2017. It is a behavioural, lifestyle-related, biofilm-mediated condition that can affect all dentate humans, but the latest prevalence and incidence data indicate a predilection towards those in society who are more vulnerable, with higher socio-economic needs and poorer access to oral and dental healthcare.

1.1.2 Terminology

Primary caries is the developing pathological biochemical process in the biofilm with a subsequent physical carious lesion occurring on a previously sound tooth surface.

Root caries is primary caries on an exposed root surface (often after gingival recession has occurred), penetrating more easily into the exposed dentine. The pathological biochemical process in the biofilm for both primary and root caries is the same (Figs. 1.1 and 1.2A–C).

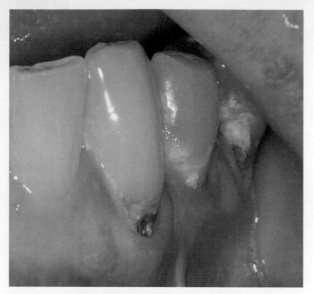

Fig. 1.1 Root surface lesions with dark, leathery dentine surfaces and stagnating surface plaque biofilm deposits, lower left quadrant (LLQ), indicative of active disease. (Courtesy B Dawett and S Young).

Caries associated with restorations and sealants (CARS) is primary caries occurring at the margin of a failing restoration. Alternative terminology includes *secondary or recurrent caries*. The aetiology is the same: metabolic activity in the stagnant plaque biofilm located at the defective margins of existing restorations and/or sealants.

Residual caries is a term sometimes used to describe that portion of caries-affected, demineralised dentine retained purposely after minimally invasive, selective caries excavation procedures have been used during cavity preparation, which is then sealed in with an overlying restoration (see later).

1.1.3 Caries: The Process and the Lesion
1.1.3.1 The Caries Process: Dental Plaque Biofilm
The caries process originates as metabolic activity within the plaque biofilm resident on the tooth surface. This biofilm begins to form just a few minutes after a tooth surface has been brushed and is adsorbed initially as the *acquired pellicle* containing an admix of salivary proteins and glycoproteins. Within a short time, oral bacteria colonise the pellicle, forming the early dental

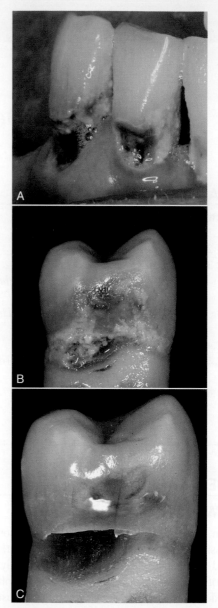

Fig. 1.2 (A) Potentially active root carious lesions in lower right quadrant, with overlying plaque deposits in an area of stagnation associated with poor oral hygiene *(courtesy P Mylonas)*. (B) A stagnant plaque biofilm present on the proximal root surface, which when removed, reveals an active root lesion (C).

Q1.2: What differences in clinical appearance are there between the coronal and root surface carious lesions in Fig. 1.2C and how may these relate to lesion activity?

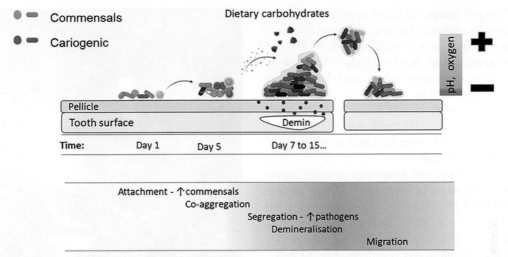

Fig. 1.3 A schematic diagram showing the stages of plaque biofilm development on a tooth surface if left undisturbed. This simulates the ecological plaque hypothesis for dental biofilm development.

plaque biofilm, associated closely with bacterial extra-cellular polysaccharides (EPS) and salivary proteins. The increased density of this developing biofilm and EPS, changing microbial population (*dysbiosis*), pH and oxygen tension combines to eventually create a cariogenic environment on the tooth surface over time (Fig. 1.3). This ubiquitous, natural metabolic process cannot be *prevented*. However, disease progression can be *controlled* by the patient, with the help of the dentist and the oral healthcare team, so that a clinically visible initial enamel lesion never forms. The de- and remineralisation (perhaps more accurately described as mineral loss and crystallisation) cyclical metabolic processes can be modified by regular disturbance of the plaque biofilm with a toothbrush or other oral hygiene aids and use of a fluoride-containing toothpaste. If the biofilm is partially or totally removed at regular close intervals, mineral loss may be stopped or even reversed towards mineral regain (especially in early or *incipient* lesions). The fluoride in toothpaste delays lesion progression primarily by resisting demineralisation and encouraging remineralisation.

1.1.3.2 The Carious Lesion: Dental Hard Tissues

The carious lesion forms within the superficial tooth structure as a direct consequence of the caries process, the metabolic imbalance described earlier, in the overlying plaque biofilm. When factors tip the de-/remineralisation metabolic balance towards mineral

> **Q1.3:** What are the different plaque development hypotheses that have been described in the literature?

loss (microbial dysbiosis, diet, salivary factors, mineral ion concentrations in saliva and time), the histological stages of progressive lesion formation, which if left unchecked ultimately lead to cavitation, can eventually be detected clinically and dealt with accordingly (secondary or tertiary prevention).

1.1.4 Aetiology of the Caries Process

Occurring in the plaque biofilm, the main factors that interplay in the aetiology of the caries process are the presence of:

- *Bacteria*: With colonisation within the plaque biofilm, several hundred different species exist within a complex ecology, dependent on the age and relative stagnancy of the plaque on the tooth surface. *Mutans streptococci* are considered to have an associative (as opposed to causative) role in the caries process and may act as a potential microbiological marker for caries. *Lactobacillus* and *Bifidobacteria* species have been shown to be significant in the caries process, and it is likely that species interaction within the dysbiotic biofilm will instigate and cause carious lesion progression. The latest research also focuses on the roles of fungi (*Candida albicans*) in the potential cariogenicity of a dysbiotic biofilm, its hyphal filaments potentially acting as a structural scaffold for and assisting migration of the developing biofilm, along with the complex multikingdom interplay with the plaque microbiome (Fig. 1.3).

- *Susceptible tooth surfaces (see Chapter 2, Section 2.5.2):* Carious lesions occur on tooth surfaces that have accumulated plaque biofilm for a prolonged period of time; these may include:
    - The depths of pits and fissures on posterior occlusal/buccal surfaces of those teeth which a patient cannot clean effectively with a toothbrush or other oral hygiene aids. These areas on newly erupting molars are particularly susceptible to caries as they are more difficult to access with oral hygiene aids.
    - Proximal surfaces (mesial and distal) *cervical* to the contact points of adjacent teeth (where patients may not floss regularly or at all). These surfaces of particularly imbricated (crowded) teeth can be more susceptible due to the lack of access for oral hygiene aids.
    - Smooth surfaces adjacent to the gingival margin (again an area that patients may often miss with their toothbrush), especially of those teeth that are imbricated, rotated or in-standing in the dental arch.
    - Ledged, overhanging or defective margins of restorations (a plaque trap is created, often not evident to the patient and inaccessible to a toothbrush or floss) (Fig. 1.4).
- *Fermentable carbohydrates:* Plaque bacteria are capable of metabolising certain dietary carbohydrates (including sucrose and glucose; see Table 1.1), producing various organic acids (lactic, acetic, propionic acids) at the tooth surface causing plaque pH to fall within 1 to 3 minutes and initiating mineral loss if the pH drops below 5.5 (critical pH of enamel). The pH can take up to 60 minutes to climb back to normal levels, with this normalisation being aided by the protective buffering capacity of saliva (pH 7.0; Fig. 1.5A–B). This demineralisation/remineralisation cycle occurs continuously on any tooth surface.
- *Time:* Even though the drop in pH commences rapidly, sufficient time is required for the plaque biofilm to produce a *net* mineral loss equating to histological hard tissue damage at the tooth surface. This is due

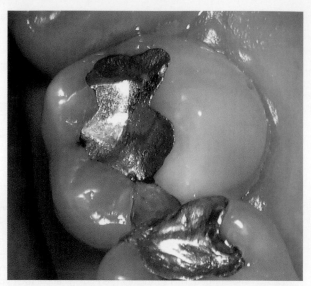

Fig. 1.4 Caries associated with restorations and sealants (CARS - secondary caries) with plaque stagnation in the mesial box of the failed Class II dental amalgam restoration in the UR7.

TABLE 1.1 Simple Classification of Dietary Sugars, with Examples

Mono- and disaccharides	Glucose, galactose, fructose, sucrose, maltose, lactose
Added sugars	All added mono- and disaccharides. Sometimes includes honey and syrups (e.g., maple syrup, agave nectar).
Natural *(intrinsic)* sugars	Sugars physically located in the cellular structure of grains, fruits and vegetables plus those naturally present in milk and milk products
Free sugars *(non-milk extrinsic)*	All sugars added by manufacturers, cook or consumer plus those naturally present in honey and syrups, fruit juices and concentrates

to the metabolic demineralisation–remineralisation cycle that occurs naturally within the biofilm.

These four causes within the oral cavity environment are then influenced by several other indirect factors to ultimately affect the disease pattern experienced by each individual patient. These include:

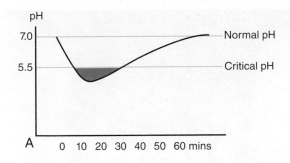

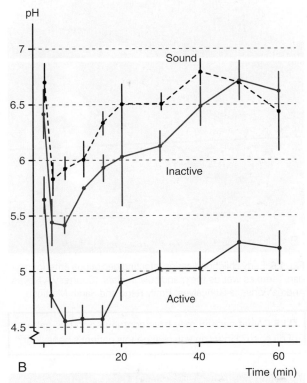

Fig. 1.5 (A) The Stephan curve, showing the changes in plaque pH over time after an oral glucose rinse at time 0 minutes. The critical pH of hydroxyapatite (5.5) is that below which the hydroxyapatite crystals begin to dissociate into its constituent ions. Note that this critical pH varies, depending on an inversely proportional correlation with the concentration of available calcium and phosphate ions in the plaque biofilm fluid at the tooth surface. The grey-shaded portion of the graph indicates the 20-minute period in which the tooth surface is under threat of mineral loss. The critical pH of dentine is 6.2, which again is not fixed. (B) The Stephan curve, showing the changes in plaque pH over time after an oral glucose rinse at time 0 minute, in a healthy patient, a patient with inactive lesions and one who is caries active. These real-time graphs indicate how the oral environment and saliva play an important part in regulating the plaque pH and its rebound back to normal, as mentioned in above.

- Individual-level influences:
  - Personal health behaviours and practices (affected by an individual's capability, opportunity and motivation; see later)
  - Physical and demographic attributes
  - Biologic and genetic endowment
  - Use of dental care provision
  - Dental insurance
- Family-level influences:
  - Health behaviours, practices and coping skills of the family unit/upbringing
  - Culture
  - Family function
  - Parental health status
  - Physical safety
  - Social support
  - Socio-economic status
- Community-level influences:
  - Culture
  - Social capital
  - Community oral health environment
  - Physical environment/safety
  - Characteristics of the healthcare system
  - Characteristics of the oral and dental care system

The relative importance of these factors for a patient can be determined during verbal history taking (*anamnesis*) and oral examination (see Chapter 2, Sections 2.3 and 2.4.2) and help form the basis of determining the individual's susceptibility and likelihood of developing caries in the future; that is, their longitudinal caries risk assessment, susceptibility and likelihood analysis (see Chapter 3, Section 3.3). It is controlling and/or modifying these factors in combination with the collective skills of the oral healthcare team that will help the patient overcome or even 'cure' their condition of dental caries.

1.1.5 Speed and Severity of the Caries Process

The caries process in a normal oral environment, when biofilm metabolism is tipped in favour of mineral loss, will take several weeks to become detectable clinically as a lesion (*signs*) with no patient-reported *symptoms* at this stage. This is because the overall process, with its continuously fluctuating ionic metabolic balance, is relatively slow and can be moderated by oral hygiene techniques used to disrupt biofilm build-up, dietary modification and the use of fluoride or other chemical mineralising agents. The presence of saliva, with its capacity to buffer plaque acids, provides a source of remineralising calcium and phosphate ions to the tooth and/or lesion surface, helping to remove food debris and lubricate or protect tooth surfaces, as well as helping to modulate this balance. Therapeutic radiation in the region of the salivary glands, used in the treatment of orofacial malignant tumours and Sjögren's syndrome, an autoimmune condition which may involve the salivary glands, is the most common cause of severe xerostomia. In addition, a large number of therapeutic drugs, such as antidepressants, tranquillisers, antihypertensives and diuretics (amongst others), can retard salivary flow and affect its quality, especially when taken together (*polypharmacy*). This commonly affects older adults. Physiological ageing can also disrupt the quality and quantity of saliva produced.

However, clinical scenarios exist where the caries process is accelerated and many biochemically active lesions form rapidly, often involving surfaces of teeth ordinarily expected to be caries-free, described historically as 'rampant' caries. This condition affects the primary dentition where it is termed *early childhood caries* (Fig. 1.6A–B), teenagers, or young adults with a highly cariogenic diet (frequent sugar episodes; Fig. 1.7) and/or addiction to recreational drugs, or in adult patients with dry mouth (*xerostomia*), for example.

Early childhood caries A child's oral health begins *in utero*. Poor maternal oral health, malnutrition and exposure to environmental factors (such as alcohol, smoking, certain types of antibiotics and other medications) during pregnancy may lead to preterm birth or low birth weight, disruptions in enamel formation and a predisposition to early childhood caries (ECC) (Fig. 1.6A–B). In addition, societal and economic factors often influence health behaviours and practices of the main caregivers and might lead to poor oral health and ECC development in offspring.

ECC, like other forms of caries, is a biofilm-mediated, sugar-driven, multifactorial, dynamic disease that is determined by biological, behavioural, psychosocial and economic factors linked to an individual's environment. ECC is commonly characterised by its rapid development, its diversity of risk factors and its control. ECC shares common risk factors with other non-communicable diseases (NCDs) associated with excessive sugar consumption, such as diabetes and obesity. According to the Global Burden of Disease

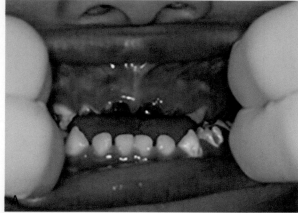
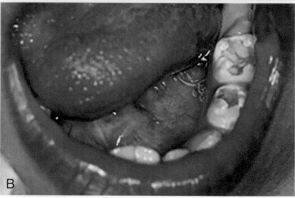

Fig. 1.6 Early childhood caries affecting deciduous anterior maxillary teeth as well as the mandibular molars. (Courtesy A Neves, Andréa Fonseca-Gonçalves, Emily Rêgo and Sarah Martins).

Q1.6: What habit(s) may have contributed to this pattern of disease? How can you change this patient's behaviour?

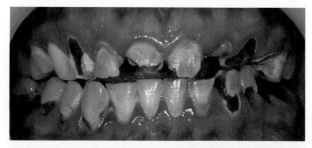

Fig. 1.7 "Rampant" caries in a young adult patient with cavities affecting sites not normally associated with caries due to their adequate accessibility for adequate oral hygiene. (Courtesy M Thomas).

Q1.7: What aetiological factors may have contributed to this pattern of disease?

study in 2017, more than 530 million children globally have dental caries of the primary teeth.

When left untreated, ECC can lead to pain and infection, as well as difficulty in eating, speaking and learning. These difficulties can influence a child's cognitive development, school readiness and self-esteem, reducing their quality of life. Children 0 to 6 years of age are entirely dependent on parents or caregivers, so early oral healthcare interventions that facilitate behaviour changes, successful prevention of caries and management of oral disease, are essential.

1.1.5.1 Definitions

Perinatal care: Medical and nursing care of a woman and her offspring 'around' the natal period; that is, preceding, during and for a short time after childbirth.

Early childhood caries (ECC): The presence of one or more decayed (non-cavitated or cavitated carious lesions), missing or filled (due to caries) surfaces in any primary tooth of a child under 6 years of age.

Primary health care: A whole-of-society approach to health and well-being focused on the needs and preferences of individuals, families and communities. It addresses the broader determinants of health and focuses on the comprehensive and interrelated aspects of physical, mental and social health and well-being.

Arrested or inactive caries In distinct contrast to "rampant" caries, the term *arrested caries* describes those lesions which have stopped progressing and are inactive biochemically. It is observed when factors in the oral environment have changed from conditions predisposing to caries to conditions that tend to slow or even reverse lesion progression. These 'arrested' lesions often have a dark, hard, shiny exposed dentine surface (Fig. 1.8; Table 1.2).

It is important to appreciate that descriptions of carious lesions as being active or inactive really refer to the manifestation of metabolic activity within the overlying plaque biofilm which drives the caries process. This metabolism needs to be appreciated longitudinally over time, and not as a single snapshot in time, in each patient. Any particular lesion will have active demineralisation and inactive periods, depending on when and how the lesion is examined and the oral factors present at that time. It is the job of the clinical practitioner and their team to elucidate, over time, the factors that will influence the overall

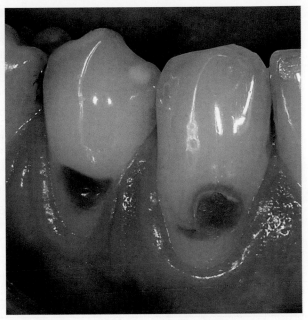

Fig. 1.8 A hard, shiny and stained arrested root surface lesion is present on the buccal cervical aspect of the LR4. The lesion on the LR3, however, has a matte, stippled surface appearance indicative of lesion activity. (From Banerjee A, Watson TF. *Pickard's Guide to Minimally Invasive Operative Dentistry*, 10th ed. Oxford University Press, 2015. Courtesy L Mackenzie).

Q1.8: Why might the lesion on the LR3 appear active whereas the adjacent lesion on the LR4 in the same patient appears arrested?

metabolic balance in the biofilm and therefore the relative activity, or not, of the caries process and the carious lesion. This information then colours the care offered to the patient.

1.1.6 The Carious Lesion

Having summarised the caries process as an ongoing, metabolic de-/remineralisation imbalance occurring at the interface between the plaque biofilm and the tooth surface, it is important to understand that the resulting carious lesion is a progressive initial alteration through to ultimate destruction of the hard tissues (mineral and organic matrix) from the enamel surface to the pulp over time. While the lesion is confined within enamel, it can be arrested and possibly reversed with net mineral gain in its earliest stages. Once into dentine, the process

TABLE 1.2   Differences in Characteristics Between Active and Inactive Carious Lesions in Enamel or Dentine

	CHARACTERISTICS OF THE CARIOUS LESION	
	Active	**Inactive (arrested)**
Enamel	• Frosty white or pale yellow in colour (white spot lesion) • Opaque, loss of lustre • Feels rough when the tip of the ball-ended probe is moved gently across the surface • Lesion in a plaque stagnation area (e.g., pits and fissures, near gingivae, proximal surface below the contact point) • Lesion covered by plaque biofilm prior to examination	• Off-white, brown or black (brown spot lesion) • Shiny • Feels hard and smooth when the tip of the ball-ended probe is moved gently across the surface • On smooth surfaces, lesion typically located at some distance from the gingival margin • Lesion not covered by plaque biofilm prior to examination
Dentine	• Moist and matte • Feels rough • Soft and wet (caries-infected) or leathery (caries-affected) on gentle probing with a dental explorer	• Shiny • Often dark brown • Hard and scratchy on gentle probing with a dental explorer

can be inactivated (arrested), but if extensive proteolytic destruction of the organic collagen matrix has already occurred, this tissue damage cannot be reversed. This section will take the reader through key features of the histological and clinical development of a lesion from its earliest enamel stages through to cavitation into the pulp chamber.

An understanding of the histological features of healthy enamel and dentine is an essential prerequisite to appreciate the changes that occur within a carious lesion, and an outline of these is presented in Chapter 7, Table 7.2. Further information can be gathered from sources offered in the Appendix. The relationship between lesion histology and its clinical appearance has been used in a caries detection and assessment index outlined and detailed in Chapter 2, Table 2.3.

1.1.6.1 Within Enamel

Plaque-acid demineralisation causes porosities within the enamel prism structure, initially beneath the outer surface of enamel, termed *sub-surface demineralisation*. The developing pore volumes through the depth of the enamel lesion, caused by a longer exposure to reduced pH, have been measured using polarised light microscopy (outermost surface zone (<1% pore volume), body (5%–25%), dark (2%–4%) and innermost translucent zone (1%) (Fig. 1.9).

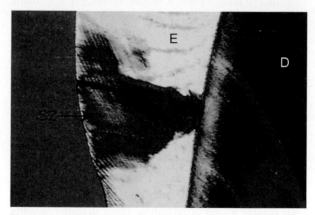

Fig. 1.9 Longitudinal ground section through a carious lesion on a smooth surface (polarised light and water; E, enamel; D, dentine). The enamel lesion is shaped as an inverted cone—widest at the tooth surface, narrowing towards the enamel–dentine junction—with a relatively intact surface zone *(SZ)*. (From Banerjee A, Watson TF. *Pickard's Guide to Minimally Invasive Operative Dentistry*, 10th ed. Oxford University Press, 2015).

Q1.9: What ions have contributed to the creation of the intact surface zone and where have they come from?

The existence of the enamel lesion surface zone may be due to increased extrinsic fluoride ion deposition in this area or as a consequence of net mineral crystal deposition, occurring cyclically at the interface with the overlying biofilm. It is essential that this intact surface is not cavitated iatrogenically (i.e., a hole created by the operator sticking a sharp dental probe or explorer into the lesion surface; see Chapter 2, Fig. 2.9B), as it still has the potential to heal if the biofilm can be regularly and effectively disrupted by the patient and remineralising agents, including toothpastes containing higher concentrations of fluoride, calcium and phosphate ions, are used periodically (see Chapter 4, Section 4.2.3).

Histologically, smooth surface primary lesions have a cross-sectional shape of an inverted cone (widest superficially, apex towards the enamel–dentine junction (EDJ); see Figs. 1.9 and 1.13A–B). Occlusal fissure lesions can be considered to take the form of two opposing smooth surface lesions (Fig. 1.10).

Clinical manifestations (Table 1.2): The active white spot lesion (WSL) is initially smooth, frosty white or opaque and non-cavitated clinically (Fig. 1.11). This can be detected more easily if the tooth surface is air-dried for a few seconds using a 3-1 air-water syringe. As the lesion develops over time, it becomes somewhat chalky, its surface eventually becoming roughened or micro-cavitated

(the roughness is detected by gently running a rounded or ball-ended probe *across* the lesion surface). This surface irregularity can encourage further plaque deposition (Fig. 1.12). There are no symptoms at this stage, but histological reactions from the dentine–pulp complex may be mediated by cytokines and bacterial breakdown products within the dentine matrix and tubules (see later).

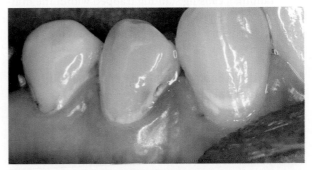

Fig. 1.11 Early white spot enamel lesions on the cervical-gingival margins of mandibular right canine and premolars. Note the more advanced lesion on the LR4.

Q1.11: What clinical sign is visible on the lesion on the LR4 to indicate its relative progression in comparison to the adjacent teeth?

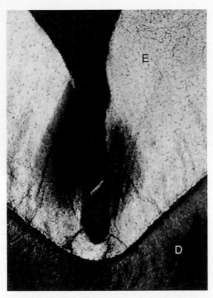

Fig. 1.10 A longitudinal ground section (polarised light with water) through an occlusal fissure showing an enamel lesion forming on the two adjacent walls of the fissure (dark regions; E, enamel; D, dentine). (From Banerjee A, Watson TF. *Pickard's Guide to Minimally Invasive Operative Dentistry*, 10th ed. Oxford University Press, 2015).

Q1.10: How might this be managed in a high caries risk patient?

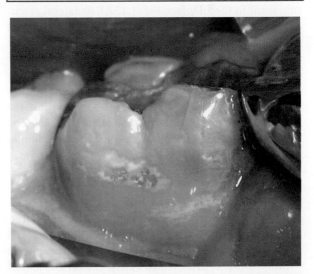

Fig. 1.12 Active white spot enamel lesion on the mid-buccal surface of the LL7. This lesion, which is more developed than that shown in Fig. 1.11) has a rough surface, acting as a plaque trap.

Q1.12: What features of this lesion will help the dentist conclude that it is active, how might these be detected and how might the patient be managed?

If the overlying plaque biofilm is disturbed regularly, the metabolic process can rebalance, allowing lesions to arrest. The subsurface porosities can be eliminated gradually by abrasive toothbrushing and/or tooth-wear, resulting in the hard, smooth, shiny surfaces of such arrested lesions. Porosities may also be filled with deposited mineral crystals and other dietary molecules (e.g., tannins), causing staining trapped within the mineral lattice. This process creates an arrested brown spot lesion (BSL) with a hard, shiny overlying smooth surface (Fig. 1.13B).

1.1.6.2 At the Enamel–Dentine Junction (EDJ)/ Amelo-dentinal Junction

Histologically, the effect of the active caries process often reaches into dentine before any signs of clinical cavitation are detectable (also described as a *closed lesion*). Histological defence reactions in the dentine–pulp complex are stimulated at this stage with evidence of translucent dentine formation at the advancing lesion boundary and tertiary dentine deposition at the dentine–pulp border beneath the advancing lesion (see later). Again, significant patient symptoms are unlikely at this stage of lesion development.

As the lesion extends into dentine, immediately subjacent to the EDJ (see Fig. 1.13A), its lateral extension along the EDJ coincides with the spread of the overlying enamel lesion at the surface of the tooth, which in turn is dependent on the extent of the resident plaque biofilm at the tooth surface. The relatively hypomineralised mantle dentine layer, with greater branching of dentine tubules or defects within the EDJ, may contribute to this spread laterally. The lesion will also penetrate in depth, along the dentine tubules towards the pulp.

1.1.6.3 Within Dentine

Once the lesion has spread histologically (and radiographically) to and beyond the middle third of dentine, it is often cavitated (open) clinically on both occlusal and smooth surfaces with plaque now able to accumulate within the exposed, protected cavity. The further spread of the lesion in dentine will undermine the overlying enamel, creating an associated visible underlying grey shadow or opacity, which becomes brittle and prone to fracture under occlusal loading. This undermined and unsupported enamel, which can act as a further plaque trap protecting the stagnating biofilm from the patient's

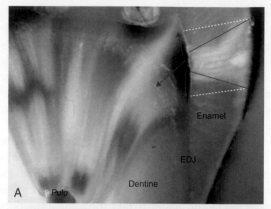

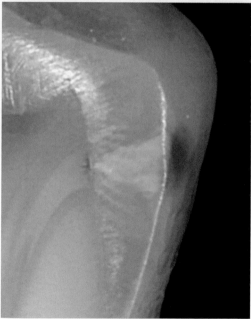

B

Fig. 1.13 (A) A mesio-distal section through a carious tooth highlighting a proximal lesion. The red lines outline the 'inverted cone' cross-sectional histological shape of the enamel lesion and the blue lines outline the direction of spread of the lesion having crossed the enamel–dentine junction (EDJ) into dentine. The white dotted lines show how the extent of the spread of the dentine lesion subjacent to the EDJ is associated with the same lateral extent of the enamel lesion on the tooth surface, both governed by the presence of the plaque biofilm at the tooth surface. (B) The surface lesion shown is an arrested brown spot lesion, its boundaries clearly aligned with the inverted cone of the enamel lesion beneath.

Q1.13B: How might the patient have arrested this once-active lesion?

oral hygiene procedures, may need to be modified and/
or removed during minimally invasive cavity preparation (see Chapter 5, Section 5.9.3).

The patient may begin to experience initial symptoms
of acute pulpitis—a poorly localised sharp pain of a few
seconds' duration provoked by hot, cold or sweet stimuli
(see Chapter 3, Section 3.2.1). The histological components of carious dentine to be considered are the mineral,
collagen, bacterial penetration and tubule structure. Both
degenerative and reparative processes act on these components simultaneously in different parts of the lesion.
The histological changes of the carious dentine biomass
through its depth (from EDJ to pulp) are described as
follows, but note that these descriptive zones are not discrete biological entities, as they blend into one another
without defined, detectable boundaries (Fig. 1.14).

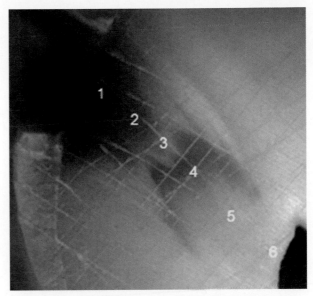

Fig. 1.14 A mesiodistal section through a proximal lesion showing a cavity in the enamel and the histological colour changes
through the dentine lesion (zone 1, caries-infected dentine;
zones 2, 3 and 4, caries-affected dentine; zone 4, translucent
dentine; zones 5 and 6, sound dentine). The crisscross surface scratches were placed to act as reference markers during
microscopy analysis of the sample.

> **Q1.14:** What are the potential causes for the colour
> change in carious dentine?

- *Caries-infected (contaminated) dentine* (zone 1,
  Fig. 1.14): The outermost, superficial, irreparable
  necrotic zone of destruction often distinguished clin-
  ically as a dark brown, soft, wet, 'mushy' layer.
  - Mineral component has dissociated extensively
    due to bacterial acid attack.
  - Collagenous matrix has been denatured (irreparably
    damaged) by proteolytic enzymes intrinsic to the
    dentine itself (zinc-dependent, acid-activated matrix
    metalloproteinases (MMPs) and cathepsins), as well
    as some from bacteria, activated by those bacterial
    acids produced during the caries process.
  - Bacterial contamination in this zone is highest.
  - Dentine tubule structure is destroyed.

This zone of 'necrotic' infected or contaminated dentine
should be removed clinically when preparing a cavity as it
cannot be repaired histologically, provides a poor-quality
bonding substrate for adhesive materials to achieve an
adequate seal and, due to its relative softness, provides
inadequate physical support to any overlying restoration.

- *Caries-affected (demineralised) dentine* (zones 2, 3,
  and 4 combined; Fig. 1.14): The inner zone of carious dentine which can be repaired by the dentine–
  pulp complex, often distinguished as paler brown,
  harder, 'sticky and scratchy' or leathery dentine
  (the surface texture is elicited from tactile feedback using a sharp dental probe, dragged across
  the surface of the dentine; care needs to be taken

when used directly over the pulpal floor of a deep
cavity).
  - Mineral dissolution is still evident but to a lesser
    extent than in infected dentine, as the pH gradu-
    ally rises towards the advancing front of the lesion
    and the ionic equilibrium rebalances.
  - Collagen is still damaged by proteolysis but to a
    lesser extent, therefore permitting dentine repair
    and/or mineral gain as the proteinaceous scaffold
    for mineral crystal deposition now exists.
  - Bacterial load lessens but anaerobic bacteria are
    still present.
  - Dentine tubule structure returns gradually within
    the depths of this zone.

The deepest layer of caries-affected dentine (zone 4,
Fig. 1.14) can be described as hypermineralised translucent dentine (due to its glassy appearance in histological cross-sections), one of several reparative

reactions of the dentine–pulp complex to the caries process (see later). As can be seen in Figs. 1.13A–B and 1.14, the lesion in dentine often has a dark brown discolouration within the caries-infected zone which then pales gradually through the depth of the lesion, towards the pulp. The aetiology of the colour changes is not clear, but a biochemical reaction between proteins and carbohydrates in a moist, acidic biological environment, the *Maillard reaction*, may play a part in this. Not all lesions are uniformly dark brown; some rapidly advancing lesions may have a pale discolouration within the caries-infected zone, and there is no definable link between the colour of dentine and the bacterial load present within these zones.

1.1.7 Carious Pulp Exposure

If the caries process cannot be modified by preventive and/or controlling measures (one of the four clinical domains of the minimum intervention oral care (MIOC) delivery framework; see Chapter 2, Section 2.1) and the lesion is not treated operatively in time with appropriate minimally invasive selective caries removal techniques and a sealed adhesive restoration, then the deeper, advancing front of the lesion will eventually approach the pulp. By this point, bacteria and/or toxins will have penetrated the pulp tissues, causing an acute inflammatory response. Depending on the timescale over which this has happened, an initial acute pulpitic response (poorly localised short, sharp pain on hot, cold or sweet stimuli) will evolve into a more chronic response, changing the symptoms experienced to a dull, prolonged ache that may last several minutes, is spontaneous and is nonspecific in origin (see Chapter 3, Section 3.2.5). The cavity will probably have enlarged due to the weakened, undermined enamel having been broken away (including marginal ridges of proximal lesions) during function and will be noticeable to the patient as 'a hole in the tooth' or *cavity*.

If the pulp chamber is breached physically by the lesion, a *carious exposure* may be created when excavating deep carious dentine and the exposed inflamed pulp tissue will bleed uncontrollably for several minutes before cotton wool pledgets can achieve haemostasis. In many cases with a carious pulp exposure, where the pulp tissue shows signs of necrosis, root canal treatment is the management option of choice (as long as the tooth is restorable with a worthwhile prognosis), but this will depend on the size of the exposure, the age of the patient

(a younger, well-vascularised pulp may have a better survival prognosis) and the ongoing nature of the caries process including whether it has been brought under control by patient preventive measures (see Chapter 4, Section 4.2). In rarer cases, on very late presentation the pulp soft tissues undergo a hyperplastic cellular reaction and appear to herniate through the exposure and into the cavity itself.

If minimally invasive selective caries removal principles and techniques are used to carefully excavate the deeper aspects of the carious lesion, the risk of a carious exposure is reduced significantly (see Chapter 5, Section 5.9). In cases where the pulp is deemed vital, with positive sensibility tests on initial clinical examination, it is a best practice to retain leathery, demineralised caries-affected dentine as an 'indirect pulp cap', sealing the cavity with a suitable long-term adhesive restoration and then reviewing the pulp status at subsequent planned recall appointments. Many clinical trials and systematic reviews of such data to date have showed this to be an effective minimally invasive method to maintain the pulp viability of teeth, therefore reducing the need for root canal treatment (see later).

1.1.8 Dentine–Pulp Complex Reactions

Dentine is a vital tissue containing the cytoplasmic extensions of odontoblasts within the tubules and must be considered together with the pulp since the two tissues are so intimately connected (see Fig. 1.15). The dentine–pulp complex, like any other vital tissue in the body, is capable of defending and repairing itself. The state of the tissue at any time will depend on the balance between the attacking forces and the host defence reactions. The defence reactions include deposition of *translucent dentine*, *tertiary dentine* and *pulp inflammation*.

1.1.8.1 Translucent Dentine

Historically and inaccurately referred to as 'sclerotic' dentine, this glassy zone of dentine (zone 4, Fig. 1.14) is caused by a tubular infill with plate-like whitlockite mineral crystals (β-octocalciumphosphate) at the advancing front of the lesion in an attempt to wall off the advancing lesion. Its appearance is due to the parity of refractive indices of intertubular and intratubular minerals, allowing light photons to pass through the sectioned boundaries with little interference when viewing and imaging them.

The whitlockite crystal deposits originate from a combination of two possible processes:

- A physico-chemical reprecipitation of calcium and phosphate ions released from the low pH heart of the lesion, diffusing towards the increasing pH environment of the lesion's deeper advancing front
- A vital process of new and rapid mineral deposition from the pulp via the odontoblast processes within the patent dentine tubules ahead of the advancing front of the lesion.

Even though hypermineralised, this zone of translucent dentine (zone 4, Fig. 1.14) is actually softer than its deeper, sound counterpart (zones 5, 6, Fig. 1.14) due to the weaker plate-like crystalline orientation of whitlockite compared to conventional hydroxyapatite crystals within the tubules (analogous to stacking dinner plates; too tall a stack and they topple over!) (Fig. 1.16).

1.1.8.2 Tertiary Dentine

Also known as reactionary, reparative, irritation or atubular dentine, this is the tissue that is laid down at the

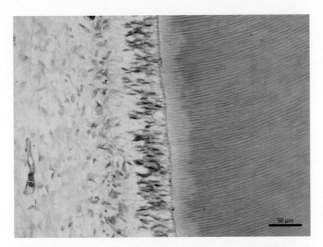

Fig. 1.15 Haematoxylin and eosin (H&E) stained histological section of the normal dentine–pulp complex; the darker pink secondary dentine is on the right-hand side of the image, with visible tubular structure, and the pulp cells are on the left. The polarised odontoblasts can be observed in the mid-section of the image, with the paler stained predentine zone visible at the interface. This zone will undergo mineralisation as part of the physiological ageing process as secondary dentine. (Courtesy Charlotte Jeanneau and Imad About, School of Dental Medicine, Marseille, France).

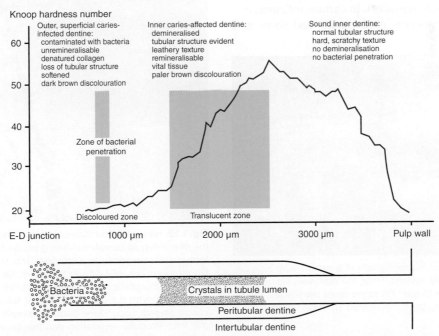

Fig. 1.16 Diagram showing the changes in hardness of carious dentine (y-axis) from the enamel–dentine junction towards the pulp (x-axis) and relating this to the histological changes that occur through the dentine lesion. The translucent zone is softer than the deeper, less mineralised, sound dentine. The diagram below the graph equates the bacterial content and mineral deposition within the tubule lumen through the progressive zones of carious dentine. (Adapted from Ogawa K, Yamashita Y, Ichijo T, Fusayama T. The Ultrastructure and Hardness of the Transparent of Human Carious Dentin. *Journal of Dental Research*. 1983;62(1):7–10. doi:10.1177/00220345830620011701)

dentine–pulp border in response to a noxious stimulus (e.g., caries or those causing toothwear) in an attempt to wall off and distance the pulp from the advancing noxious stimuli (Fig. 1.17). It may resemble secondary dentine histologically but has an irregular tubular or atubular structure, depending on the speed of its creation. *Reactionary dentine* is deposited as a result of a mild irritant where original odontoblasts survive and are metabolically upregulated (Fig. 1.18). *Reparative dentine* is deposited in response to a stronger irritant which compromises the vitality of the original odontoblasts. Progenitor cells from the sub-odontoblastic layer then differentiate and are upregulated to produce an atubular defence reaction (Fig. 1.19).

1.1.8.3 Pulp Inflammation

This is the fundamental response of all vascular connective tissues to injury. Inflammation of the pulp (*pulpitis*) may, as in any other tissue, be acute or chronic. In a slowly progressing carious lesion, toxins reaching the pulp may provoke chronic inflammation. However, once the organisms actually reach the pulp, acute inflammation may supervene. Inflammatory reactions have vascular and cellular components. In chronic inflammation the cellular components predominate and there may

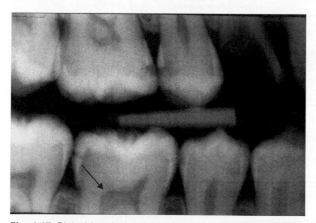

Fig. 1.17 Right bitewing radiograph of a patient with high caries rate and multiple lesions. Note the dentine–pulp complex reparative response of the LR6 to the distal dentine lesion; the distal pulp horn has been obliterated by deposits of tertiary dentine *(arrow)*.

Q1.17: How many other carious lesions can you detect and how would you classify them radiographically?

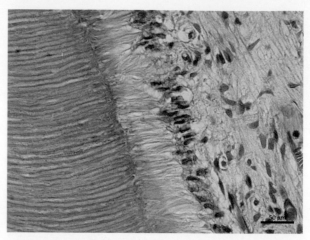

Fig. 1.18 Haematoxylin and eosin (H&E) histological section of the dentine–pulp complex showing reactionary tertiary dentine formation in response to a milder irritant on the pulp cells. Existing odontoblasts *(purple stained line of cells)* are metabolically up-regulated to form new dentine with a similar histological tubular structure to secondary dentine *(pink stained cells on the left)*. (Courtesy Charlotte Jeanneau and Imad About, School of Dental Medicine, Marseille, France).

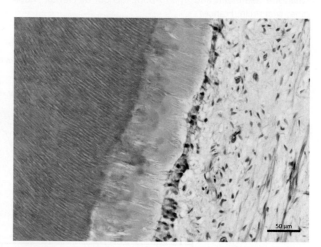

Fig. 1.19 Haematoxylin and eosin (H&E) histological section of the dentine–pulp complex showing reparative tertiary dentine formation in response to a stronger irritant on the pulp cells. Odontoblast-like cells differentiate from the sub-odontoblastic cell layer *(purple stained line of cells)* to form new irregular dentine with no clear histological tubular structure. The image shows secondary dentine *(purple stained cells on the left)*, irregular reparative dentine *(pale pink stained tissue in the centre)*, and odontoblast-like cells (purple stained cells aligned along the interface). (Courtesy Charlotte Jeanneau and Imad About, School of Dental Medicine, Marseille, France).

be increased collagen production, leading to fibrosis but without immediately endangering the vitality of the tooth. In acute inflammation, the vascular changes predominate.

Infection is the most common cause of pulp inflammation and caries is the most common microbial source. Dentine caries will result in pulp inflammation, and chronic inflammatory cells (macrophages, lymphocytes and plasma cells) will infiltrate the pulp near the odontoblast layer. Indeed, this cellular infiltration has been detected in response to initial enamel caries. This chronic inflammatory reaction is due mainly to the movement of bacterial toxins through the dentine tubules. Secretory immunoglobulins travel in the dentine fluid, up the remaining patent tubules. With increasing carious involvement of enamel and dentine, the area of chronic inflammation increases in size but is believed to remain localised until pulp exposure. Bacteria may enter the pulp with polymorphonuclear leucocytes predominating and acute inflammation can supervene, spread throughout the pulp and result in necrosis.

1.2 TOOTHWEAR

'The irreversible surface loss of dental hard tissues caused by factors other than caries or trauma'. Toothwear can be *physiological*, occurring slowly and naturally throughout life, or *pathological*, occurring at a much faster rate and usually caused by combinations of erosion, attrition, abrasion and abfraction (Table 1.3).

Erosion can be defined as the irreversible loss of dental hard tissues by a chemical process (acid attack) not involving bacteria. It is often the common denominator in the multifactorial aetiology of toothwear. Sources of acid can be either intrinsic (stomach acid regurgitation) or extrinsic (dietary, environmental). Involuntary gastro-oesophageal reflux disease (GORD) is a common cause of intrinsic stomach acids entering the oral cavity on a regular basis and occurs primarily due to transient relaxation or incompetence of the lower oesophageal sphincter. Certain factors in combination often predispose to GORD, and these factors may include:

- Diet; fatty, spicy foods consumed in large quantities, especially late at night
- Alcohol
- Certain medications (e.g., diazepam)

- Causes of increased gastric pressure including obesity, pregnancy, posture (lying down increases pressure on the sphincter) and even excessive exercise
- Gastro-oesophageal reflux predisposes to further GORD symptoms
- Neuromuscular conditions

Treatment for GORD will depend on the aetiology. As well as conservative management involving diet and lifestyle modifications and the use of sugar-free chewing gums, stomach acids can be neutralised using conventional antacids (e.g., Gaviscon) or their production limited with oral medications including proton pump inhibitors (e.g., omeprazole (Losec)) or H_2 antagonists (e.g., cimetidine). Surgical procedures can be carried out to repair physical damage to the gastro-oesophageal system. Once this is done, any dental damage can be repaired as required. A carefully taken history from the patient will highlight any functional, aesthetic or sensitivity concerns that would indicate minimally invasive operative dental intervention in the first instance. More long-term extensive toothwear damage may require more invasive indirect restoration. The patient's oral health clinician may often be the first to notice the problem through the dental manifestations and appropriate referral to medical colleagues may be required.

Intrinsic acids can also enter the oral cavity through voluntary or involuntary vomiting, causes of which include:

- Psychosomatic:
  - Eating disorders:
    - Bulimia nervosa (affects 1%–2% of the adolescent population; F:M ratio, 10:1)
    - Anorexia nervosa (affects 0.1%–1% of the teenage population; F:M ratio, 10:1)
  - Rumination (voluntary regurgitation followed by redigestion of stomach contents)
  - Stress-induced psychogenic vomiting
- Metabolic/endocrine:
  - Pregnancy
- Gastro-intestinal disorders:
  - Peptic ulcer/gastritis
  - Hiatus hernia
  - Achalasia, a condition associated with a narrowed lower oesophageal sphincter and reduced oesophageal motility leading to stagnation and fermentation of ingested food within the oesophagus and concomitant regurgitation
  - Cerebral palsy

TABLE 1.3   Toothwear: Common Aetiology, Features and Simple Classification

Aetiological Factors		Comments
Erosion	Intrinsic, regurgitation (GORD, vomiting)	Common cause of erosion; affects palatal surfaces of maxillary anterior teeth, occlusal/buccal surfaces of lower molars. Stomach hydrochloric acid originates from: • Involuntary GORD • Involuntary or voluntary vomiting
	Extrinsic, dietary	Affects labial surfaces of maxillary anterior teeth. ↓ pH due to excess acidic food and/or drink intake: • Citrus fruit and fruit juices • Pickles, vinegar-containing foodstuffs • Carbonated drinks (including diet drinks and health drinks) • Some mouthwashes have a low pH Drinking habits: Through straw and frothing around mouth. Acids include citric, carbonic, acetic, hydrochloric and phosphoric acids. Often associated with a healthy lifestyle; patient understanding required to modify erosive potential of the diet.
	Extrinsic, environmental	Labial surfaces of maxillary anteriors/pitting. Rare nowadays due to stringent health and safety regulations in the workplace. Historically industrial processes where acid was vaporised and inhaled (battery manufacturers, tanning factories).
Attrition		Toothwear caused by occlusal tooth–tooth contact; occlusal facets match with opposing teeth; usually in combination with erosion. Often caused by grinding/parafunctional habits.
Abrasion		Toothwear caused by tooth-on-tooth contact; hard toothbrushing with coarse toothpastes, dish- or V-shaped, smooth buccal cervical lesions; incisal wear or grooves from long-term habitual behaviour (e.g., pipe smokers, milliners holding pins between their teeth, builders holding nails, etc.)
Abfraction		Buccal or lingual cervical V-shaped enamel–dentine lesions with no history of abrasion. Aetiology not clear, but masticatory flexural stresses may concentrate at cervical margins of teeth and perhaps open up pre-existing cracks or weaknesses in the enamel structure. Little/no evidence exists.

GORD, Gastro-oesophageal reflux disease.

• Drug-induced:
  ▪ Primary – cytotoxics
  ▪ Secondary – gastric irritation, alcohol, aspirin, and other nonsteroidal antiinflammatory medications

Again, in the preceding cases, the initial cause of the vomiting must be determined from the patient's history and examination and the cause itself treated first before restoring any damaged dentition (see Chapter 2, Section 2.6), with close cooperation with the patient's medical practitioner.

The aetiology and features of abrasion and attrition have been outlined in Table 1.3. Patients suffering from dry mouth with reduced and/or chemically or physically altered saliva may also be at greater risk of dental erosion. This is because they will lack the protective features of saliva which include the ability to neutralise or buffer intraoral acids and to supply mineral ions for

potential mineral deposition, including statherins and proline-rich proteins. The mucin component of saliva may also help to protect the tooth surfaces from dietary acids, with contributions to the formation of the surface pellicle and biofilm. Erosion is often a contributory factor in the overall pattern of clinical toothwear. Acid-softened tooth surfaces are more susceptible to long-term 'wear' forces from opposing teeth (attrition) or other external influences (abrasion). Clinical examples of these are shown in Chapter 2, Section 2.6.2.

1.3 DENTAL TRAUMA

While caries and toothwear have a relatively slow onset, traumatic injuries, by definition, are acquired suddenly. When these involve the hard dental tissues and the pulp, they usually require immediate operative management

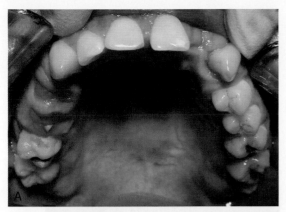
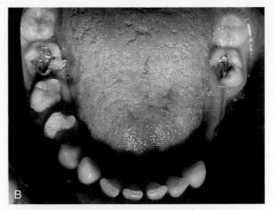

Fig. 1.20 (A) and (B) Maxillary and mandibular occlusal views of a patient having sustained multiple facial blows in a fight. Note the decoronated UR4,5 and large enamel and dentine fractures sustained on the UR6, UL7, LR4,5,6, and LL6. The UL2 and LL45 were avulsed in the incident.

Q1.20: What might have been the presenting dental complaints from the patient in Fig. 1.20A–B?

to stabilise the traumatised tissues, provide pain relief and restore function and appearance if possible. Trauma to the mouth can produce any combination of the following local injuries with varying degrees of severity:

- Lacerations to the lips, tongue, buccal and gingival tissue
- Alveolar fractures so that a number of teeth become mobile within a block of bone
- Complete or partial subluxation of a tooth
- Root fracture
- Damage to the apical blood vessels without fracture
- Fracture of the crown of the tooth involving enamel alone, enamel and dentine, or exposure of the pulp (see Chapter 2, Fig. 2.27).

1.3.1 Aetiology

Trauma is commonly caused by:

- Falls
- Sports/athletics injuries
- Blows from heavy objects
- Fights
- Car/bicycle accidents
- Injuries sustained during convulsive seizures (e.g., epilepsy)
- Child abuse (the most difficult and yet the most important to diagnose)

Detection and management will be discussed in subsequent chapters. Examples of dental trauma can be seen in Figs. 1.20A–B and 1.21A–D.

In some cases, untreated traumatic injury can lead to the development of long-term pathology (see Fig. 1.21A–D).

1.4 DEVELOPMENTAL DEFECTS

Teeth do not always develop normally, and a number of defects in tooth structure or shape occur during development and become apparent on eruption. Such teeth are often unsightly or prone to excessive toothwear or loss of clinical crowns, and thus they may require restoration to improve appearance or function or to protect the underlying tooth structure. These defects, their aetiology and their clinical appearance are outlined in Chapter 2, Table 2.8, with examples, and include the acquired conditions of enamel hypoplasia, molar-incisor hypomineralisation and intrinsic staining (fluorosis and tetracycline) as well as the hereditary conditions of hypodontia, amelogenesis imperfecta and dentinogenesis imperfecta.

1.5 CAUSES OF TOOTH DISCOLOURATION

The previous sections have summarised some of the more common pathologies affecting teeth. They all can affect the physical structure and strength of the functioning dentition as well as their appearance or aesthetics. There are many causes of tooth discolouration which may need some form of operative management in the long term. These are summarised in Table 1.4.

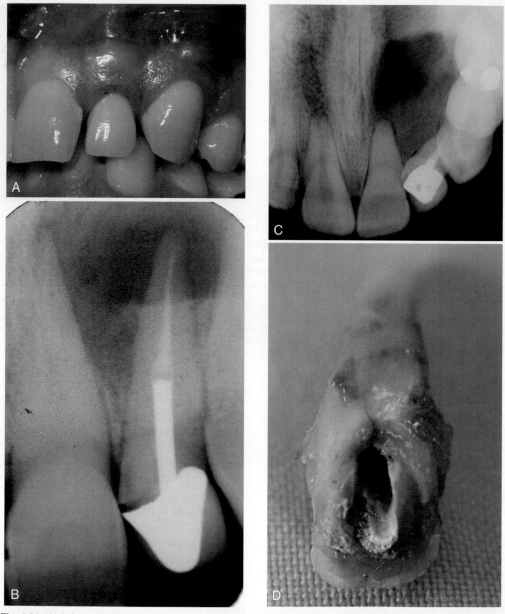

Fig. 1.21 (A) A fit and well young adult has sustained an accidental blow to the teeth in the UL123 area several months earlier. (B) Periapical and (C) upper standard occlusal radiographs of the UL123 shown in (A). Note the large, well-demarcated pathological radiolucency originating from the root apex of the fractured and displaced root, post-core and crown complex in the UL2. The lesion is tracking in the overlying mucosa to the swelling pointed out in (A). (D) The extracted UL2 root with the post-core and crown removed showing the crack sustained from the impact.

Q1.21A: Can you detect any abnormal clinical findings from Fig. 1.21A (clue: check the mucosae)?

Q1.21C: What other findings are evident from the USO radiograph?

TABLE 1.4 Summary Classification of Potential Causes of Dental Discolouration, Including Aetiology, Clinical Appearance and Possible Management Options

Cause of Discolouration		Pathology	Visual Changes	Possible Management Options
Developmental defects				
	Hereditary defects			
	Amelogenesis imperfecta	Fourteen different subtypes. Disturbance of mineralisation or matrix production during enamel formation.	Yellow-brown to dark yellow appearance ± pitting/surface irregularities	Bleaching Micro-abrasion Resin composite bonding
	Dentinogenesis imperfecta	Type I: Disorder of type I collagen	Bluish or brown in appearance, opalescence on transillumination	Bleaching Resin composite bonding Veneers
		Type II: Hereditary opalescent dentine	Opalescent primary teeth. Enamel chips away to expose enamel–dentine junction. Once dentine is exposed, teeth show brown discolouration, wear rapidly.	Resin composite bonding Veneers Full-coverage indirect crowns
		Type III: Brandywine isolate hereditary opalescent dentine	Similar outward appearance to types I and II. Multiple pulpal exposures in primary dentition. Dentine production ceases after mantle dentine has formed.	Resin composite bonding Veneers Full-coverage indirect crowns Replacement of teeth may be required if severe

Continued

TABLE 1.4   Summary Classification of Potential Causes of Dental Discolouration, Including Aetiology, Clinical Appearance and Possible Management Options—cont'd

Cause of Discolouration		Pathology	Visual Changes	Possible Management Options
Metabolic disorders				
	Alkaptonuria	Incomplete metabolism of tyrosine and phenylalanine. Promotes buildup of homogentisic acid.	Brown discolouration	Bleaching Resin composite bonding Veneers
	Congenital hyperbilirubinaemia	Deposition of bile pigments in the calcifying dental tissues	Purple or brown discolouration	Bleaching Resin composite bonding Veneers
	Congenital erythropoietic porphyria	Accumulation of porphyrins in teeth	Red-brown discolouration Red fluorescence under ultraviolet light	Bleaching Resin composite bonding Veneers
	Vitamin D-dependent rickets	Defects in enamel matrix formation	Pitting and yellow-brown discolouration	Bleaching Micro-abrasion Resin composite bonding
	Epidermolysis bullosa	Pitting of enamel, possibly caused by vesiculation of the ameloblast layer	Pitting and yellow-brown discolouration	Bleaching Micro-abrasion Resin composite bonding
	Ehlers-Danlos syndrome	Areas of hypoplastic enamel and irregularities in region of enamel–dentine junction	Pitting and brown or purple-brown discolouration	Bleaching Micro-abrasion Resin composite bonding
	Pseudo-hypoparathyroidism	Defects in enamel matrix formation	Pitting and yellow-brown discolouration	Bleaching Micro-abrasion Resin composite bonding
	Molar-incisor hypomineralisation	Unknown aetiology. Hypomineralised enamel affecting incisors and permanent first molars.	Asymmetrical appearance in arch. Enamel defects vary from white to yellow to brown areas.	Bleaching Micro-abrasion Resin composite bonding

TABLE 1.4 **Summary Classification of Potential Causes of Dental Discolouration, Including Aetiology, Clinical Appearance and Possible Management Options—cont'd**

Cause of Discolouration		Pathology	Visual Changes	Possible Management Options
Intrinsic discolouration				
Acquired defects				
	Trauma	Pulpal haemorrhage may lead to accumulation of haemoglobin or other iron-containing haematin molecules within the dentine tubules	Grey-brown to black	Bleaching
	Internal resorption	Increased volume of pulp space and pulp tissue	Pink	Extirpation and obturation of pulp space
	Systemic infectious disease (e.g., rubella)	Generalised hypoplasia due to disturbance of the developing tooth germ	Pitting or grooving leading to yellow-brown discolouration	Bleaching Micro-abrasion Resin composite bonding Veneers
	Localised infection	Localised hypoplasia due to disturbance of the developing tooth germ	Pitting or grooving leading to yellow-brown discolouration	Bleaching Micro-abrasion Resin composite bonding
	Excessive fluoride intake (fluorosis)	Enamel most often affected. Change in mineral matrix from hydroxyapatite to fluorapatite.	Flecking to diffuse mottling. Colour changes range from chalky white to dark brown appearance.	Bleaching Micro-abrasion Resin composite bonding
	Administration of tetracycline	Chelation to form complexes with calcium ions on the surface of hydroxyapatite crystals, mainly in dentine but also in enamel	Depends on type of tetracycline used, dosage and duration of administration. Yellow or brown-grey discolouration.	Bleaching Resin composite bonding Veneers

Continued

TABLE 1.4 Summary Classification of Potential Causes of Dental Discolouration, Including Aetiology, Clinical Appearance and Possible Management Options—cont'd

Cause of Discolouration		Pathology	Visual Changes	Possible Management Options
	Dental amalgam	Migration of tin ions into the dentine tubules	Grey-black discolouration to dentine	Bleaching Bonding using opaque materials
	Eugenol and phenol containing endodontic materials	Staining of the dentine	Orange-yellow discolouration	Bleaching
Extrinsic discolouration	**Direct stains**			
	Food and drink (e.g., tea, coffee, red wine), smoking	Usually multifactorial. Chromogens incorporated into the plaque or acquired pellicle.	Varies from mild yellow to more severe brown-black discolouration	Good oral hygiene May benefit from bleaching
	Chromogenic bacteria	Incorporated into plaque	Varies from yellow to green-black discolouration	Good oral hygiene May benefit from bleaching
	Indirect stains			
	Chlorhexidine and other metal salts in mouthrinses	Precipitation of chromogenic polyphenols onto tooth surface	Brown to black discolouration	Good oral hygiene May benefit from bleaching
Dental caries		Cariogenic bacteria, fermentable carbohydrate, susceptible tooth surface, time	Demineralisation and eventual proteolytic destruction of organic matrix	White spot lesion to black arrested carious dentine	Micro-abrasion Resin composite bonding Direct or indirect restoration

Adapted from: M Thomas. Common Clinical Conditions Requiring Minimally Invasive Esthetic intervention. In: Banerjee A, ed. *Minimally Invasive Aesthetics.* Elsevier, 2015.

1.6   ANSWERS TO SELF-TEST QUESTIONS

Q1.2: What differences in clinical appearance are there between the coronal and root surface carious lesion in Fig. 1.2C and how may they relate to lesion activity?

A: See Table 1.2.

Q1.3: What are the different plaque development hypotheses that have been described in the literature?

A: Investigate the traditional nonspecific plaque hypothesis (1890), specific plaque hypothesis (1976), updated nonspecific plaque hypothesis (1986), ecological plaque hypothesis (1994) and keystone-pathogen hypothesis (2012).

Q1.6: What habit(s) may have contributed to this pattern of disease? How can you change this patient's behaviour?

A: This child was allowed to suck a bottle of sweet drink frequently. Advice needs to be given to the caregiver with alternative healthy options and behaviours.

Q1.7: What aetiological factors may have contributed to this pattern of disease?

A: In a young adult patient factors might include the obvious causes of a long-term poor diet, poor oral hygiene, but consideration also has to be given to other human factors including recreational drug abuse or other social and environmental factors.

Q1.8: Why might the lesion on the LR3 appear active whereas the adjacent lesion on the LR4 in the same patient appears arrested?

A: If you look closely at the lesion on the LR3, you will notice an undermined periphery of enamel. Plaque stagnation has occurred beneath this lip, therefore activating the lesion metabolically. It was difficult for the patient to manually disrupt this biofilm, which stagnated and underwent dysbiosis, thus reactivating the caries process in this lesion specifically.

Q1.9: What ions have contributed to the creation of the intact surface zone and where have they come from?

A: Fluoride, calcium and phosphate ions in particular help to form a more acid-resistant fluoride-substituted hydroxyapatite. These ions will have come from the saliva as well as from the biofilm, in higher concentrations, thus creating a positive equilibrium with the tooth surface.

Q1.10: How might this scenario be managed in a high caries risk patient?

A: Instruct the patient regarding their oral hygiene procedures, and if this does not improve, then carry out debridement/air abrasion followed by application of a fissure sealant.

Q1.11: What clinical sign is visible on the lesion on the LR4 to indicate its relative progression in comparison to the adjacent teeth?

A: If you look carefully, you can see signs of early cavitation with enamel surface breakdown and some brown discolouration towards the mesial aspect of the tooth.

Q1.12: What features of this lesion will help the dentist conclude that it is active, how might these be detected and how might the patient be managed?

A: The lesion has surface roughness (detectable as vibrations in the handle of the ball-ended explorer as it is gently run across the lesion surface) and is covered with plaque (detected visually, disclosing agent). This patient was under preventive therapy including modifications in their oral hygiene, possibly diet, and application of fluoride varnish to arrest the lesion.

Q1.13B: How might the patient have arrested this once-active lesion?

A: By judiciously removing the plaque biofilm regularly using proper oral hygiene methods including floss. This, combined with the use of a fluoride dentifrice over time, will inactivate the incipient white spot lesion into the brown spot lesion seen in the image.

Q1.14: What are the potential causes for the colour change in carious dentine?

A: Although not conclusive, this colour change may be due to the Maillard reaction, a biochemical reaction between proteins and carbohydrates in a moist, acidic biological environment.

Q1.17: How many other carious lesions can you detect and how would you classify them radiographically?

A: Distal/mesial (d/m) UR6, d/m UR5, m LR7, d/m LR6, d/m LR5, not including the grossly broken down UR4!

Q1.20: What might have been the presenting dental complaints from the patient in Fig. 1.20A–B?

A: Pain, difficulty chewing, sharp fractured teeth or fillings against the tongue or cheeks, not being able to bite properly, poor appearance, difficulty in brushing the teeth due to sensitivity, and tooth fractures.

Q1.21A: Can you spot or detect any abnormal clinical findings from Fig. 1.21A (clue: check the mucosae)?

A: It's difficult, but did you notice the mucosal swelling level with the mucogingival junction adjacent to the UL3?

Q1.21C: What other findings are evident from the USO radiograph?

A: The near-complete obliteration of the pulp chamber and root canal spaces in the UL1.

Minimum Intervention Oral Care (MIOC) – Clinical Domain 1

Minimum Intervention Oral Care (MIOC) – Clinical Domain 1

MIOC Domain 1: Identifying Clinical Problems

CHAPTER OUTLINE

2.1 INTRODUCTION: MINIMUM INTERVENTION ORAL CARE AND MINIMALLY INVASIVE DENTISTRY

Minimum intervention oral care (MIOC) describes a universal primary oral healthcare delivery framework in which the oral healthcare team (comprising dentists, nurses, oral health educators, dental hygienists, dental therapists, clinical dental technicians, reception staff and practice managers), often guided by the dentist, act as one to provide individualised person-focused care, advice and treatment to encourage and help the patient take responsibility of, value and maintain their own oral health throughout life. The MIOC delivery framework is based on four broad, interlinking clinical domains (Fig. 2.1):

- Identify: Methods of detection/diagnosis/prognosis of oral disease; risk/susceptibility assessment of the patient; use of investigations to formulate personalised care plans

- Prevent lesions and control disease: Non-operative and/or micro-invasive primary and secondary prevention of diagnosed conditions
- Restore: *Minimally invasive* operative (surgical) interventions/dentistry (MID) to repair or replace tissue damage/loss (tertiary prevention)
- Re-assess: Review/maintenance/recall of patient behaviours; treatment outcomes including the advice/care offered by the dentist/oral healthcare team; active surveillance of early lesions, tooth-restoration complexes.

The underpinning tenet behind the MIOC delivery framework is prevention.

- *Primary prevention*: Aims to prevent disease or injury before it has occurred in susceptible patients/populations; essentially, keeping healthy people healthy by instituting risk-limiting behaviours/practices in daily life through universal or targeted measures.

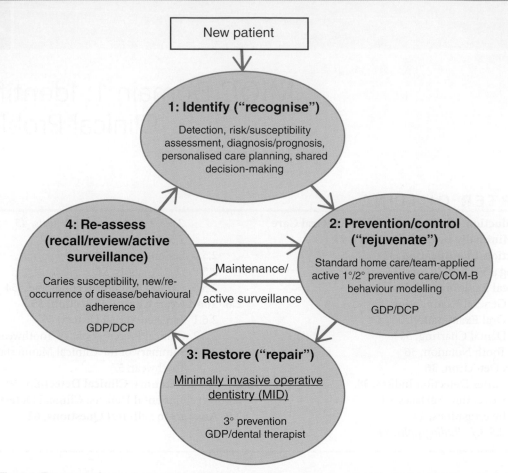

Fig. 2.1 The person-focused, prevention-based, risk-related, team-delivered minimum intervention oral care delivery framework. The arrows indicate the direction of the patient journey through this care delivery framework, and within each domain an indication is given of the members of the oral healthcare team who might be involved, including a general dental practitioner (GDP) and dental care professionals (DCPs, including oral health educators, extended duties dental nurses (EDDNs), dental hygienists, dental therapists, practice managers, clinical dental technicians and reception staff).

- *Secondary prevention*: Emphasises early disease detection, targeting those with the earliest, often sub-clinical, manifestations of the disease/condition. Once detected and diagnosed, these can be reversed with appropriate measures, guiding the patient back to full health.
- *Tertiary prevention*: Targets both the clinical and outcome stages of a disease. It is implemented in symptomatic patients and aims to reduce the severity of the disease as well as of any associated adverse sequelae. While secondary prevention seeks to prevent the onset of illness, tertiary prevention aims to reduce the effects of the disease once established in

> **Q2.1:** Can you research any other categories of prevention that have been classified in the recent literature?

> **Q2.2:** What are examples of primary, secondary and tertiary prevention measures used for managing dental caries?

an individual. It softens the impact of an ongoing illness or injury that has lasting effects.

As you can see, operative *minimally invasive dentistry* (MID) fits in as the third of the four clinical domains of the MIOC delivery framework. It is that aspect of restorative dentistry which repairs, restores and/or replaces damaged and defective tooth tissues to maintain pulp sensibility, oral and dental function and aesthetics throughout the life course of the patient. The primary goal of MID is to respect tooth tissues during the surgical intervention, preserving viable and biologically repairable tissue histology to maintain pulp sensibility and clinical function for as long as possible.

The process of *personalised care planning* involves patient and/or caregiver input in all the MIOC domains, including disease control and lesion prevention, by instilling behaviour/attitude change throughout the patient's life course. It is not just listing in order those operative procedures offered to restore damaged or defective teeth in isolation, which is outdatedly termed a "treatment plan". The personalised care plan can be phased, will adapt to patient behaviours and attitudes, and adapts as the care is delivered by members of the oral healthcare team. It must be well reasoned and justified from the outset and throughout its execution. It

must be understood from the outset that, even though operative minimally invasive dentistry has a pivotal role in the "surgical" repair of damaged teeth, it alone does not provide the actual cure for dental disease. *"Drilling, filling and billing does not cure caries!"*

Fig. 2.2 shows how the MIOC framework can be used to deliver better oral health across several disciplines in restorative dentistry, including periodontology, prosthodontics and paedodontics, as well as cariology. It is an all-encompassing approach to improving patient care and well-being, placing the patient as the focal point of the process and delivering phased care through an integrated team approach.

The primary oral healthcare team (dentist, nurse, extended duties dental nurse, dental hygienist, dental therapist, oral health educator, laboratory technician, receptionist, practice manager), led by the principal dental practitioner, should be involved in the decision-making processes and oral health management of the patient, as part of delivering the MIOC framework (see Figs. 2.1 and 2.2A–E). This care rationale is person-focused: engaging with the patient to

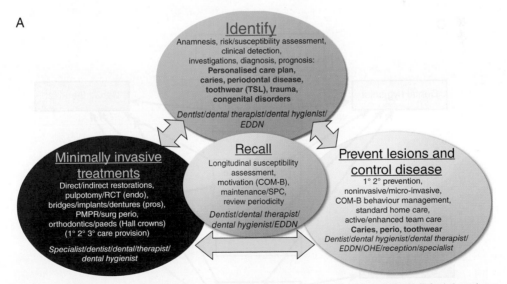

Fig. 2.2 A to E Diagram (A) showing how the MIOC framework with its four interlinked clinical domains can be applied across many disciplines in restorative dentistry. (B) to (E) The roles of the oral healthcare team members in each of the four MIOC clinical domains. Teamwork is essential in delivering the MIOC framework to patients throughout their life course; *TSL,* tooth surface loss; *Perio,* periodontology; *COM-B,* capability, opportunity, motivation behaviour modelling; *RCT,* root canal treatment; *PMPR,* professional mechanical plaque removal; *Pros,* prosthodontics; *SPC,* supportive periodontal care. (From Young S, Dawett B, Gallie A, Banerjee A, Deery C. Minimum intervention oral care delivery for children – developing the oral healthcare team. *Dent Update.* 2022;49(5):424-430. doi:10.12968/denu.2022.49.5.424.)

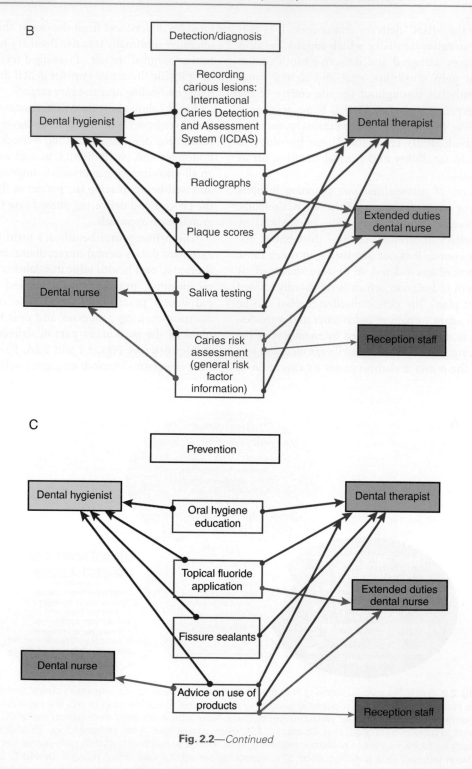

Fig. 2.2—*Continued*

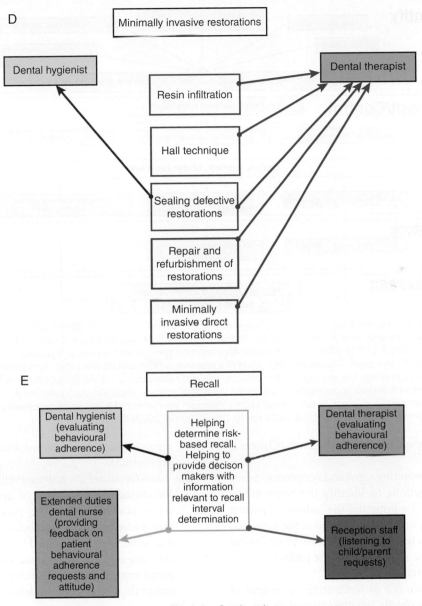

Fig. 2.2—*Continued*

encourage them to take responsibility of their own oral health, a concept known as shared decision-making. The role of the oral healthcare team is to provide advice and guidance to help the patient maintain oral health as well as providing operative treatment to repair damaged hard and soft tissues. Sometimes the dentist will refer difficult cases to a specialist clinician for their opinion as to what the diagnosis and personalised care plan should be, as well as its execution in some cases.

To successfully manage the patient's journey through the MIOC framework, key stages must be completed within the four clinical domains (Fig. 2.3):

1. Detecting clinical problems and their aetiology Chapter 1:
   • This involves team detective work to help gather clinically relevant and useful information primarily using the skills of verbal history taking (anamnesis), oral examination and the interpretation of relevant investigations.

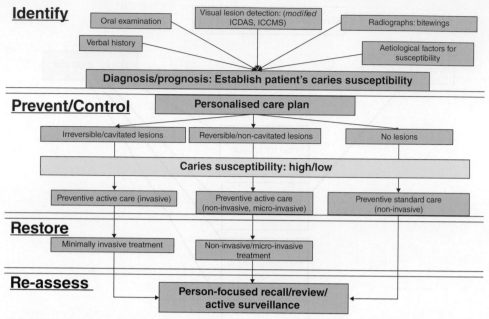

Fig. 2.3 MIOC implementation flowchart showing how the clinical domains of *identify* (discussed in this chapter), *prevent and control* (Chapter 4), *MI restore* (Chapters 5–8) and *re-assess* (Chapter 9) link to one another (see also Fig. 2.1). Note how the person-focused care plan centres on risk and susceptibility (caries management in this case). The medium-risk grade at a practical patient contact level often is managed as part of the high-risk strategy. The key factor is that patients' risk and susceptibility are monitored over time longitudinally and not as a simple single snapshot during the treatment episode. (Adapted from Banerjee A, Doméjean S. The contemporary approach to tooth preservation: minimum intervention (MI) caries management in general practice. *Primary Dent J.* 2013 Jul;2(3):30-37. doi:10.1308/205016813807440119.)

2. Risk/susceptibility assessment and diagnosis (Chapter 3, Section 3.3):
   - The art of interpreting signs and symptoms, results from investigations to identify the cause of the problem and the potential the individual patient has of developing further disease in the future, or responding to treatment. Both aspects are critical to planning the overall care of the patient.
3. Prognosis (Chapter 3):
   - The art and science of forecasting the course of a disease or problem, whether treated or not, for that particular patient.
4. Formulation of a personalised care plan (Chapters 3 and 4):
   - This must be underpinned by the non-invasive/ micro-invasive control of disease and lesion prevention, following the principles of minimum intervention oral care (primary and secondary prevention).
   - The personalised risk-related care plan will also include relevant itemised, costed and justified minimally invasive operative treatments as required to

repair/replace damaged/lost tooth tissue (tertiary prevention).
5. Re-assess (recall/review, active surveillance) (Chapter 9):
   - Reviewing the outcomes of any care provided, active surveillance of the patient's response to assess whether knowledge/behavioural adaptations and adherence have helped to control and/or prevent disease reoccurrence and developing adaptive recall strategies/intervals that are person-focused, rather than generically guideline driven.

2.2 DETECTION/IDENTIFICATION

This clinical domain of patient management involves gathering the relevant information based on which sound clinical judgments can be made as to the best course of care for the individual patient. Clinical detection works on two levels:

- Detecting the immediate clinical problem (i.e., trauma or the physical manifestation of the disease process, such as carious lesions, toothwear lesions)

- Detecting and understanding the complex interplay of aetiological factors that have *caused* the problem for that particular patient over time

It is critical that detailed notes are made for all stages of the MIOC patient management pathway and that they are documented at every visit. These notes can be made using electronic patient recording systems or they can be handwritten. Each patient will have their own notes with their name, date of birth, address, contact details, occupation and updated medical history listed. It is essential to check that the correct notes have been called up for the attending patient and that the date and time of the appointment have been noted for each visit. All members of the oral healthcare team are responsible for this.

2.3 TAKING A VERBAL HISTORY

The art of verbal history taking (anamnesis) is the first and most important way to obtain information about any problems the patient may present with and their aetiology. The answers to a series of carefully planned and sequenced questions will help shed light on the nature, cause and severity of any presenting problem(s). A generic structured interview with the clinical relevance of each question is presented in Table 2.1. This, of course, is not the only format of interviewing that can be used, and with experience, these should be adjusted to the specific needs and conditions and modified to assess the aetiological factors of the presenting conditions (see later). Please remember, the best clinician always asks, "Why?".

This information should be ascertained using a relaxed, non-judgmental, conversational and empathetic approach. The clinician should be sitting at the same eye level as the patient, using eye contact whilst also observing non-verbal cues from the patient, including their posture, body movements, tone of voice and level of directness of their responses (see Chapter 5, Section 5.2). These cues help the clinician begin to build a psychological picture of the patient that they can use when planning any advice and care to be offered.

2.4 PHYSICAL EXAMINATION

Once the verbal history has been taken and duly noted, a physical examination follows, divided into a general and oral examination.

2.4.1 General Examination

This will commence as soon as the patient enters the clinic/surgery and whilst the clinician is in the process of interviewing the patient. The demeanour and movement of the individual, facial/optical asymmetries, facial nerve palsies, pallor, tremors or mental/physical disabilities can be noted and followed up on if relevant to the oral/dental care required.

2.4.2 Oral Examination

A common error made by inexperienced clinicians is to dive into an oral examination, focusing all attention on the teeth and the immediate acute problem raised in the presenting history. It is better to have a systematic approach that encompasses all aspects of the head and neck (*extra-oral*) as well as the oral cavity (*intra-oral*), including the mucosal soft tissues, periodontal tissues as well as teeth and any prostheses (see Table 2.2). When examining the oral mucosae, learn and use a system which ensures that all aspects of the oral cavity are included; that is, anterior to posterior (lips to tonsils), posterior to anterior or clockwise/anticlockwise around the oral cavity. Once learnt and practised, this is never forgotten, even during the stress of time pressure and undergraduate/postgraduate clinical examinations! Ensure adequate time has been set aside for the examination along with suitable dental instrumentation and lighting (Chapter 5, Section 5.2). Clinical digital photography can often assist in the documentation of any notable findings during the examination, but appropriate informed and written consent must be taken prior to any images being captured and stored securely. Data to be recorded along with the image must include patient details, the date the image was captured, a report of any clinical findings and, where appropriate, a linear scale to help the viewer assess the size of any lesion that has been imaged. The camera settings and ambient lighting should also be noted in case comparative images are taken at a later date to enable standardisation between them. The assisting staff member can be trained to document accurately and faithfully all the information gathered during this part of the examination. The practising clinician, however, has ultimate responsibility to check and authorise any records taken during the examination.

The intra-oral examination can be greatly assisted for the clinical operator by the use of magnification loupes with accompanying focused lighting. This will be discussed further in Chapter 5, Section 5.6.

TABLE 2.1　Relevant Questions to Help Diagnose Presenting Problem and Formulate Personalised Care Plan

Structured Verbal History	Comments
Patient complains of (PCO, C/O)…	Document in the patient's own words the presenting symptom(s)/problem(s).
History of presenting complaint(s) (HPC)	*Commencement*: When did it (they) start? *Location*: Ask patient to describe or to point to or outline the area with one finger. *Type*: Description of symptoms. Avoid putting words in the patient's mouth. *Incidence*: How long ago did the episodes start? *Duration*: How long do they persist? Frequency? Are they getting better, staying the same or deteriorating? *Initiating or relieving factors*: Does anything make the symptoms worse or better? Answers to the above will often provide the clues to help focus the clinician towards the correct diagnosis.
Past dental history (PDH)	What previous dental treatment have they experienced (orthodontics, extractions, periodontal treatment, fillings, etc.)? How regularly do they visit the dentist? What previous preventive advice have they received/do they follow? Answers will help create a picture of the attitude and motivation of the patient towards dentistry and their own oral health, without asking them directly about these issues.
Relevant medical history (RMH)	Most oral healthcare teams use a preformatted checklist, which will include information regarding: • Cardiac problems, disease, rheumatic fever, blood pressure • Respiratory disease, asthma, shortness of breath • Diabetes, epilepsy, jaundice, hepatitis history • Current or recent past medications • Allergies • Bleeding, haemorrhage, clotting defects • Other illnesses, operations, hospital admissions • Pregnancy • HIV/AIDS, communicable disease risk Relevant information regarding drug interactions with local anaesthetic, allergies to latex, resins or dental materials. Bleeding problems/anticoagulant therapies relevant for periodontal surgery, subgingival professional mechanical plaque removal (PMPR), extractions. Check medication in the Dental Formulary or equivalent. Medications causing dry mouth, gingival overgrowth, or vomiting (emesis) should be noted.
Social history (SH)	Occupation, family members, availability for appointments Relevant when considering appointment logistics to deliver the personalised care plan.
Habits	Oral hygiene (procedures, frequency), use of fluoride, diet (amount and frequency of sugar intake, balanced diet, erosive potential for toothwear), smoking, alcohol intake, parafunctional habits (bruxism [teeth grinding], clenching) Relevant when planning care, preventive advice. What the patient says might be checked/verified during the oral examination to follow. Helps to ascertain the possible aetiology of the presenting problem.

TABLE 2.2 Steps Involved in a Comprehensive Clinical Examination

Examination Site	Comments
Extra-oral (head, neck and face)	Facial swellings, asymmetries, lesions Lips: form and seal, lesions Facial and neck lymph nodes TMJ: pain on palpation, crepitus, clicking (unibilateral/on opening, closing, both) Mandibular movement (opening gape, deviations [check dental centre lines], lateral/ protrusive excursions) Operator stands behind the patient for the TMJ/LN exam. Remember to notify the patient of what you are about to do prior to starting!
Intra-oral	
Oral mucosae	All internal buccal, labial, alveolar mucosae Vermilion border of lips Tongue (dorsum, lateral borders and ventral surfaces) Retromolar areas, hard and soft palate, floor of mouth Palpation of the pterygoid muscles Saliva quality and quantity (see below) Checking for white or erythematous patches/plaques indicative of trauma, lichenoid reactions, neoplastic change – referral to an oral medicine specialist might be appropriate. Tenderness in the pterygoid muscles – possible sign of TMD? Dry mucosae and frothy, viscous sparse saliva indicative of dry mouth (see Section 2.5.4).
Periodontium	Marginal gingivae (colour, contour, consistency) Gingivitis (BPE score) Recession, loss of attachment, probing depths Tooth mobility Presence of supra-/subgingival calculus Plaque indices Relevant to assess periodontal status which will affect the overall restorative status of the mouth and of the individual tooth.
Teeth	Missing teeth, mobility, restoration status, caries (mICDAS/ICCMS; see later), toothwear (site, enamel ± dentine, BEWE), malpositioning (tilting, rotation, overeruption/submerged)
Dental prostheses	Crowns, removable partial or complete dentures, fixed bridges, implant-retained crown and bridge work, orthodontic appliances (fixed and removable), obturators Relevant regarding oral hygiene procedures, plaque-retentive margins, aesthetics, status of abutment teeth, quality of fit/seal/stability
Dental occlusion	Angle's classification (Class I, II, III) Incisor relationship (Class I, II division 1/2 and Class III) Intercuspal position (ICP), retruded contact position (RCP) Protrusive, retrusive, lateral excursive movements – working and nonworking side contacts Skeletal discrepancies Relevant to the restoration of individual/groups of teeth to conform to the existing occlusal harmony or to assess changes in a reorganised approach in more complex operative personalised care plans (Chapter 5, Section 5.13).

Continued

TABLE 2.2   Steps Involved in a Comprehensive Clinical Examination—cont'd

Examination Site	Comments
Saliva (cross-reference with Table 2.5)	*Quality:* Normal, frothy, viscous *Quantity:* Normal, reduced output, buccal mucosae/tongue sticks to mirror head, limited/ no pooling in floor of mouth, shiny mucosae lobulated/fissured tongue, altered gingival architecture, glassy appearance of oral mucosae, cervical caries, food debris present Challacombe Scale of Clinical Oral Dryness Relevant regarding the protective effects of saliva for teeth and the oral mucosae. Low saliva output/poor quality increases patient risk of caries and oral infections.

Note: A full examination should not be rushed and careful recording of findings is essential both clinically and dento-legally. *BEWE,* basic erosive wear examination; *BPE,* basic periodontal examination; *ICCMS,* International Caries Classification and Management System; *LN,* lymph node; *mICDAS,* modified international caries detection and assessment system; *TMJ,* temporomandibular joint; *TMD,* temporomandibular dysfunction.

The examination of the oral cavity must also include an assessment of the quantity and quality of the patient's saliva. As has been previously mentioned, saliva plays a critical role in the control of dental disease risk, especially caries and erosion (see Section 2.5.4).

2.4.3 Dental Charting

When examining the dentition, the clinician must relay certain features to their assistant to record accurately in a written or electronic dental chart (Fig. 2.4A–B). This chart is interpreted as though the dentist is looking at a patient face-to-face and the notation is communicated from the patient's perspective. These features are:

1. Which tooth, side, position; For example, upper left 6 (UL6) or upper left first permanent molar, rotated/tilted/space-closed
2. Presence of existing restoration(s): Location (mesio-occlusal, buccal, cervical, etc.), number of tooth surfaces involved and type of material (amalgam, tooth coloured, gold, ceramic, etc.).
3. Status of the existing tooth-restoration complex: Sound, or deficient margins/fractured/missing portions of the restoration or adjacent tooth structure
4. Presence of carious lesion(s): Location, mICDAS/ICCMS classification (see Table 2.3), lesion activity
5. Presence of toothwear: Location (buccal, occlusal, incisal) and extent (in enamel or dentine, exposing pulp, BEWE score [see Table 2.7])
6. Presence of other abnormalities: For example, fluorosis, hypoplastic enamel, cracks

With practice, this can be done with a series of abbreviated responses, and good teamwork with the nurse/assistant can expedite this process. Of course, if features 2 to 6 do not apply after careful examination, then a summary of 'sound' will usually suffice and a dot is placed on the

relevant tooth in the chart. It is important to check all five surfaces of each tooth either with direct vision or using the dental mirror and good illumination of a clean, dry tooth. It might be necessary in some patients, before the visual examination (but after checking any relevant medical history), to clean the teeth with a periodontal hand/ultrasonic scaler to remove supragingival plaque and calculus deposits that might be obscuring the clear view of the tooth surfaces beneath. These deposits would of course need to be recorded in the notes, prior to their removal before the underlying tooth surfaces could be properly examined.

2.4.4 Tooth Notation

In the UK, the notations used most commonly are the Palmer system and a two-letter coding system. Both are shown in Fig. 2.5, dividing the mouth into four quadrants with the teeth in each numbered 1 to 8 from central incisors to third molars.

Two other numerical notation systems exist: the FDI (Fédération Dentaire Internationale, favoured in mainland Europe; Fig. 2.6) and the Universal notation system (favoured in the United States; Fig. 2.7). Users tend to credit these systems for crossing language boundaries, but confusion can occur with these solely numerical notations; for example, FDI 16 (Fig. 2.6) represents UR6 (upper right first permanent molar, 6⏌) whereas Universal 16 (Fig. 2.7) represents UL8 (upper-left third permanent molar, ⌊8).

2.5 CARIES DETECTION

Visual detection of carious lesions in enamel and dentine relies on several operator-controlled factors:

- Using 'sharp' eyes and the recommended use of magnification in the form of dental loupes with their

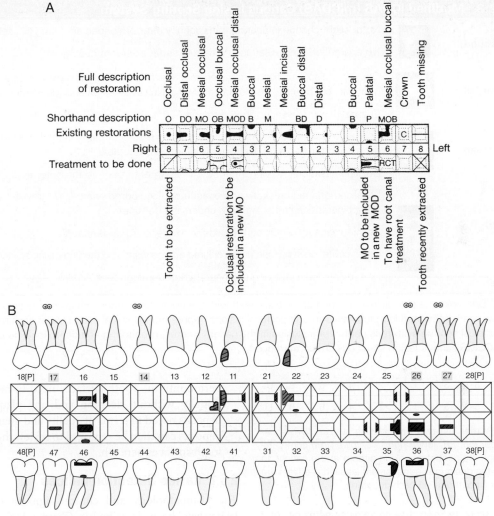

Fig. 2.4 Conventions for recording restorations, lesions/teeth requiring restoration, teeth to be extracted and other conditions on a dental chart (A). An example of a commercially available digital electronic dental charting system allowing more detailed annotations to be made about each tooth (B).

additional focused illumination (see Chapter 5, Section 5.6).
• Using good illumination from the overhead dental chair light or a more focused light from an LED headlight (usually coupled with the use of magnification loupes).
• Having clean tooth surfaces to examine both wet and dry (using a three-in-one air/water syringe; Fig. 2.8A, B and E). If surface debris (plaque/calculus) is present, this will have to be removed prior to any tooth surface examination taking place (Chapter 1, Fig. 1.2B–C; Fig. 2.8C–D).

• Using rounded/ball-ended dental explorers on tooth surfaces. The use of sharp dental probes/explorers is contraindicated for carious lesion surface detection as they can, with injudicious use, cause cavitation in a previously non-cavitated lesion surface (Fig. 2.9B).
• Separating teeth may be beneficial to assess proximal surfaces of adjacent teeth visually, ideally with magnification. Wedges or orthodontic separators can be placed interproximally for a few minutes prior to the examination of the field to gently displace the gingiva apically and part the teeth slightly through

TABLE 2.3　Modified ICDAS (mICDAS) Carious Lesion Scoring System

0 **(ICCMS sound)**		No or slight change in enamel translucency after prolonged air drying (>5 secs). No enamel demineralisation or a narrow surface zone of opacity.
1 **(ICCMS initial)**		Opacity or discolouration from the enamel (white spot lesion) hardly visible on a wet surface, but distinctly visible after air-drying. No cavitation on occlusal / smooth surfaces. Enamel demineralisation limited to outer 50%.
2 **(ICCMS initial)**		Enamel opacity (white spot lesion) or greyish discolouration distinctly visible without the need for air-drying. No clinical cavitation detectable. Demineralisation involving inner 50% of enamel through to the outer third of dentine.
3 **(ICCMS moderate)**		Localised enamel breakdown in opaque or discoloured enamel,+/- greyish discolouration/shadowing from underlying dentine. Demineralisation involving the middle to inner third of dentine.
4 **(ICCMS extensive)**		Gross cavitation in opaque or discoloured enamel exposing the underlying stained dentine. Demineralisation involving the inner third of dentine towards pulp.

Note: The mICDAS links the clinical lesion appearance (black text) with the equivalent underlying lesion histology (red text). Images show teeth sectioned longitudinally through occlusal lesions, representing clinical examples of each mICDAS score. This clinical scoring system is useful for inclusion in the patient's notes, monitoring and dento-legal purposes. The equivalent ICCMS carious lesion staging is cross-referenced.

UR	8 7 6 5 4 3 2 1	1 2 3 4 5 6 7 8	UL
LR	8 7 6 5 4 3 2 1	1 2 3 4 5 6 7 8	LL

Fig. 2.5 The Palmer and two-letter coding system *(UR, upper right; UL, upper left; LR, lower right; LL, lower left)* communicated as though the dentist is looking directly at the patient. In both systems the deciduous dentition are labelled a–e from the midline, moving posteriorly in each quadrant.

UR	18 17 16 15 14 13 12 11	21 22 23 24 25 26 27 28	UL
LR	48 47 46 45 44 43 42 41	31 32 33 34 35 36 37 38	LL

Fig. 2.6 The FDI tooth notation system with the teeth in each quadrant prefixed by a number from 1 to 4.

UR	1 2 3 4 5 6 7 8	9 10 11 12 13 14 15 16	UL
LR	32 31 30 29 28 27 26 25	24 23 22 21 20 19 18 17	LL

Fig. 2.7 The Universal tooth notation system, with each individual tooth being allocated a number from 1 to 32 in the permanent dentition.

movement within their periodontal ligament spaces. In this way, proximal incipient or cavitated lesions may become more evident.

• Allowing sufficient time for the examination of all tooth surfaces as well as the soft tissues and periodontium. Tooth surfaces need to be examined initially without cleaning and any plaque biofilm deposits noted in terms of quality and quantity. These deposits can then be removed to review the clean, dry tooth surfaces beneath.

2.5.1　Caries Detection Indices

The histopathology and clinical signs of the carious lesion have been described in Chapter 1, Section 1.1.6. The clinical manifestation of the caries process occurring within the overlying dental plaque biofilm is the progressive carious lesion created within the dental hard tissues. The clinical practitioner must be able to link the visual clinical appearance of the lesion surface with the underlying histological damage that has occurred in the tooth (and possibly link this to lesion activity status) at a particular moment in time. In this way, they can then diagnose problems and decide how to manage the lesion/disease process in that individual patient through the development of a suitable prevention-based personalised care plan. In an attempt to do this, as well as for active surveillance of the relative success or failure of previous treatment at recall consultations and to help with dento-legal documentation, several clinical visual indices

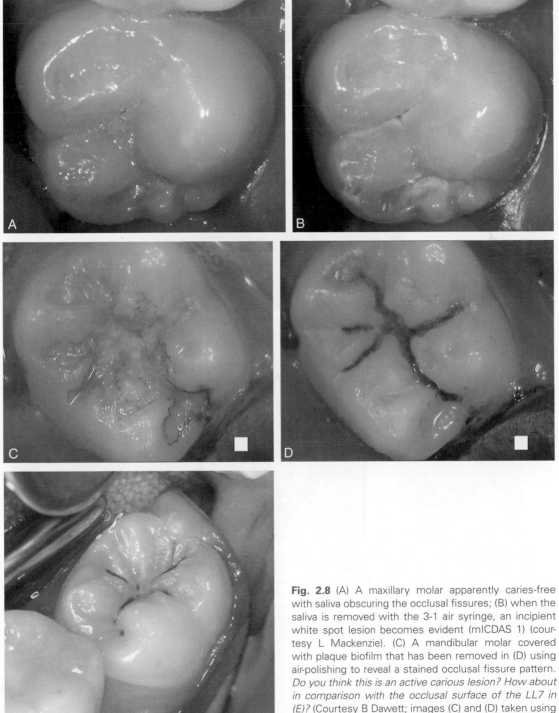

Fig. 2.8 (A) A maxillary molar apparently caries-free with saliva obscuring the occlusal fissures; (B) when the saliva is removed with the 3-1 air syringe, an incipient white spot lesion becomes evident (mICDAS 1) (courtesy L Mackenzie). (C) A mandibular molar covered with plaque biofilm that has been removed in (D) using air-polishing to reveal a stained occlusal fissure pattern. *Do you think this is an active carious lesion? How about in comparison with the occlusal surface of the LL7 in (E)?* (Courtesy B Dawett; images (C) and (D) taken using Acteon's intraoral Soprocare camera system.)

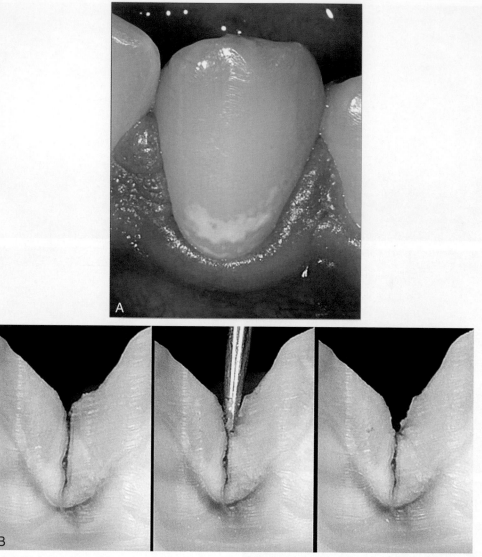

Fig. 2.9 (A) A smooth surface incipient white spot lesion (WSL) associated with the cervical aspect of a mandibular canine. (B) A cross-section through an occlusal fissure WSL showing the classic shape of the non-cavitated enamel lesion (see Chapter 1, Fig. 1.9). This lesion has been probed in a vertical direction using firm finger pressure with a sharp dental explorer, resulting in operator-induced (iatrogenic) cavitation of the lesion that should have been managed non-operatively. The use of a sharp dental probe to elicit 'sticky fissures or surfaces' in this way is contraindicated for caries detection. (Courtesy Mackenzie L, Banerjee A. The minimally invasive management of early occlusal caries: a practical guide. *Primary Dent J.* 2014 May;3(2):42-49. doi:10.1308/205016814812143987.)

> **Q2.9:** What hand instrument should be used instead for carious tooth surface detection and for what purpose?

have been described over the years. In 2004, the ICDAS (International Caries Detection and Assessment System) Foundation was convened to produce an evidence-based clinical caries assessment system to be used primarily for epidemiological and research studies, as well as for use in general dental practice (www.icdas.org). A simpler, modified version is presented in Table 2.3 with clinical examples (Figs. 2.11–2.13), which permits the clinician to clinically examine the tooth surface and appreciate the underlying

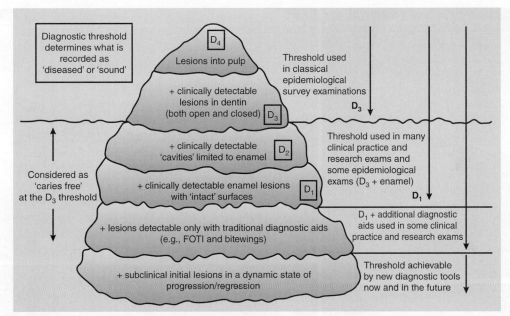

Fig. 2.10 The caries iceberg classifying clinically detectable lesions with regard to their level of tissue invasion and degree of cavitation most often used in population-based epidemiological surveys. (From Pitts NB. Diagnostic tools and measurements – impact on appropriate care. *Community Dent Oral Epidemiol.* 1997 Feb;25(1):24–35. doi:10.1111/j.1600-0528.1997.tb00896.x.)

histological damage that has developed. Then, depending on the individual's caries risk/susceptibility assessment, the most relevant treatment option can be chosen. This index requires that the clinical examination detail listed and discussed earlier is carried out judiciously and its use permits an objective numerical record to be made in the dental chart to permit longitudinal, dento-legally appropriate assessment of the particular lesion over time.

Alternative indices exist which classify carious lesions. The Nyvad classification is a visual-tactile caries classification system devised to enable the detection of the activity and severity of carious lesions with special focus on low caries risk populations. The criteria behind the classification reflect the entire continuum of the carious lesion, ranging from clinically sound surfaces through non-cavitated and micro-cavitated lesions in enamel, to open cavitation in dentine. Lesion activity at each severity stage is discriminated by differences in surface topography and lesion texture. The International Caries Classification and Management System (ICCMS) has also been published and is cross-referenced in Table 2.3 (https://www.acffglobal.org/resources/icdas-iccms/).

The "caries iceberg", developed in collaboration with cariologists and epidemiologists, is an index used by many experts to study the incidence and prevalence of dental caries in different populations (Fig. 2.10). This permits the development of strategies to manage caries at a population level as well as at a patient level. Clinically detectable lesions are divided into four groups, D_1 to D_4, depending on the depth of tissue invasion and the degree of cavitation. Note that careful selection of caries detection thresholds is required or else this index may lead to threshold bias when interpreting data for caries prevalence in a population. For example, if the D_3 detection threshold (dentine lesions, cavitated or not (open or closed)) is selected to establish the presence/absence of caries, patients with early-stage lesions within enamel, cavitated or not, will not be included in the final data, thus incorrectly reducing the caries prevalence for that particular population.

2.5.2 Susceptible Surfaces

Carious lesions occur on tooth surfaces that have accumulated a stagnant, dysbiotic plaque biofilm over a prolonged period of time. During the clinical examination, it would be prudent to carefully examine the following areas for early signs of lesions, using magnification and focused illumination:

- The depths of pits and fissures on posterior occlusal surfaces (which the patient cannot clean effectively

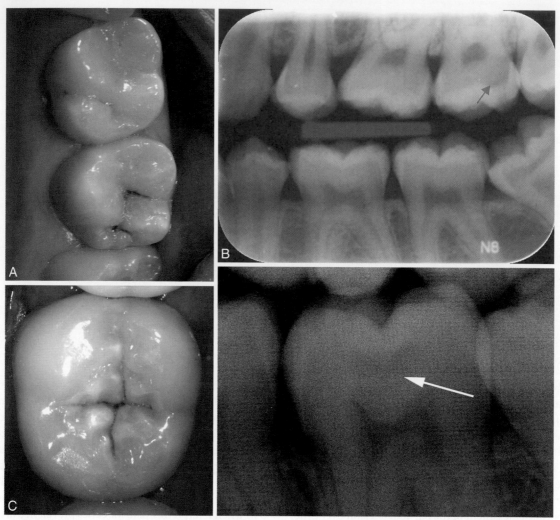

Fig. 2.11 (A) The brown, non-cavitated fissures with underlying grey discolouration on the occlusal surface of the UL7 are caused by demineralised, discoloured dentine shining through intact, wet enamel (a closed lesion, visible in dentine on (B) the bitewing radiograph *(right, blue arrow)* (mICDAS 2/ICCMS initial-moderate). (C) Mandibular molar, clinically non-cavitated but with fissure staining and an underlying greyish shadow and the radiograph showing demineralisation into the outer third of dentine *(arrow)* (mICDAS 2/ICCMS late initial). (Courtesy Mackenzie L, Banerjee A. The minimally invasive management of early occlusal caries: a practical guide. *Primary Dent J.* 2014 May;3(2):42-49. doi:10.1308/205016814812143987.)

> **Q2.11:** What treatment may be required for these teeth?

with a toothbrush). These areas on newly erupting, partially erupted or submerged molars are particularly susceptible to caries attack. These surfaces may need to be debrided before examination can be carried out.

- Proximal surfaces (mesial and distal) *cervical* to contact points of adjacent teeth (where patients may not floss effectively, regularly or at all). The surfaces of particularly imbricated (crowded) teeth can be more susceptible due to their poor accessibility to oral hygiene aids.
- Smooth surfaces adjacent to the gingival margin (areas patients often miss with their toothbrush).

- The ledged, overhanging or deficient margins of existing restorations (a plaque trap often inaccessible to a toothbrush and/or floss).

Of course, these are not the only sites at which carious lesions occur. The site and distribution of lesions in a patient's mouth might give an indication to underlying

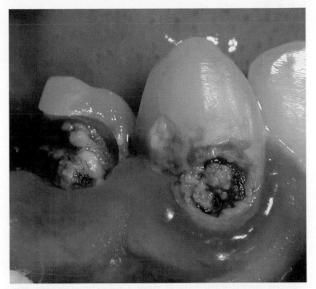

Fig. 2.13 Grossly cavitated buccal carious lesions on the LR3 and LR4 with copious quantities of stagnant, dense, cariogenic, dysbiotic plaque on the exposed dentine surfaces (mICDAS 4/ICCMS extensive).

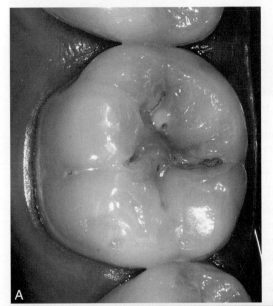

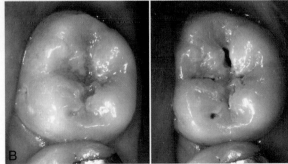

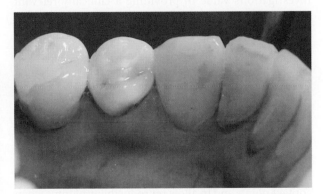

Fig. 2.14 A patient with an eating disorder, anorexia nervosa, with carious cavitated lesions on the lingual aspects of LL124 (mICDAS 2,3/ICCMS initial-moderate).

Fig. 2.12 (A) A small cavity is just clinically detectable within the whitish opacity/brown discolouration on the occlusal surfaces of this LR6, appearing as a widened fissure and a cavitated pit, respectively. They can easily be missed clinically unless the surfaces are clean and vision aided by the use of magnification and good illumination. (B) An LR7 with plaque obscuring the occlusal distal fissure cavity, which has been removed using bioactive glass air-abrasion. Histologically, both lesions extended into dentine, visible on radiographs; (mICDAS 3/ICCMS moderate). (Courtesy Mackenzie L, Banerjee A. The minimally invasive management of early occlusal caries: a practical guide. *Primary Dent J.* 2014 May; 3(2): 42-49. Doi:10.1308/205016814812143987.)

aetiological factors. For example, patients with xerostomia (dry mouth) due to intrinsic salivary gland disease or extrinsic damage (e.g., from radiotherapy when treating head and neck cancers) can develop lesions on the incisal surfaces of anterior teeth and lesions that circumvent the neck of the crown at the gingival margin. Patients with eating disorders may present lesions on the lingual-cervical aspect of the mandibular teeth (Fig. 2.14).

2.5.3 Investigations

To aid the process of clinical detection and information gathering—the first clinical domain of the MIOC framework—other investigations may be required, the results of which must be interpreted clinically to help verify or make the final diagnosis of the problem and possibly its aetiology. Investigations have a cost implication to the patient or the health service provider and, depending on the test, may be invasive or even potentially harmful in nature. It is imperative that information gathered using multiple investigations must not be interpreted individually, but in conjunction with all the clinical methods described in this chapter, to help formulate the diagnosis for the patient. All investigations are prone to false-positive and false-negative outcomes. By analysing the relative proportions of these outcomes, statistical measures of *sensitivity* (how effective an investigation is at detecting true disease) and *specificity* (how effective an investigation is at detecting true health) as well as the *positive predictive value* (ppv;– true positives divided by the sum of true and false positives) can be developed and used to assess the investigation's value in providing a clinically relevant diagnostic yield. For caries detection, these include intra-oral radiographs, pulp sensibility tests and percussion tests.

2.5.3.1 Radiographs

Horizontal bitewing radiographs should be used to aid carious lesion detection on proximal surfaces of posterior teeth, especially when adjacent teeth are present and direct vision is not possible. A film holder and beam-aiming device should be used routinely to obtain the optimal angulation of the beam perpendicular to the contact points and to allow reproducibility of films when monitoring lesions over a period of time (Fig. 2.15).

Incipient occlusal lesions are difficult to detect and only later-stage occlusal lesions are clearly visible on these radiographs. Periapical radiographs may be used to assess the depth of proximal lesions in anterior teeth. Dental panoramic tomograms (sometimes also called DPTs, OPTs or OPGs) should not be used routinely for caries detection due to their limited resolution, potential for distortion and increased radiation dose when compared with small intra-oral films. The radiographic appearance of carious lesions (radiolucency in enamel or dentine) is often described as being up to 6 months behind the actual histological spread of the lesion in the

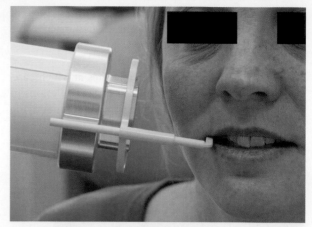

Fig. 2.15 Right bitewing radiograph being taken with film holder and beam-aiming device *(yellow arm)* enabling optimal alignment of the radiographic beam at right angles to the teeth and intra-oral film.

tooth. Therefore a lesion radiographically encased within enamel may have actually spread histologically across the enamel–dentine junction (EDJ) into the outer third of dentine. This is because intra-oral radiography, at the conventional clinical radiation dose, has only sufficient sensitivity to detect relatively gross changes in mineral density. As the beam passes through quantities of potentially sound, highly mineralised tissues in a tooth, zones of early demineralisation will be masked and therefore become undetectable on the film, plate or sensor. Thus conventional radiography can detect only the demineralisation in more extensive enamel lesions and the caries-infected dentine of the deeper lesion (refer to Chapter 1, Section 1.1.6). Remember, radiographs are two-dimensional representations of the change in radiodensity of a three-dimensional object, taken at a snapshot in time. Studies have shown that once a carious lesion has progressed radiographically into the middle third of dentine and beyond, the enamel is likely to be grossly demineralised and cavitated. Radiographically shallower lesions show a tendency towards less or no cavitation.

Table 2.4 shows how the mICDAS scores for the visual and histological lesion appearance correlate with the radiographic appearance and depth of enamel and dentine lesions. Examples of lesions detected from right and left bitewing radiographs of a high caries risk patient are shown in Fig. 2.16A and B. Once experience has been gained in interpreting radiographs, other clues can often be found to help with the diagnosis and potential activity status of the lesion(s). These might include the

TABLE 2.4   Association Between Radiographic Lesion Depth (E1–D3) and mICDAS Scores

Enamel Lesion		mICDAS
E1	Outer half of enamel	0,1
E2	Inner half of enamel	1
Dentine Lesion		**mICDAS**
D1	Outer third of dentine	2
D2	Middle third of dentine	3
D3	Inner third of dentine	4

outline of the pulp horns that form the roof of the pulp chamber; often, tertiary dentine has been laid down in response to past active disease, and this can be observed by the relative shrinkage of the radiolucent pulp horn subjacent to the spreading lesion. Also, the 'moth-eaten' appearance of the advancing edge of the radiolucency is a clue that, at the time when the film was taken, the lesion was in a state of relative activity, causing active demineralisation. If the dentine–pulp complex has had a chance to lay down extra mineral to wall off the lesion (a more defined radio-opaque boundary), this implies a relative tip in the metabolic balance towards inactivity in the biofilm and relative healing or remineralisation within the advancing front of the lesion itself.

It is imperative that the clinician does not immediately jump into operatively treating a radiolucency on a radiograph alone, without considering all the other clinical findings, signs and symptoms. A diagnosis must be made using all of the preceding information prior to any operative intervention. Radiographic radiolucencies and radio-opacities in teeth may be caused by:

- Pathology (e.g., caries, internal resorption, pulp calcifications)
- Natural anatomy (e.g., pulp chamber morphology, rotations or malpositioning of teeth, anatomical superimposition, canine fossae in first premolars)
- Artefacts (e.g., cervical burnout in the proximal region of the tooth close to the alveolar crest, where the enamel thins out, mimicking a proximal carious lesion; Fig. 2.16C)
- Restorations (e.g., radiolucent or opaque restorative materials; Fig. 2.16C–E)

Fig. 2.16C–E show examples of potential conundrums that a clinician may encounter when interpreting the causes of differing radiodensities in bitewing or other radiographs. An 'obvious' initial diagnosis of active caries made from detecting the well-demarcated hemispherical radiolucency in Fig. 2.16C does not correlate with the clinical findings from the same tooth (Fig. 2.16D). So what is the cause of the radiolucency? (See answer to self-assessment question 2.16C). The diffuse radiolucency just subjacent to the restoration in the maxillary left first molar in Fig. 2.16E poses an interesting dilemma. This laminate or layered restoration was placed after minimally invasive, selective carious dentine excavation (see Chapter 5, Section 5.9) and the digital radiograph taken at the 1-year recall consultation. What might cause such an appearance?

- Residual, inactive caries retained during the minimally invasive caries excavation procedure
- Active caries due to microleakage at the proximal restoration margin
- The presence of a radiolucent pulp protection material (see Chapter 5, Section 5.10)
- The possible effect on dentine of the restorative adhesive process (e.g., adhesive procedure, dental adhesive (see Chapter 7, Section 7.2.3) or even the direct effect of a biointeractive restorative material on dentine (e.g., tricalcium silicates, Chapter 7, Section 7.7)

In such cases, it is imperative to examine the tooth-restoration complex carefully and to check for signs and symptoms from the patient. The findings from other investigations may be required (see later). Collectively, this information will help the clinician ascertain the cause of the radiographic finding and therefore the necessity to manage the situation operatively or preventively. Examination of the patient notes and any previous radiographs and their radiographic reporting will also be useful in this regard.

Just taking and filing radiographs in the patient's notes is not acceptable. It is essential that a comprehensive report of all radiographic findings are dated and duly noted in the patient's notes for long-term scrutiny, active surveillance and dento-legal reasons.

2.5.3.2 Pulp Sensibility Tests

Technically, the term *pulp vitality* refers to the status of pulpal blood flow. This can only be measured, strictly speaking, using laser Doppler flowmetry, with a limited

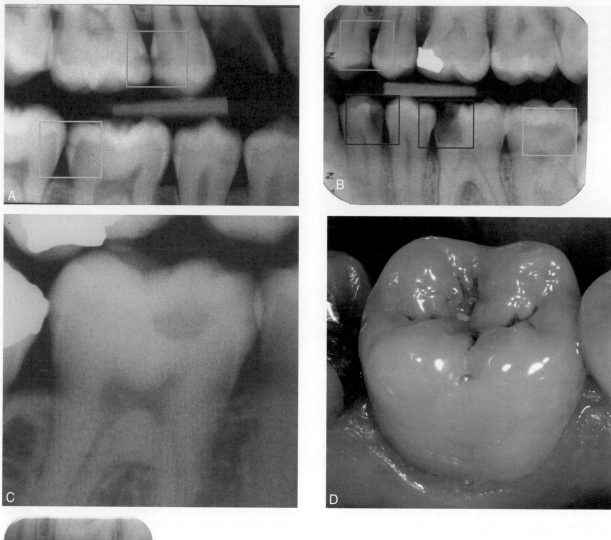

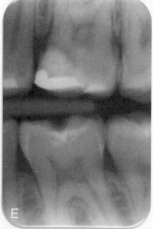

Fig. 2.16 (A) Right and (B) left bitewing radiographs from two different patients, both with high caries experience, showing carious lesions within enamel and outer third of dentine (E2–D1, *blue square*), approaching middle third of dentine (D2, *amber square*) and very close to the pulp (D3, *red square*). Note that other lesions can be detected on these films. (C) Well-defined radiolucency in the occlusal aspect of the mandibular molar and radiolucencies present at the cervical aspects both mesially and distally. (D) Clinical image of the mandibular molar whose radiograph is shown in (C) (Fig. 2.16C–D courtesy L Mackenzie). (E) Left bitewing radiograph focusing on the maxillary and mandibular first molars. Note the radio-opacity associated with the occlusal aspect of the mandibular first molar. The maxillary left first molar has received a mesio-occlusal proximal restoration to treat a large carious lesion. Note the differences in radiodensity between the different restorative materials, enamel and dentine. Note also the diffuse radiolucency between the deepest aspect of the restoration and the pulp chamber (see text for explanation).

Q2.16A and B: Can you find more lesions and radiographically classify them? Can you comment on the radiographic changes of the pulp chambers in those teeth?
Q2.16C: What is the cause of the radiolucencies in Fig. 2.16C? (Clue: Examine Fig. 2.16D very carefully for the answer!)
Q2.16E: i. Can you work out which materials have been used to restore the left maxillary first molar?
ii. What other information would you need before deciding whether to operatively intervene to manage the diffuse radiolucency subjacent to the restoration?
iii. What might be the cause of the radio-opacity in the mandibular first molar?

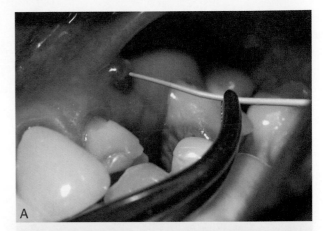

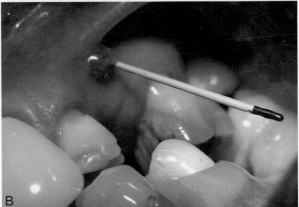

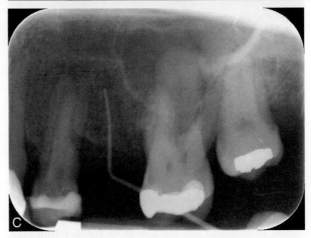

research use only. Clinical signs of a non-vital, necrotic pulp may include:

- Discolouration and darkening of the tooth due to the breakdown products of haemoglobin in the pulp chamber. Greying and reduced translucency of the crown of the tooth might also be noticed. These changes may be difficult to detect if the tooth is heavily restored or has an extra-coronal restoration covering it.
- Over time, a necrotic pulp may give rise to a sinus tract, tracking from the periapical tissues to the mucosal surface usually adjacent to the apex of the tooth in question. A gutta percha point inserted gently into the endodontic sinus and then radiographed will show the direction of the sinus track and ultimately the periapical origin of the infection (Fig. 2.17A–C).

The status of pulp innervation (sensibility) can be assessed to ascertain the effect of the caries process on the pulp using a:

- *Thermal test*: Heat from warm gutta percha sticks (rarely used) or, more commonly, cold from cotton wool pledgets soaked in ethyl chloride or ice sticks may be used to ascertain the status of pulp innervation. Unrestored tooth surfaces to be assessed must be dry and clear of surface debris (plaque and calculus; Fig. 2.18A–B). Check equivalent teeth on the contralateral side to the tooth in question and then the adjacent teeth (acting as an internal control), ensuring that the cotton wool, ice stick or gutta percha stick is placed on a clean, dry, sound tooth surface. Ask the patient to raise a hand when they feel a sensation in the tooth being tested. Vital teeth tend

Fig. 2.17 (A) A soft, non-tender fluctuant swelling on the dentoalveolar mucosa adjacent distally to the periapical region of the broken-down UL4. This is the orifice of a chronic sinus into which a sterile gutta percha point has been carefully inserted (B) and a periapical radiograph taken to show the exact location of the source of infection (C). The UL6 is vital with no symptoms.

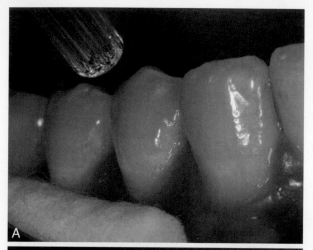

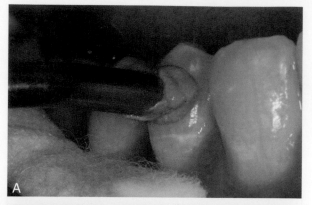

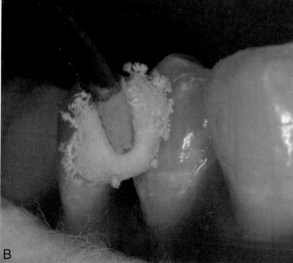

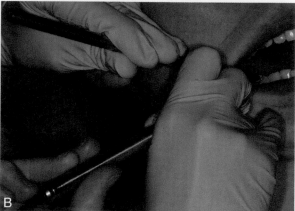

Fig. 2.19 (A) The probe tip of the electric pulp tester is placed on the clean, dry tooth surface, coupled with prophypaste. (B) Note the patient's fingers (ungloved) touching the probe handle, thus completing the electrical circuit. The patient should let go to break the circuit when a sensation is felt in the tooth.

Fig. 2.18 (A) Pulp sensibility testing of cleaned and air-dried LR4 using a cold ethyl chloride-soaked cotton wool pledget (B). Avoid direct contact with restorations and the gingival margin as false-positive readings may ensue.

to respond quickly whereas false-positive readings respond more slowly (conduction through dentine or metallic restoration into the periodontal membrane).

- *Electrical test*: A mono-polar electric pulp test unit passes a small current (direct or alternating) through the patient and the tooth it is in contact with. The patient's hand must be in contact with the metal handle of the handpiece to complete the circuit with some commercial systems. The probe is placed on a clean, sound tooth surface (contralateral and adjacent equivalents are tested first as an internal patient control) using an electrolytic coupling agent on the tooth surface to ensure completion of the circuit (usually a

small amount of prophylaxis paste; Fig. 2.19A–B). The current is increased gradually by the dentist until the patient feels a tingling sensation in the tooth. At this point they are instructed to let go of the handpiece and the circuit is broken. The numerical value can be recorded and is useful for monitoring purposes for a particular tooth but is not equivocal as the readings can vary from the same patient. False-positive responses may be elicited through stimulation of nerve fibres in the periodontium, and in posterior multirooted teeth a mixture of vital and non-vital pulp tissue may confound the interpretation of the reading.

- *Test cavity preparation without local anaesthesia*: This is a rarely used, invasive last resort test that checks the innervation of the dentine–pulp complex by drilling into potentially vital dentine. If the patient feels pain, then at least partial innervation of the pulp remains.

It is important to note in these cases that a positive response from the pulp does not necessarily mean all is well. There is no clinical way to know whether there is partial necrosis or denervation in the dental pulp, and multirooted teeth can present with partially diseased pulp tissues. Indeed, the clinical assessment of histological pulp status is not a pure, objective science and requires careful interpretation of all clinical findings associated with the tooth in question.

2.5.3.3 Percussion Tests

Percussion tests (gently tapping the crown axially and then obliquely with a probe or mirror handle) assess the physical condition of the periapical tissues and periodontal membrane, not the pulp directly. If periapical periodontitis is present, the piston-like effect of the tooth being pushed into the inflamed periapical tissues will elicit acute tenderness to percussion, denoted as TTP. The inflammation in the periodontal tissues might be caused by the toxins from a necrotic pulp. This clinical finding is also of interest when interpreting reported patient symptoms. If a patient describes a pain on biting and can point to the specific tooth in question, the diagnosis is more likely to be a periapical or periodontal problem or a cracked tooth (see later). The pain caused by the caries process will often not be specific to a single tooth, and patients will often describe an area or region of the jaws or face that is affected (see Chapter 3, Section 3.2.1).

2.5.4 Lesion Activity

As has been emphasised in Chapter 1, the caries process is driven within the stagnant, dysbiotic plaque biofilm at the tooth surface. The histological tooth tissue damage that gradually ensues is a direct consequence of this surface biofilm's metabolic processes. So when discussing caries activity, one has to distinguish between the biofilm metabolic activity and the lesion activity that is being considered. As the metabolic activity of the biofilm is continually dynamic, it is safely assumed that the presence of a stagnant, dense and more tenacious biofilm is indicative of an ongoing active metabolic caries process. This is why in the clinical examination, it is important to identify and describe any such surface biofilm deposits in the clinical notes before removing them to view the underlying tooth surfaces directly (see Section 2.5). Within the carious lesion itself, it is important to ascertain whether the biochemical conditions within the lesion lead to:

- Net tissue breakdown (demineralisation and proteolytic organic breakdown – lesion progression)

- Net balance (inactivity or arrested lesion)
- Ideally, net healing with a tendency towards mineral crystal deposition (lesion regression or reversal)

Gathering this information is critical to develop the correct personalised care plan which can then be implemented. However, this can be difficult to intraorally define and measure objectively at present, especially as clinical examinations occur at a single moment in time whereas metabolic biofilm and lesion activity will clearly fluctuate over time and will not be constant. There is therefore a clinical need in the future for longitudinal, intra-oral, ionic-level monitoring to help solve this problem of measuring activity accurately. In the meantime, certain clinical indicators of activity can be gleaned from the:

- *Colour and surface texture of a cavitated lesion*: An arrested lesion is often darker in colour and the exposed dentine has a flint-like, hard, shiny outer surface when probed (see Chapter 1, Table 1.2).
- *Presence of gingival bleeding around the tooth*: The presence of gingival inflammation implies poor oral hygiene in that area which will increase the risk of dental plaque accumulation, thus making it more likely for the adjacent lesion to be in an active state of metabolic transition.
- *Presence of dense plaque*: If a thick biofilm overlies the lesion, it can reasonably be assumed that it is in a state of activity as it is the presence of the plaque biofilm that is critical to the development of the carious lesion (Fig. 2.20A). If plaque can be found on non-retentive sites, again this implies poor oral hygiene measures and therefore an increased risk of caries incidence.
- *Accessibility to OH procedures*: If lesions are present in uncleansable sites (see earlier), then again it is likely that the lesions will be active as a biofilm will collect and stagnate on their surfaces.
- *Use of plaque indicators* (Fig. 2.20B–E): Dental manufacturers have produced two- and three-tone plaque disclosing solutions and gels which can give the practitioner and patient an indication not only on which surfaces the plaque biofilm is stagnating, but also for how long, as well as the plaque density and even the acid levels present in specific areas on the tooth surface. The bacterial population (and the cariogenicity) of the biofilm develops in a structured manner in correlation with its age: the older the plaque is, the more anaerobic and acidic the conditions on the enamel surface are likely to be (see Chapter 1, Sections 1.1.3 and 1.1.4).

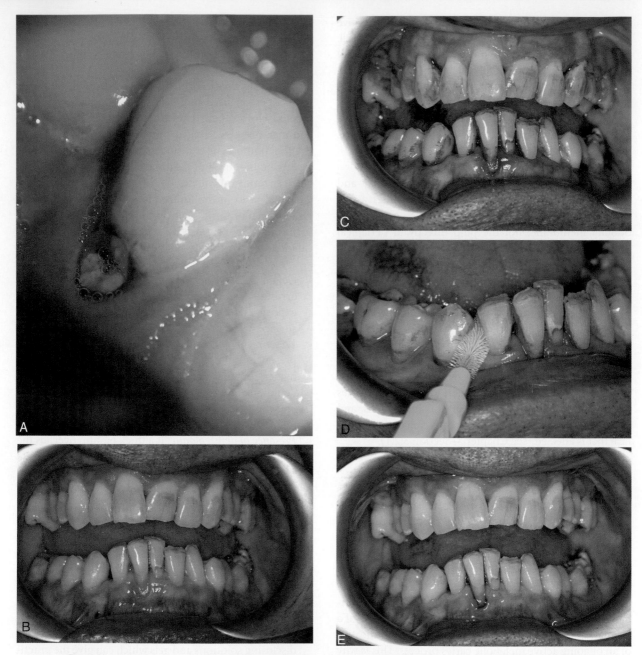

Fig. 2.20 (A) Dense plaque biofilm sitting on the surface of a buccal cervical carious lesion indicating a high potential for caries activity. (B) Anterior view of dentition in a patient on initial presentation. (C) A three-tone plaque indicator gel applied *(dark blue, pink, pale blue; GC Corp)*, highlighting the differing densities of plaque accumulated on the labial and gingival margins of the same teeth in (B) and highlighting areas of increased acid presence *(pale blue)*. (D) oral hygiene procedures are taught and practised by the patient and (E) the final result after air-polishing. (Courtesy B Dawett.)

Q2.20A: How could you manage this case?

These proprietary kits assess neither absolute lesion activity nor overall patient susceptibility to caries from the relative quantities, age and acidogenicity of plaque, but can usefully add to all the other information gathered from the history and examination, thus helping to formulate an overall picture of the individual's susceptibility and likelihood to suffer from caries in the future. They also can be helpful as strong motivators for patients, coupled with the use of intra-oral clinical photographs, to show them their problems directly and to help improve their own oral health with better oral hygiene procedures that can be easily demonstrated by members of the oral healthcare team. Indeed, mobile phone apps are now being developed using augmented reality technology to allow patients to disclose plaque and then help guide their oral hygiene practice to remove it in the comfort of their own bathrooms.

- *Use of saliva test kits*: The lack or absence of saliva is an important aetiological factor in increasing the susceptibility of patients to caries and toothwear, more specifically dental erosion. More individuals are taking multiple medications (polypharmacy) with the synergistic negative side effect of increased dry mouth (xerostomia), thus leading to a prevalence of this condition of approximately 20% of the older adult UK population currently. Volumetric and flow rate analyses can be carried out using simple chairside kits assessing unstimulated and stimulated salivary flow and volume as well as crude levels of *Streptococcus mutans* (as a broad indicator of the caries process) can also be calculated from saliva samples. The quality of the saliva can also be documented and monitored clinically using the clinical oral dryness index (Table 2.5). This includes a clinical assessment of the viscosity, colour and frothiness of the saliva. If the results from volumetric and flow rate analyses indicate low salivary output and there are high levels of *Streptococcus mutans* in a sample of the patient's saliva, then, *in conjunction with the results of other clinical investigations and observations*, the clinician may collate evidence that points to the patient having a higher caries risk or susceptibility, with any lesions present having an increased chance of being active over a period of time.

To make effective use of the data, all of the preceding assessments need to be carried out periodically over time, as opposed to a simple single snapshot. After initial recorded baseline investigations in patients deemed at risk of caries, follow-up tests may be carried out at predefined, patient-specific recall intervals, a process known as *active surveillance*. This will help to evaluate a patient's change in risk or susceptibility over time and thus make suitable, evidence-based adjustments to their personalised care plan. Patients categorised at low risk do not necessarily need continuous testing, apart from at the routine examination, as this may prove expensive with no positive clinical benefits gained. Do not forget that in primary care, this latter group will form the majority of the patients you provide care for.

2.5.5 Diet Analysis

The primary, mouth-level aetiological factors for dental caries, as described in Chapter 1, include a susceptible tooth surface, presence of bacteria, fermentable carbohydrates and enough time for the combination to start demineralising the tooth surface beneath the thickened dysbiotic plaque biofilm. The surfaces of the teeth can be examined for carious lesions, as can the bacterial levels in plaque and saliva (see earlier). The other main aetiological factor that can be assessed during this detection phase of patient management is the dietary intake of refined carbohydrate and sugar levels of patients, especially those exhibiting signs of high caries susceptibility (multiple lesions (>2) developed within the previous 2 years). This is done by asking the patient to fill out a diet analysis sheet (an example is given in Fig. 2.21) usually over a period of at least 3 days, encompassing the weekend. They should be advised to write down everything that passes between their lips in that time (including water, carbonated and non-carbonated drinks, numbers of spoons of sugar in tea and/or coffee, sauces used during meal preparation and consumption, etc.) and to note when they brush their teeth and the type of brush and dentifrice used.

Dietary sugars can be classified into (see Chapter 1, Table 1.1):

- Mono- and disaccharides (e.g., glucose, galactose, fructose, sucrose, maltose, lactose)
- Added sugars (all added mono- and disaccharides including honey and syrups, such as maple syrup and agave nectar)
- Natural (intrinsic) sugars (those sugars located physically in the cellular structure of grains, fruits and vegetables plus those naturally present in milk and milk products)
- Free (non-milk extrinsic) sugars (those sugars added by manufacturers, chefs or consumers plus those present naturally in honey and syrups, fruit juices and concentrates)

TABLE 2.5   Challacombe Scale of Clinical Oral Dryness (QR code)

The Challacombe Scale
of Clinical Oral Dryness

KING'S *College* LONDON

The Challacombe Scale was developed from research conducted at King's College London Dental Institute under the supervision of Professor Stephen Challacombe*. The purpose of this scale is to be able to visually identify and quantify whether your patient has xerostomia (dry mouth) and if so, how it changes over time and the most appropriate therapy options. This scale is applicable whatever your profession.

The Challacombe Scale works as an additive score of 1 to 10 : 1 being the least and 10 being the most severe. Each feature scores 1 and symptoms will not necessarily progress in the order shown, but summated scores indicate likely patient needs. Score changes over time can be used to monitor symptom progression or regression.

1   ☐ Mirror sticks to buccal mucosa

2   ☐ Mirror sticks to tongue

3   ☐ Saliva frothy

An additive score of 1 - 3 indicates mild dryness. May not need treatment or management. Sugar-free chewing gum for 15 mins, twice daily and attention to hydration is needed. Many drugs will cause mild dryness. Routine checkup monitoring required.

4   ☐ No saliva pooling in floor of mouth

5   ☐ Tongue shows generalised shortened papillae (mild depapillation)

6   ☐ Altered gingival architecture (ie. smooth)

An additive score of 4 - 6 indicates moderate dryness. Sugar-free chewing gum or simple sialogogues may be required. Needs to be investigated further if reasons for dryness are not clear. Saliva substitutes and topical fluoride may be helpful. Monitor at regular intervals especially for early decay and symptom change.

7   ☐ Glassy appearance of oral mucosa, especially palate

8   ☐ Tongue lobulated / fissured

9   ☐ Cervical caries (more than two teeth)

10 ☐ Debris on palate or sticking to teeth

An additive score of 7 - 10 indicates severe dryness. Saliva substitutes and topical fluoride usually needed. Cause of hyposalivation needs to be ascertained and Sjögrens Syndrome excluded. Refer for investigation and diagnosis. Patients then need to be monitored for changing symptoms and signs, with possible further specialist input if worsening.

© King's College London 2011

* S Osailan et al "Investigating the relationship between hyposalivation and mucosal wetness" (2011) Oral Diseases volume 17, Issue 1, Pages: 109–114

Printing supported by:

A.S Saliva Orthana - fast relief for dry mouth
www.aspharma.co.uk   ■   info@aspharma.co.uk   ■   01264 332172

A.S SALIVA ORTHANA

Note: Assessing 10 common clinical signs in no particular clinical order, the clinician can assign an additive score, dependent upon the number of signs observed (1–10). Each has a score of 1; the total score helps direct likely management outcomes. Total scores can change over time and can be used to monitor and document changes in the oral environment.

	Thursday			Friday			Saturday			Sunday		
	Time	Item	⑧	Time	Item	⑧	Time	Item	⑧	Time	Item	⑧
Before breakfast	7.30	(Tea*)		7.0	(Tea*)		7.30	(Tea*)		7.05	(Tea*)	
Breakfast	8.00	2 Wheat slices 2 Crisp bread 1 Apple (Coffee*)		8.00	2 Wheat slices 2 Crisp bread 1 Apple (Coffee*)		8.30	2 Wheat slices 2 Crisp bread 1 Apple (Coffee*)		8.05	2 Wheat slices 2 Crisp bread 1 Apple (Coffee*)	
Morning	9.00	(Polo)		10.00 11.30	(Murray mint) (Tea* Biscuit)		11.15	(Tea*)		10.00 12.30	(Lemon Barley) (Tea*)	
Mid-day Meal	12.30	Meat roll (Tea*)		2.00	Steamed fish Parsley sauce Boiled potatoes		1.45	Sausage, onion, Boiled potatoes (Ice Cream tinned fruit)		1.40	Roast lamb, potatoes, cabbage, carrots	
Afternoon	2.00 5.30	2 Cream crackers 1 Dairy Lea (Tea*) (2 Short bread biscuits Tea*)		2.45 6.00	(Tea*) (Tea*)		2.30 5.45	(Tea*) (Tea*)		2.00 4.00	(Tea*) (Tea*)	
Evening Meal	8.00	Chop, leeks, boiled potatoes (Choc-ice Tea*)		8.30	Bacon sandwich (Tea*)		7.30	Fried kipper bread and butter		8.15	Ham salad, bread and butter (Tea*)	
Evening and night	1.00	(Horlicks* Biscuits)		10.00 1.30	Peanuts (Horlicks* Biscuits)		9.15 1.45	(Chocolate) (Horlicks* Biscuits)		1.15	(Horlicks* Biscuits)	

Fig. 2.21 Diet analysis sheet filled in by a middle-aged man with a high incidence of caries.

> **Q2.21:** What stands out as the main issues regarding this patient's dietary sugar intake?

The World Health Organization (WHO) has issued guidelines recommending that intake of free sugars should provide ≤10% of energy intake and suggesting further reductions to <5% of energy intake to protect dental health throughout life.[1] The quantity of total free sugar consumption and frequency of intake per person across most age groups has, however, increased significantly over the past four decades in the UK and in many countries throughout the world. These are the two key parameters that are being checked with a diet history or diet diary. No indication of the relevance of the diet analysis should be revealed to the patient at the first appointment so as not to bias the patient or allow them to manipulate data by

writing down a diet intake they perceive is an improvement on what they are actually doing! These data could be collected in real time using an online form that directly uploads the information into the patient's clinical notes in the dental practice. The results should then be analysed by the dentist and/or trained members of the oral healthcare team, possibly beforehand and an appointment made to discuss them with the patient and/or caregiver. This consultation could also be carried out remotely, using online video technology at times to suit the patient, utilising the skill sets of different members of the oral healthcare team. In this way, availability and access to care might be improved for those patient groups most in need of the advice and attention, but less likely to actually attend physical appointments. Issues to highlight include frequency of meals and sugar intake, quantity of hidden sugar content (e.g., many sauces, ingredients and condiments are high in sugar), quantity, oral medications and drinks consumed (which have additional sugar, high sugar content and/or erosive potential due to their high titratable acidity). It is imperative that the whole team works with the patient to *modify* their existing dietary habits pragmatically. Chastising or criticising the patient and telling or ordering them to change will have the opposite effect! Work with positive reinforcement and motivational interviewing techniques and offer suggestions or, even better, encourage the patient to make sensible suggestions themselves to lower their sugar intake, frequency and duration. Remember, goal setting and positive encouragement to instigate small, simple changes over time are most likely to result in positive adherence to behavioural change in the long term. Motivational interviewing skills are a valuable asset in helping to alter patient attitudes and adherence to advice. COM-B psychological behaviour change modelling with goal setting has been proven to help in this regard (enlightening, facilitating, enhancing and encouraging patients' capability, opportunity and motivation, all leading to positive behaviour change; see Chapter 4, Section 4.2.2).

2.5.6 Caries Detection Technologies

As an adjunct to the investigations and examinations described earlier, many other technologies are available to help the clinician detect carious lesions. Examples of some of these are shown in Table 2.6. Most detection technologies work on four basic physics principles affecting macroscopic and microscopic changes in mineralised dental tissues:

- Optical light scattering effects
- Mineral density changes
- Fluorescent characteristics
- Tissue porosity

It is evident from the list in Table 2.6 that the currently available caries detection devices all work by assessing levels of tissue damage that have already occurred due to the active caries process in the overlying biofilm. It is arguable that these technologies do not go far enough in terms of early detection—the ideal detection device perhaps is one that detects biochemical and metabolic activity changes that would lead to clinical tissue damage if left unchecked; that is, detecting lesions before they actually present. Indeed, a technology exists that is capable of assessing the release of free calcium ions from a tooth surface by detecting the bioluminescent signal emitted from a photoprotein that binds to such ions: Calcivis. However, the counter-argument to this degree of lesion detection is what would the clinician do with the information gathered using such a device? How would the clinical care change or be enhanced from the primary preventive advice already advocated? If clinical data are to be collected, however non-invasive the process is, it is essential

TABLE 2.6	**Modern Technologies to Help Detect and Characterise Carious Lesions**		
	Light Scattering	**Mineral Content/ Density**	**Fluorescence/ Luminescence**	**Ionic/Tissue Porosity**
In-vivo	Vision/magnification DIFOTI UV illumination Quantitative laser fluorescence (QLF) DiagnoDent	Radiography RVG Computer Tomography MRI Tactile surface hardness	QLF Canary Dye-enhanced Laser fluorescence (DELF) UV illumination Calcivis DiagnoDent	ECM AC Impedance (ACIST) DELF Dye penetration (iodide) Ultrasound Bioluminescence
In-vitro	Polarised, transmitted light microscopy (PTLM)	SEM Quantitative BSE-SEM Microradiography Microfocal CT X-ray microtomography X-ray microanalysis	Confocal laser-scanning fluorescence microscopy	PTLM Acoustic microscopy Iontophoresis

Note: The four columns indicate the basic physics principle on which each technology relies. The second row gives the technologies useful in the research laboratory.

that the patient derives from the process a clear clinical outcome benefit. Collection of clinical data per se is not acceptable unless it is perhaps part of a clinical research project in which some other outcome will be achieved.

It is important to understand the physics of how a particular technology works so as to be able to accurately interpret the information it is providing. An example of such an ambiguity is the DiagnoDent laser-fluorescence caries detection system. Note that in Table 2.6, this system has been placed into two categories, optical light scattering and fluorescence, as clinical research has shown the unit is affected by both properties to a varying degree. Therefore the clinical interpretation of results—that is, whether to prepare a cavity or not—must be assessed with caution in the clinical environment, again in conjunction with all the other information gathered for the particular patient and tooth. Remember, the best detection technology is a combination of your keen eyes and cerebral processing of all the information gathered, using your clinical experience gained over time! Ultimately the use of such adjunctive detection technologies can be beneficial, but only if the clinician is experienced enough to understand the device limitations. It is the responsibility of the operator to do their own research and critically read any published papers, especially those highlighting the sensitivity (the ability of the device to detect true lesions and disease) and specificity (the ability of the device to detect true health) measurements of such technologies. Be aware that many such studies are carried out in controlled in-vitro laboratory experiments and the results are difficult to extrapolate into the clinical setting. No clinical detection devices are perfect—they will always provide false-positive and false-negative readings—so always interpret any information with clinical caution.

2.6 TOOTHWEAR: CLINICAL DETECTION

2.6.1 Targeted Verbal History

In patients with lifestyle-related toothwear lesions or pathological tooth surface loss, it is critical that not only are these detected, noted carefully and a putative cause attributed (i.e., erosive, attritive, abrasive or abfraction lesions from their clinical presentation; see later), but also that the aetiology of the erosion, attrition, abrasion or abfraction is appreciated by both the patient and the oral healthcare team (see Chapter 1, Section 1.2 and Table 1.3). In this way, the overall clinical problem can be managed successfully. It is all too easy to try to treat the tissue damage alone as a quick fix for the patient, but without addressing and managing the cause of the problem, a cure will not

be found. Coupled with the general information obtained from the presenting history as described and discussed previously, more specific questions may be targeted to assess the aetiology of the specific type of toothwear, often after the initial clinical examination has been completed:

- Relating to *erosive* toothwear:
  - Past and present diet (using a diet analysis sheet (Fig. 2.21); questions regarding quantity and frequency of specific acidic food and drink intake using a risk factor questionnaire (Fig. 2.22)
  - Digestive disorders causing intrinsic regurgitation erosion or pregnancy sickness
  - Past or present slimming habits, eating disorders, periods of weight loss
  - Past or present alcohol intake
  - Past or present oral medications (e.g., vitamin C, iron preparations)
  - Past or present occupation (environmental conditions and/or industrial erosion can be associated with certain occupations, but thanks to more stringent workplace safety regulations and risk assessments, these causes are rare nowadays)
- Relating to *attrition*:
  - Clenching or grinding habits during the day or at night (often, information might be gleaned from a partner)
  - Levels of stress or anxiety in personal or professional life, linked to clenching or grinding habits
  - Evidence of masseteric hypertrophy
- Relating to *abrasion*:
  - Past or present oral hygiene techniques (toothbrushing, flossing, abrasive toothpastes)
  - Habits causing dental abrasion, such as pipe smoking, pen chewing and fingernail biting (Fig. 2.26)

2.6.2 Clinical Presentations of Toothwear

The causes of pathological toothwear (erosion, attrition, abrasion and abfraction) have been outlined and discussed in Chapter 1, Section 1.2. The clinical examination described previously will help guide the clinician towards the visual detection of some characteristic features (site and shape of facets or presence of facets on opposing teeth) of the different presentations of toothwear. However, these are often combined as the cause, and therefore the clinical manifestations of toothwear lesions are multifactorial (Fig. 2.23).

- *Erosion*: Depending on the direct cause, affects the labial (extrinsic dietary acids) and palatal smooth

Risk factor questionnaire

Thank you for taking the time to fill in this questionnaire. Please read the following questions and answer in the space provided giving details where possible. All answers will be kept **strictly confidential** and will serve to give you advice in reducing the risk of tooth wear and caries.

What are your concerns regarding your mouth? (please tick where appropriate).

Pain	
Sensitivity	
Shape or size of your teeth	
Grinding/Clenching your teeth	
Fractured/sharp teeth	
Wear of teeth	
Bad breath	

Other (please detail):

Please tell us how much of these foodstuffs do you eat per *week* in the numbers of units outlined in brackets.

Chocolate (1 bar)	
Cakes, biscuits, sweet buns, pastries and /or fruit pies (1 slice)	
Sweet puddings (1 medium pudding)	
Sugared breakfast cereals (1 bowl)	
Jams and preserves (1 tablespoon)	
Ice cream (1 scoop)	
Dried fruits and fruit in syrup (1 tablespoon)	
Sweet syrups and sweet sauces (1 tablespoon)	
Honey (1 tablespoon)	
Sugar (1 tablespoon)	

Do you hold or swill drinks in your mouth before swallowing?	Yes: ☐ No: ☐
Do you use a glass, a straw or do you drink straight from the can/carton?	Glass:☐ Straw:☐ Can/Carton:☐
Do you suffer or have you ever suffered from an eating disorder? i.e. anorexia or bulimia	Yes: ☐ No: ☐
How many units of alcohol do you consume per week? (on average): A pint of lager, beer or cider contains 3 units. A small glass of wine (175 ml) contains 2 units. A double shot of spirits (50 ml) contains 3 units.	

Please tell us how much of these drinks do you drink per *week* (average number of cans, glasses or bottles).

Fizzy cola drinks (diet or regular)	
Fizzy lemonade/orangeade	
Energy drinks and other fizzy drinks	
Apple juice	
Orange juice	
Grapefruit juice	
Cranberry juice	
Fruit smoothies	
Other fruit juices	
Squash	
Sweetened milk drinks	

Other acidic or sweet drinks (please specify):

Please tell us how much of these fruits do you eat per *week* in the number of units outlined in brackets.

Lemons (1/2 fruit)	
Oranges / Tangerines / Clementines (1 medium fruit)	
Grapefruit (1/2 fruit)	
Pineapple (1 slice)	
Apples/Pears (1 medium fruit)	
Peaches/Apricots/ Plums (1 fruit)	
Kiwi fruit (1 fruit)	
Berries, Grapes (1/2 cup)	

Other acidic fruits (please specify):

Have you suffered or do you currently suffer from the following (please circle frequency: *yearly (Y); monthly (M); weekly (W), daily (D) or more than once per day (M).*

Heartburn	(Y) (M) (W) (D) (+1)
Regurgitation	(Y) (M) (W) (D) (+1)
Vomiting	(Y) (M) (W) (D) (+1)
Acid taste in your mouth	(Y) (M) (W) (D) (+1)
Clenching your teeth	(Y) (M) (W) (D) (+1)
Grinding your teeth	(Y) (M) (W) (D) (+1)
Aches or pains around your jaw	(Y) (M) (W) (D) (+1)
Sensitivity of teeth	(Y) (M) (W) (D) (+1)

What is your occupation?	
Gender:	M: ☐ F: ☐
Age:	
How many times a day do you brush your teeth?	
Inter-dental cleaning? (floss or brushes)	Yes: ☐ No: ☐

THANK YOU FOR TAKING THE TIME TO FILL IN THIS QUESTIONNAIRE. PLEASE HAND IT TO THE CLINICIAN WHEN YOU COME TO YOUR APPOINTMENT.

Fig. 2.22 An example of a risk factor questionnaire for use when taking a targeted history for dental caries/dental erosion. (Courtesy of Jose Rodriguez.)

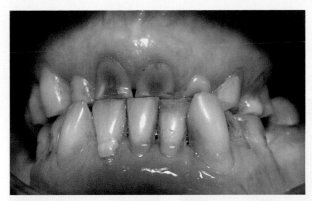

Fig. 2.23 A clinical case of toothwear showing the multifactorial aetiology including incisal attrition, labial erosion and buccal cervical abrasion in a middle-aged patient.

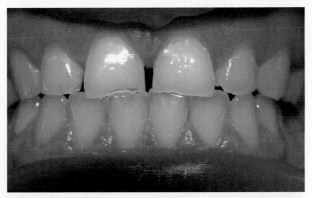

Fig. 2.24 A clinical anterior view of a patient with labial erosion. Note the reflective, smooth, featureless labial enamel surfaces of the UR2 to the UL2. There are early signs of incisal attrition and the resulting blue-grey, enamel translucency at the chipped incisal edges as the enamel has thinned.

> **Q2.23:** What would be the most obvious cause of the buccal cervical abrasion?

> **Q2.24:** What might be the presenting complaint of this patient?

surfaces and/or mandibular buccal or occlusal surfaces (extrinsic and intrinsic gastric regurgitation acids). Enamel loses its histological surface characterisation and becomes smooth and featureless (Figs. 2.24 and 2.25) and eventually dissolves completely to expose dentine. Erosion can cause smooth-cupped lesions on posterior occlusal surfaces (Fig. 2.25B). Existing restorations, especially dental amalgams, may appear to stand proud from the occlusal surface as the enamel and dentine erodes around them (Fig. 2.25B).

- *Attrition*: Often produces sharp, well-defined, interdigitating toothwear lesions on the incisal edges of anterior teeth that meet together precisely in occlusion (Figs. 2.23 and 2.24). Can also affect the occlusal surfaces of the molars but to a lesser extent.
- *Abrasion*: Lesions caused by repetitive foreign body contact, such as from toothbrushing (classic v-shaped notching on the buccal cervical aspect of mainly anterior teeth and premolars, but can sometimes affect molar teeth also). Can you guess the cause of the incisal wear lesions in Fig. 2.26?

2.6.3 Summary of the Clinical Manifestations of Toothwear

- The clinical features of faceting and/or loss of mineralised tissues highlighted in the previous section, cuspal wear (Fig. 2.25B).
- Dental sensitivity or pain caused by active toothwear as dentine tubules are freshly exposed and pain is elicited on hot and cold stimulation (physiological principles of Brannström's hydrodynamic theory). This is a surprisingly uncommon presenting complaint as toothwear occurs over a longer period and therefore tertiary or reparative dentine deposition will often prevent pulp symptoms from occurring.
- Weakened and chipped incisal edges causing trauma to or pain from the anterior tip of the tongue (due to roughness) and poor aesthetics (Figs. 2.23 and 2.24).
- Blue-grey appearance of the thinned enamel incisal edges and possible darkening of teeth due to the change in the optical qualities of the remaining mineralised tissues, again affecting overall aesthetics (Fig. 2.24).
- Loss of tooth structure and/or fractured teeth or restorations possibly leading to difficulties in chewing due to changes in the occlusion (loss of occlusal contacts, changes in vertical dimension of the bite) and aesthetics (Fig. 2.26).
- Increased risk of marginal fracture or defects of existing restorations as the surrounding hard tissues wear away more rapidly, leaving restorations standing proud.
- Pulpitis, exposure or even loss of sensibility attributable to the extent of tissue loss.
- Active toothwear lesions will often have a clean, fresh appearance whereas those lesion surfaces where the aetiology has been controlled and the process arrested, may pick up exogenous stains (dietary, smoking).

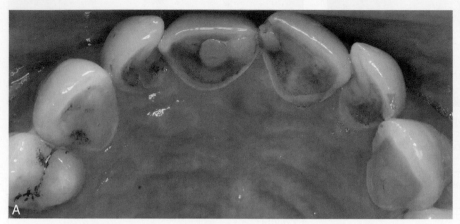
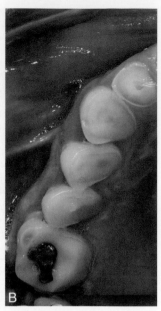

Fig. 2.25 (A) A mirrored clinical palatal view of an anterior dentition with erosion caused by excessive consumption of dietary acidic drinks. Note the smooth surfaces and peripheral rims of enamel on the UL3 to the UR3 as well as the resin composite restorations in the central incisors standing slightly proud of the eroded tooth surfaces. There was no evidence of gastro-oesophageal reflux from this patient's history. (B) A clinical occlusal view of the maxillary right quadrant of a patient showing the extensive and occlusal cupped lesions (UR6) associated with dental erosion and a dental amalgam restoration that seems to be standing proud from the eroded occlusal tooth surface (with an attritive component also). (Courtesy P Mylonas.)

Q2.25A: What clinical clues are present to indicate the relative activity of erosion?
Q2.25B: What might be the cause of such extensive erosion affecting these particular surfaces?

Some of these features may need operative management to gain immediate relief of acute symptoms or to restore overall dental form and function. However, without the aetiological factor(s) of toothwear being discovered, it will never be cured for that particular patient and the problems will return (see later). Toothwear also needs careful reviewing over a prolonged period to be able to assess its relative progress or stasis (see Chapter 9, Section 9.1.3). As with caries and periodontal disease, several clinical screening indices exist to enable practitioners to ascertain:

- The grade and stage of progress of the lesions
- Help in deciding on the intervention level required
- Prognosis of any such treatment provided
- Enabling medium to long term monitoring with careful documentation (also for dento-legal considerations)

One such clinical screening tool, the basic erosive wear examination (BEWE), can be used to stage toothwear in a similar way that the BPE (basic periodontal examination) does for periodontal disease (see Table 2.7).

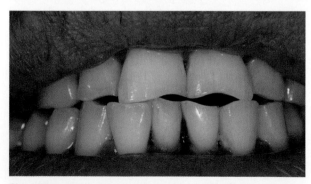

Fig. 2.26 An intriguing case of anterior, incisal, undulating lesions affecting both the mandibular and maxillary incisors. As they do not interdigitate in occlusion, they cannot be caused by attrition.

Q2.26: What do you think might be the cause of these incisal wear lesions?

TABLE 2.7 BEWE Index Table

A: Clinical sequence when using the BEWE
1. Diagnose the presence of toothwear; eliminate teeth with trauma and developmental defects from the score.
2. Examine all teeth and all surfaces of teeth in the mouth for toothwear.
3. Identify in each quadrant the most severely affected tooth with wear.
4. Conduct BEWE score.

B: Criteria for grading erosive wear

Score	Features
0	No erosive tooth wear
1	Initial loss of surface texture
2	Distinct defect, hard tissue loss <50% of the surface area
3	Hard tissue loss ≥50% of the surface area

C: Complexity levels as a guide to clinical management

Complexity Level	Cumulative Score of All Sextants	Management
0	Less than or equal to 2	Conduct routine maintenance and observation. Repeat at 3-year intervals.
1	Between 3 and 8	Provide oral hygiene and dietary assessment and advice, routine maintenance and observation. Repeat at 2-year intervals.
2	Between 9 and 13	Provide oral hygiene and dietary assessment and advice, identify the main aetiological factor(s) for tissue loss and develop strategies to eliminate respective impacts. Consider fluoridation measures or other strategies to increase the resistance of tooth surfaces. Ideally, avoid the placement of restorations and monitor erosive wear with study casts, photographs, or silicone impressions. Repeat at 6- to 12-month intervals.
3	14 and over	Provide oral hygiene and dietary assessment and advice, identify the main aetiological factor(s) for tissue loss and develop strategies to eliminate respective impacts. Consider fluoridation measures or other strategies to increase the resistance of tooth surfaces. Ideally, avoid restorations and monitor toothwear with study casts, photographs or silicone impressions. Especially in cases of severe progression, consider special care that may involve restorations. Repeat at 6- to 12-month intervals.

From Bartlett D. A proposed system for screening tooth wear. *Brit Dent J*. 2010 Mar 13;208(5):207-209. doi:10.1038/sj.bdj.2010.205

2.7 DENTAL TRAUMA: CLINICAL DETECTION

For patients presenting to a general dental practice after having sustained facial, oral or dental trauma, it is imperative that before any clinical examination is performed, a thorough history is taken of the incident leading to and causing the trauma. Any suspicions of a head injury including facial fractures (from the history, patient behaviour, general physical examination) should be dealt with by immediate referral to a hospital accident and emergency unit for medical investigation.

Other dentally relevant points to consider are:

- *Patient's age*: Stage of tooth or root and soft tissue development and patient compliance issues.
- *Direction of impact, blow or injury*: Relevant to the possible direction of displacement of tissues or restorations.
- *Extra-oral soft tissue injuries*: Examination of the full face, cheeks and lip lacerations before investigating

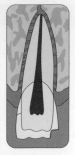
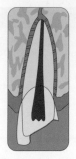
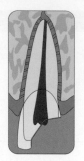
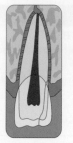
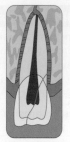
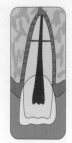

| Enamel infraction
Enamel fracture | Enamel + dentine
fracture | Enamel + dentine
+ pulp fracture
(complicated fracture) | Uncomplicated
crown-root fracture
(enamel + dentine
+ cementum) | Complicated
crown-root
fracture (enamel +
dentine + cementum + pulp) | Root fracture |

Fig. 2.27 Classification of traumatic dental tooth fractures.

intra-orally. Make clear clinical records with a date and time stamp alongside diagrams and clinical photographs (after gaining the appropriate consent).

- *Teeth*: Can the patient occlude their teeth? Have any teeth been avulsed from their sockets? If so, for how long, and has the patient managed to retrieve the tooth? Also assess tooth displacement (including intrusion), mobility (of the individual tooth or dentoalveolar complex) and bleeding from intra-oral soft tissue wounds as well as type of dental fracture sustained (see Fig. 2.27).

Note that if the interval between the injury and presentation is short, pulp sensibility testing and percussion tests will have no diagnostic value as the teeth are more than likely to have been concussed and the periodontal ligament bruised. Patient compliance for these investigations (including intra-oral radiography) may also be limited! Depending on the severity and symptoms of the injury, it might be worth cleaning up the soft tissue wounds, removing blood clots, conducting debridement under local anaesthesia where necessary and prescribing relevant and necessary pain relief medication at the first visit, and then inviting the patient to

return after 2 to 3 days to investigate the dental injuries further and initiate a suitable personalised care plan (see later). Further information on the management of dental trauma in primary care can be found at: https://www.dentaltrauma.co.uk/Guidelines.aspx.

2.8 DEVELOPMENTAL DEFECTS: CLINICAL DETECTION

As teeth develop and form they are at risk of developing defects that manifest clinically after tooth eruption, often affecting tooth size, shape, number or quality/quantity of the mineralised tissues themselves. These affected teeth can pose an aesthetic, functional problem and may also be more prone to the ravages of toothwear and/or carious attack. These defects have to be detected and diagnosed from the intra-oral dental examination and careful history taking, especially of childhood or maternal illnesses or trauma to the deciduous dentition. Even though developmental defects are relatively rare, the aetiology and clinical appearance of some of the more commonly occurring conditions have been described in Table 2.8.

TABLE 2.8 **Acquired and Hereditary Developmental Defects: Basic Aetiology and Clinical Appearance (in red)**		
Developmental Defect		**Aetiology/Clinical Appearance**
Acquired	Enamel hypoplasia (Fig. 2.28)	Ameloblast damage (systemic childhood infectious diseases, trauma/infection to deciduous predecessor). Hypoplastic – ↓ matrix, normal maturation: Pitted, thin enamel of normal hardness. Hypomineralised – normal matrix, ↓ mineralisation: Opaque, chalky-white, softened enamel? Systemic cause – defined areas, bands on all teeth developing at time of illness.

TABLE 2.8   Acquired and Hereditary Developmental Defects: Basic Aetiology and Clinical Appearance (in red)—cont'd

Developmental Defect		Aetiology/Clinical Appearance
	Molar-incisor hypomineralisation (MIH) (Fig. 2.29)	Systemic illness (high fever, respiratory illness) from 0 to 2 years affecting occlusal surfaces of the first molars and possibly maxillary incisors. Hypomineralised – White-yellow or yellow-brown opacities, easily chipped, ↑ sensitivity (exposed dentine, plaque stagnation).
	Intrinsic dental fluorosis (Fig. 2.30)	Excessive fluoride ion intake (water, toothpaste, tablets) poisons ameloblast function during enamel formation/maturation. Chalky-white flecks, confluent blotches, brown discolouration, pitted enamel.
	Intrinsic tetracycline stain (Fig. 2.31)	Broad-spectrum antibiotic with affinity for mineralised tissues. If taken by mother during pregnancy, deciduous teeth affected; if taken <12 years, permanent teeth affected. Nowadays rare as use of tetracycline is reduced. Dark, grey horizontal bands affecting all teeth.
Hereditary (genetic, familial history)	Hypodontia (oligodontia)	Some teeth do not develop; associated with microdontia (abnormal crown shape/size). Third molars, second premolars and upper lateral incisors are most affected.
	Amelogenesis imperfecta (Fig. 2.32)	Abnormalities in enamel formation (complex classification): *Hypoplastic:* Defect of matrix formation. Thin enamel, yellowish teeth (dentine showing through). Or granular, pitted, stained thin enamel. *Hypomineralised:* defective matrix maturation. Soft, friable, stained or chalky-white enamel, frequently lost due to weakness at the enamel–dentine junction (EDJ).
	Dentinogenesis imperfecta	Odontoblast defect affecting dentine matrix formation and mineralisation. Rare. Enamel lost rapidly due to defective EDJ, brown, opalescent dentine colour, prone to fracture/wear. Short roots, bulbous crowns, pulps obliterated.

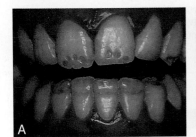 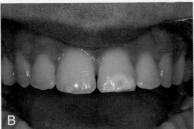 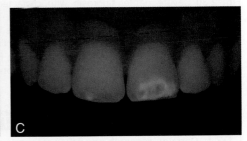

Fig. 2.28 (A) Pitted hypoplastic enamel in a patient who experienced a severe childhood illness. Note the pattern of teeth affected: maxillary central incisors and tips of maxillary canines and all mandibular incisors approximately one-third the length from the incisal edges and tips of the mandibular canines. (B) Hypomineralised enamel hypoplasia associated with the UL1. Note the localised opaque, chalky-white appearance. (C) The same tooth in (B) visualised in polarised light, with the surface reflections removed, allowing a clearer view of the hypoplastic lesion. ((A) Courtesy Banerjee A, Watson TF. *Pickard's Guide to Minimally Invasive Operative Dentistry.* 10th ed. Oxford University Press, 2015. (B) and (C) Courtesy M. Thomas)

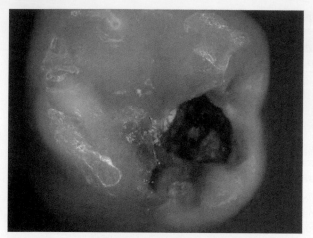

Fig. 2.29 Example of molar-incisor hypomineralisation with yellow-brown opacities on the occlusal surface of a molar tooth. There is evidence of marked post-eruptive enamel breakdown with demarcated border opacities, but the exposed dentine is hard when scratched with a sharp dental explorer.

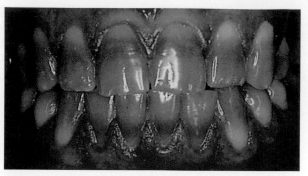

Fig. 2.31 Severe intrinsic tetracycline staining with classic horizontal banding of the stain on the labial surfaces. (From Banerjee A, Watson TF. *Pickard's Guide to Minimally Invasive Operative Dentistry*. 10th ed. Oxford University Press, 2015.)

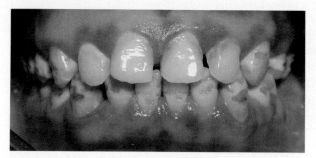

Fig. 2.30 Severe dental fluorosis with characteristic generalised enamel pitting and brown discolouration. This patient resided in a Sudanese village with natural fluoride levels in the drinking water exceeding 4000 ppm F. The maxillary central incisors have been polished by a dentist using a fine grit bur, thereby removing the superficial weakened fluorotic enamel.

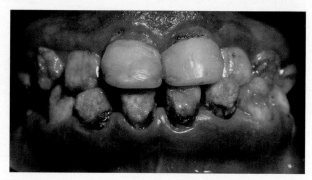

Fig. 2.32 Severe hypoplastic amelogenesis imperfecta with hard, thin and pitted enamel remaining on the teeth. The patient presented with two poor-quality acrylic crowns on the upper central incisors and buccal cervical caries on the lower incisors.

2.9 ANSWERS TO SELF-TEST QUESTIONS

Q2.1: Can you research any other categories of prevention that have been classified in the recent literature?

A: Primordial prevention consists of risk factor reduction targeted towards an entire population through a focus on social and environmental conditions. Such measures typically get promoted through laws and national policy (e.g., water fluoridation).

Quaternary prevention: An action taken to protect individuals (persons and patients) from medical interventions that are likely to cause more harm than good (e.g., dental overtreatment).

Q2.2: What are examples of primary, secondary and tertiary prevention measures used for managing dental caries?

A: Primary: Oral hygiene, diet, fluoride toothpaste and/or OTC remineralisation agents (nonoperative and/or noninvasive)

Secondary: Fissure sealants, resin infiltration, use of extrinsic remineralisation agents prescribed or administered by the team (micro-invasive)

Tertiary: Selective caries removal, cavity prep and restoration (minimally invasive)

2.9   ANSWERS TO SELF-TEST QUESTIONS—cont'd

Q2.9: What hand instrument should be used instead for carious tooth surface detection and for what purpose?
A: A ball-ended/round-headed dental explorer or periodontal probe to ensure iatrogenic cavitation cannot occur by digging into the tooth surface.

Q2.11: What treatment may be required for these teeth?
A: Initial improvement in oral hygiene to effectively remove the plaque from the occlusal surface. If the patient is not compliant, add topical remineralisation agents, then a therapeutic sealant restoration might be considered to seal the cleaned fissures. Ultimately, a minimally invasive disto-occlusal restoration may be required.

Q2.16A and B: Can you find any more lesions and radiographically classify them? Can you comment on the radiographic changes of the pulp chambers in those teeth?
A: Mesial UR6, distal UR5: D1. Note how even in these relatively superficial dentine lesions, tertiary dentine has already partly occluded the pulp chambers in these teeth, laid down in response to the closest aspect of the advancing front of the lesions.

Q2.16C: What is the cause of the radiolucencies in Fig. 2.16C? (Clue: Examine Fig. 2.16D very carefully for the answer!)
A: The well-defined ovoid radiolucency is caused by superimposition of the radiolucent resin composite restoration that is evident buccally in Fig. 2.16D. The proximal radiolucencies are cervical burnout, due to the narrowing of the tooth at this morphological junction between crown and root.

Q2.16E
i. Can you work out which materials have been used to restore the cavity in the maxillary first molar?
ii. What other information would you need before deciding whether to operatively intervene to manage the diffuse radiolucency subjacent to the restoration?
iii. What might be the cause of the radio-opacity in the mandibular first molar?

A: i. The more radio-opaque overlying material is probably a resin composite. The underlying less radio-opaque material is possibly a glass-ionomer cement or biodentine (see Chapter 7).
ii. The clinical findings are the integrity of the restoration's proximal/occlusal margins, signs and symptoms from the patient/pulp, pulp test results, caries presence elsewhere in the mouth and review of previous notes and radiographs.
iii. The presence of a resin composite restoration (preventive fissure sealant/therapeutic sealant restoration; see Chapter 8).

Q2.20A: How could you manage this case?
A: Improve oral hygiene first and review. Then consider minimally invasive restoration of the cavity to enable easier biofilm disruption by the patient.

Q2.21: What stands out as the main issues regarding this patient's dietary sugar intake?
A: The number of episodes per day and their frequency throughout each 24-hour period. This would ensure the patient's teeth were bathed in plaque with a pH below 5.5 for significant periods leading to demineralisation of the enamel (Stephan curve).

Q2.23: What would be the most obvious cause of the buccal cervical abrasion?
A: Excessive or prolonged action of horizontal toothbrushing with a hard-bristle brush head.

Q2.24: What might be the presenting complaint of this patient?
A: The appearance of the incisal edges, chipping of the front teeth, sharpness to the tongue and grey discolouration.

Q2.25A: What clinical clues are present to indicate the relative activity of erosion?
A: The appearance of brown staining and discolouration on the affected tooth surfaces. The fact that extrinsic dietary stains have formed on these surfaces is indicative that the erosive process either has not been active for a period of time or is at least very slowly progressing.

Continued

2.9   ANSWERS TO SELF-TEST QUESTIONS—cont'd

Q2.25B: What might be the cause of such extensive erosion affecting these particular surfaces?
A: The site of such aggressive dental erosion is indicative of exposure to a regular, strong intrinsic acid source (e.g., gastric reflux or gastro-oesophageal reflux disease (GORD).

Q2.26: What do you think might be the cause of these incisal wear lesions?
A: The patient plays with a large, metal tongue stud across the anterior teeth, causing a significant amount of toothwear damage.

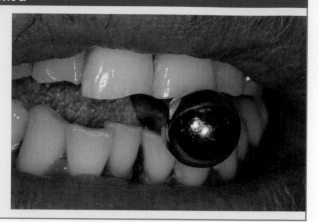

REFERENCE

1. Moynihan PJ, Kelly SAM. Effect on caries of restricting sugars intake: systematic review to inform WHO guidelines. *J Dent Res.* 2014 Jan;93(1):8–18. doi:10.1177/0022034513508954.

MIOC Domain 1: Diagnosis, Prognosis and Personalised Care Planning

CHAPTER OUTLINE

3.1 INTRODUCTION

Once a general and targeted history, examination and clinical investigations have been carried out (*information gathering*) and analysed, it is time for the dentist and their oral healthcare team to assimilate all the relevant information to formulate a diagnosis, prognosis and personalised care plan for each patient (*information processing*). Even though the detection and diagnostic phases have been separated for discussion in this book, an experienced clinician will accomplish both simultaneously as part of clinical domain 1 of the minimum intervention oral care (MIOC) pathway (see Chapter 2, Fig. 2.1). It is vital to remember that *diagnosis must precede any definitive treatment* in all cases.

3.1.1 Definitions

Diagnosis The art or act of inferring from its signs and symptoms or manifestations, the nature or cause of an illness or condition. This stage is critical to allow the oral healthcare team and the patient/caregiver to appreciate what are the nature, cause and severity of the condition suffered.

Prognosis The forecast of the course of a disease or the patient's response to treatment of the disease. This stage helps the dentist, team and patient to understand how easy or difficult the treatment will be to carry out and permit assessment of the patient's motivation to cure the problem. In dentistry, the oral healthcare team can only start the patient on the road to recovery by restoring form and function to their dentition as well as helping the patient to prevent/control the disease process, thus preventing its return. It is then up to the patient as to whether they follow this advice and maintain their oral health in the future. Therefore shared decision-making, patient behaviour management and ownership of their own health outcomes are paramount in the successful long-term care and maintenance of lifelong oral health.

Personalised care plan The formal itemised management strategy developed by the dentist and their oral healthcare team, for the individual patient and with the patient (shared decision-making), to treat the manifestations of a disease and to control/prevent it from reoccurring. Each step of the plan should be accompanied in the written notes with the clinical reasoning and evidence behind its inclusion: why is that particular item of treatment being carried out at that specific stage in the care plan? This essential piece of information is critical for several reasons:

- It elevates the personalised care plan beyond a simple fixed 'shopping list' of treatments to be carried out, commonly termed a *treatment plan*, to a clinically reasoned, evolving strategy of management, dependent upon the outcome of previous care and treatment provision.
- Each treatment item and its clinical justification should be clearly documented in the notes (also including situations where no intervention is advised) to allow other clinicians who might treat the patient an insight into the structure of the care plan as a whole and so that they can understand the reasons for its development and planned ordered execution.
- Each item of treatment plus its clinical justification must be communicated to the patient/caregiver as part of the shared decision-making process and documented carefully. This can then be referred to in cases of dispute, at a later stage. Dento-legally, it is imperative that there is evidence as to why a clinical scenario was reviewed, why a procedure was carried out, its justification at the time and the quality of the surgical outcome itself.

The personalised care plan can be divided into phases of therapy (e.g., prevention/control of disease, stabilisation/definitive treatments, review/re-assessment/active surveillance/recall) and should be adapted and modified during its execution for maximum benefit to the patient. Any changes should be clearly explained to the patient/caregiver and documented in the clinical notes. It should take into account unforeseen developments in the course of the disease or the patient's response to treatment. It should be written and made clear to all parties for discussion so that informed consent can be gained prior to implementation.

3.2 DIAGNOSING DENTAL PAIN, 'TOOTHACHE'

'Common conditions/diseases occur commonly'. Following is a list of common diagnoses of dental pain, with the various features of each summarised in Table 3.1:

- Acute pulpitis
- Acute periapical periodontitis
- Acute periapical abscess
- Acute periodontal (lateral) abscess
- Chronic pulpitis
- Chronic periapical periodontitis (apical granuloma)
- Exposed sensitive dentine
- Interproximal food-packing
- Cracked cusps/tooth syndrome

Other conditions outwith the remit of this book which may also manifest as oro-dento-facial pain include maxillary sinusitis, trigeminal neuralgia and facial arthromyalgia, amongst others. It must be understood that pain symptoms do not always fall neatly into the diagnoses in the preceding list (see Table 3.1) and that a degree of clinical experience will be required to interpret the relevant signs and symptoms to permit a diagnosis to be made. It is important to recognise that the signs and symptoms from an inflamed pulp do not necessarily correlate fully with the histological changes that are occurring within that pulp. Therefore interpretation of the signs and symptoms must be carried out with care.

3.2.1 Acute Pulpitis

- The pain is acute, severe and poorly localised.
- The pain does not cross the facial midline and might be difficult for patients to identify from which jaw it is originating. They will often present holding their face on the relevant side, rather than identifying a particular tooth.
- There are two clinical presentations (not necessarily relating to pulp histology): *reversible* and *irreversible*. Table 3.2 highlights their similarities and differences.
- Clinically, offending teeth may present with carious lesions or large restorations which may be defective, but the dentist must always check the status of all the dentition in both quadrants on the relevant side.

3.2.2 Acute Periapical Periodontitis

- Pain is often localisable to the offending tooth. The patient will be able to point to it and will complain of pain on biting onto it (due to stimulation of pain and pressure-sensitive fibres in the periodontal ligament).
- The tooth is tender to palpate/percussion. This should only entail a gentle pushing action on the suspect teeth into their sockets or laterally. It does not mean tapping the crown of the tooth with a mirror

TABLE 3.1 Classic Signs and Symptoms for Differential Diagnoses for Dental Pain

	Acute Pulpitis	Acute Apical Periodontitis	Acute Apical Abscess	Acute Periodontal Abscess	Exposed Sensitive Dentine	Food Packing	Cracked Cusp	Chronic Pulpitis	Chronic Apical Periodontitis (Apical Granuloma)
History	Recent pain with hot and cold; may be very severe; poorly localised	Tender to bite; well localised	Pain and swelling; very well localised	Localised swelling; some pain	Generalised pain to hot, cold and sweet	Pain after eating fibrous food (e.g., meat)	Vague intermittent pain usually on biting; may be poorly localised	Vague, unprovoked intermittent but increasing pain; poorly localised	May have had pain in the past; now not sensitive to hot or cold
Clinical examination	Possibly caries or recent large restoration	Possibly caries	May be extra-oral or intra-oral swelling over apex of tooth	Intra-oral swelling nearer to gingival margin; tooth may be mobile	Gingival recession; exposed dentine at the gingival margin; sensitive to probe or cold air	Open contact points; gingival inflammation; food. Usually present	Often nothing, but crack may be seen; may be painful with occlusal contact only	May have large restoration or caries	May have large restoration or caries
Sensibility (vitality) test	Hypersensitive	May still be vital, but usually non-vital	non-vital	Often vital	Vital	May be vital or non-vital	May be hypersensitive	Often normal but may be hypersensitive	non-vital
Percussion	Not tender	Tender	Tender to touch; too tender to percuss	Slight tenderness, more to lateral than axial pressure	Not tender	Not tender to percussion; may be sore with lateral percussion	Usually not tender but may be tender	Not tender	Slightly; may give dull sound on percussion
Other clinical investigations			Raised temperature; looks ill	Deep pockets; pus may be released on probing pocket		Floss passes the contact easily	Sometimes tender to lateral pressure on an individual cusp		

Continued

TABLE 3.1   Classic Signs and Symptoms for Differential Diagnoses for Dental Pain—cont'd

	Acute Pulpitis	Acute Apical Periodontitis	Acute Apical Abscess	Acute Periodontal Abscess	Exposed Sensitive Dentine	Food Packing	Cracked Cusp	Chronic Pulpitis	Chronic Apical Periodontitis (Apical Granuloma)
Radiographic findings	Probably caries close to pulp; no periapical change	Usually no periapical change in the early stage	Usually no periapical change except slight widening of apical periodontal ligament space	Alveolar bone loss; usually no periapical change	May be some alveolar bone loss	None	None	None	Periapical radiolucency
Findings on further investigations	Carious exposure of pulp	Necrotic pulp	Pus may be drained via access cavity to root canal without local anaesthetic, giving immediate relief of pain and confirming the diagnosis				Crack sometimes visible at base of cavity when old restoration is removed; if left, cuspal fracture will eventually occur	Symptoms may settle if restoration is removed and tooth is dressed with calcium hydroxide or tricalcium silicates but pulp often dies eventually	Necrotic pulp

Note: Unfortunately, not all symptoms fall into these clear categories and experience is required for their interpretation.

TABLE 3.2 **Clinical Characteristics of Acute Pulpitis**	
Reversible Pulpitis	**Irreversible Pulpitis**
• Characteristic short, sharp pain • Stimulated by hot, cold or sweet stimuli • Few seconds' duration; disappears when stimulus is removed • Pulp sensibility tests may elicit an exaggerated response compared to adjacent, opposite and contralateral control teeth • Tooth not tender to percussion (TTP; see Chapter 2, Section 2.5.3)	• Characteristic dull, throbbing pain (but may experience bouts of sharp pain) • Onset usually unprovoked or exacerbated by hot, cold or sweet stimuli • Several minutes' or hours' duration; persists when stimulus is removed • Pulp sensibility tests may elicit an exaggerated or negative response • Tooth not necessarily TTP (unless late-stage presentation)

handle (warn the patient that it may be uncomfortable and gain their permission for this examination!).

- Tenderness is felt over the root apex through mucosae in the buccal sulcus.
- Pulp may initially retain sensibility but will eventually become necrotic.
- Periapical radiographs *may* show loss of lamina dura around the root apex region during late-stage presentation. Cone-beam computed tomography (CBCT) may offer a more detailed and accurate picture of the mineral density changes at the apical tissues (see Chapter 2, Section 2.5.3).

3.2.3 Acute Periapical Abscess

- The patient may present with a large facial and/or intra-oral swelling associated with the affected relevant quadrant or a more localised swelling in the alveolar mucosa over the affected root.
- The patient may present before swelling occurs or after it has burst and subsided, with evidence of a sinus tract.
- The patient may present with pyrexia.
- The tooth will be painful to bite on. Often there will be negative results from pulp sensibility tests (if the patient permits these to be taken).
- The periapical radiograph/CBCT will usually show loss of lamina dura and widening of the periodontal ligament space around the root apex.

3.2.4 Acute Periodontal (Lateral) Abscess

- The abscess forms at the base of a deep periodontal pocket.
- The pain is well localised and associated with a vital pulp.

- If this is combined with pulp necrosis (of differing aetiology), then a "perio-endo" lesion can be diagnosed, often with poor prognosis leading to extraction of the tooth.

3.2.5 Chronic Pulpitis

- Mild, poorly localised, periodic grumbling pain (on and off) occurs over several weeks or months.
- Initially vital pulp and tooth are not tender to percussion (TTP), but if the condition progresses, eventually symptoms of periapical periodontitis may supervene.
- Initial treatment will be monitoring to assess whether the pulp has recovered after treating the cause (e.g., caries, cracked tooth).
- More severe cases will require removal of any restoration, placement of a sedative dressing over the pulp and then a provisional restoration. This may be followed by pulpotomy, pulpectomy and/or root canal treatment of the tooth and placement of a sealed definitive coronal restoration soon afterwards.

3.2.6 Chronic Periapical Periodontitis

- The patient can be symptomless or experience mild pain on biting.
- A periapical radiograph shows well-demarcated radiolucency around the root apex (Fig. 3.1A–C).
- The patient experiences a positive response to vigorous percussion or even presents with a sinus tract (Fig. 3.2A–C).
- This condition can be described as an apical granuloma.
- The apical granuloma is a chronic inflammatory response (highly vascularised granulation tissue) to toxins leaching from the necrotic pulp causing increased osteoclastic action in the subjacent bone leading to bone resorption. As the toxins dilute, the

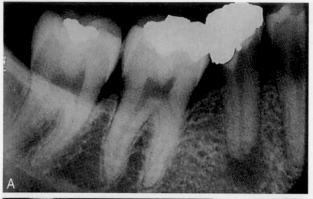

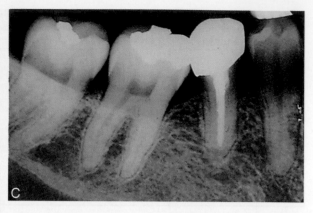

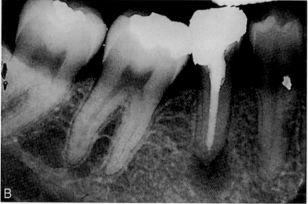

Fig. 3.1 (A) Periapical radiograph showing a well-demarcated radiolucency at the apex of the LR5 (with accompanying loss of lamina dura and relative widening of the periodontal ligament space when compared with the adjacent healthy LR7). The large restoration has contributed to pulp necrosis in this tooth and it is likely that a periapical granuloma has formed, but this could strictly only be diagnosed from histological analysis of a biopsy sample. (B) Periapical radiograph of the same tooth after the gutta percha root filling was placed. (C) Radiograph 3 years later showing healing around the root apex of the LR5, bony infill and reformed lamina dura. (Courtesy the late Professor Pitt Ford. From Banerjee A, Watson TF. *Pickard's Guide to Minimally Invasive Operative Dentistry.* 10th ed. Oxford University Press, 2015.)

extent of the resorption is naturally limited. If the necrotic pulp and therefore the source of toxins is removed, bony repair can result (Fig. 3.1A–C).

- If infection occurs, the chronic apical granuloma can flare up into an acute apical abscess with a sinus tract (Fig. 3.2A–C).
- Chronic apical granulomas may become cystic and require surgical intervention for treatment (Fig. 3.3A–B).

3.2.7 Exposed Dentine Sensitivity

- The patient experiences poorly localised short, sharp sensitivity to hot, cold or sweet stimuli caused by exposed root dentine surfaces (gingival recession). The pain response can be elicited by air-drying the exposed surface using a dental 3-1 air/water syringe.
- The patient has a positive sensibility test (perhaps slightly hyper-responsive if tested during an acute episode); teeth are not TTP.
- To reduce the sensitivity with an immediate effect, the exposed tubules may be blocked using a dentine

bonding agent or dental adhesive or a thin layer of resin composite placed on the surface of the sensitive areas. Depending on their depth of penetration into the exposed dentine tubules and site of application (and therefore exposure to abrasive or attritive forces), these topical treatments will wear away with time and symptoms might return. Use of potassium nitrate/chloride compounds (topical pastes or gels) may also help to reduce tubule conduction and pain transmission; although these may not offer immediate pain relief, they can be effective with prolonged use over time.

3.2.8 Interproximal Food-Packing

- Open contact points (drifted teeth, poor contouring of adjacent proximal restorations) enable food debris to get caught between teeth and traumatise the interdental gingival papillae leading to localised tenderness, bleeding and inflammation. If left untreated, gingivitis may ensue and eventually periodontitis and dental caries in those cases where the biofilm is left to stagnate over a prolonged period.

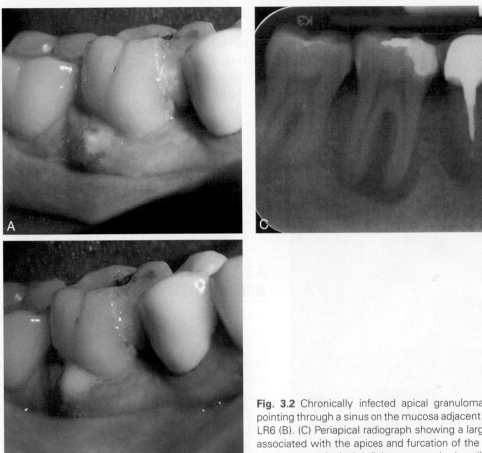

Fig. 3.2 Chronically infected apical granuloma (A) with pus pointing through a sinus on the mucosa adjacent to the non-vital LR6 (B). (C) Periapical radiograph showing a large radiolucency associated with the apices and furcation of the LR6 as well as a separate periapical radiolucency on the heavily restored (but inadequately root-treated) LR5.

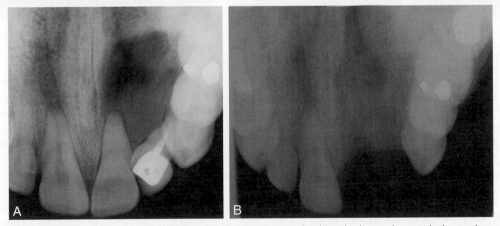

Fig. 3.3 (A) Upper standard occlusal radiographs showing large palatal cystic change in an apical granuloma associated with the UL12. (B) The same radiograph taken 3 years later after the UL12 was extracted and the cyst surgically managed. Note the near complete bony infill of the initially large defect. Implants were placed successfully into the new bone to restore the UL12.

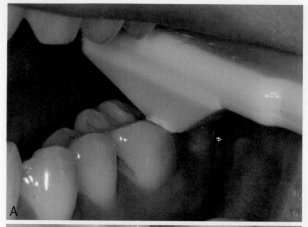

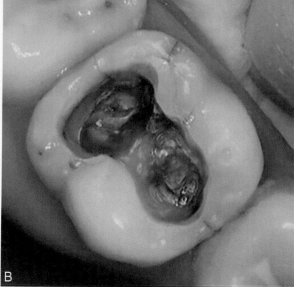

Fig. 3.4 (A) Using a Tooth Slooth to detect whether there is a cracked cusp on the disto-buccal aspect of the left mandibular first molar. The patient bites on the plastic tip, which directs the occlusal force onto the disto-buccal cusp in this case. Pain may be elicited on pressure or release as the cracked cusp flexes under occlusal strain. (B) A mandibular molar with symptoms of a cracked tooth. The large existing amalgam restoration was removed, revealing a clear fracture line mesio-distally (more easily detected using magnification; see Chapter 5, Section 5.7). As the portions of the tooth were mobile and the coronal extent of the fracture was considerable, the tooth was deemed unrestorable and was extracted. (Courtesy B Dawett.)

3.2.9 Cracked Cusp/Tooth Syndrome

- Cracks can involve enamel only (no pain; similar to those superficial cracks often found in a porcelain teacups) or both enamel and dentine (± pulp), which can cause sharp pain periodically.

- There is sometimes a sharp pain on biting, release and/or thermal stimulus. Pulp sensibility tests may be inconclusive, as can percussion and palpation tests.
- Transillumination or dyes can be used to detect cracks, but this does not necessarily link their presence to the cause of pain.
- Diagnostic tests may involve careful analysis of pain on biting. Using a cotton wool roll, wood stick (wooden tongue depressor split lengthways), rubber suction tip or proprietary kits such as a Tooth Slooth, cracked tooth/cusp pain can be elicited on specific cusps at specific angles of pressure and must be assessed both on biting and release. This helps to ascertain where and how deep the crack might be and therefore what treatment is required (Fig. 3.4A–B).

3.3 CARIES RISK/SUSCEPTIBILITY ASSESSMENT (CRSA)[1]

The aetiology, histopathology and detection methods for caries have been discussed in Chapters 1 and 2, all as part of MIOC clinical domain 1: *identifying the problem.* Once this information has been gathered through a documented targeted verbal history and clinical examination, further analysis (*information processing*) is required to:

- Understand why the individual patient presents with such disease activity
- Ascertain the risk, susceptibility and likelihood of the individual patient to develop further disease
- Aid in prognosis and clinical shared decision-making to develop a patient-focused, team-delivered, risk-related personalised care plan to manage the current and future disease experience.

This is accomplished by relating the overall risk and susceptibility status of the patient on presentation with the net longitudinal activity state of any lesions present. This is known as a caries risk/susceptibility assessment or analysis (CRSA). Without this knowledge, caries management at an individual patient level will never be successful in the long term. Risk assessments can also be carried out at a population level to help promote public health prevention strategies (e.g., water fluoridation programmes) for large numbers of people.

- It makes health, economic and practical sense to target preventive care pathways and specific treatments in practice at the appropriate risk/susceptibility

Age					
	0–2 years	**3–6 years**	**7–17 years**	**18–65 years**	**Older/vulnerable adults**
Diseases and conditions (most common)	Dental caries	Dental caries Toothwear	Dental caries Gingivitis Toothwear	Dental caries Periodontitis Toothwear Oral cancer	Dental caries Periodontitis Toothwear Oral cancer Dry mouth
Major risk factors in this age group	Diet: sugar-containing food/drinks Lack of fluoride	Diet: sugar-containing food/drinks Lack of fluoride Poor oral hygiene	Diet: sugar-containing food/drinks Low/no fluoride Poor oral hygiene Tobacco commencing Alcohol commencing	Diet: sugar-containing food/drinks Low/no fluoride Poor oral hygiene Tobacco Alcohol Polypharmacy Tooth loss Dentures	Diet: sugar-containing food/drinks Low/no fluoride Poor oral hygiene Tobacco Alcohol Polypharmacy Tooth loss Dentures
What to actively promote for everyone in this age group	Healthy diet Parental toothbrushing Fluoride toothpaste	Healthy diet Parental brushing/assistance Fluoride toothpaste Spit but don't rinse after brushing	Healthy diet Good oral hygiene Fluoride toothpaste Spit but don't rinse after brushing Avoid/stop tobacco Avoid alcohol	Healthy diet Good oral hygiene Fluoride toothpaste Spit but don't rinse after brushing Avoid/stop tobacco Avoid/minimise alcohol	Healthy diet Good oral hygiene (including dentures) Fluoride toothpaste Spit but don't rinse after brushing Avoid/stop tobacco Avoid/minimise alcohol Dry-mouth care
Monitoring and recall period	3–12 months	3–12 months	3–12 months	3–24 months	3–24 months

Fig. 3.5 The key oral diseases/conditions affecting different population age groups, with their associated risk factors and preventive management pathways/clinical advice.

group, as well as at a larger, age-related population level (see Fig. 3.5).

- Oral and dental healthcare neither begins nor ends with a single course of treatment, but is ongoing. When a course of dental treatment is complete, the dentist, team and patient decide when it would be wise to check that all is well (shared decision-making). This recall interval is based partly on an assessment of the likelihood and risk of disease progression and should not be standardised automatically at 6 months or any other period.
- Patients and caregivers must be made aware of their risk/susceptibility status. This knowledge encourages them to attend appropriately timed recall appointments, to become *motivated* and involved, taking responsibility of their own preventive care, and, if they pay for their treatment, it may help them budget for future dental bills.

Most oral healthcare professionals seem to perform an informal and intuitive caries risk/susceptibility assessment ('an educated best guess') when taking the case history and examining their patients. The most commonly used single variables are the past caries experience and

the level of oral hygiene, while the level of fluoride exposure seems to be considered less important. The CRSA methods that combine several factors can be divided into reasoning-based checklists and algorithm-based computer models. Most checklists, as well as software programmes, are available for downloading from the internet free of charge. The reasoning-based models are based on a number of age-related background factors (biological, behavioural, socioeconomic status) with demonstrated associations with caries activity. Some of the various patient factors that affect the CRSA are highlighted in Table 3.3. A chart similar to Table 3.4 might be used in the patient notes to document such findings. Formal, 'standardised' risk/susceptibility assessment systems exist which help the oral healthcare team *calculate* their patients' risk status (e.g., Cariogram, Caries Management by Risk Assessment (CAMBRA); search these systems online for further information). In some cases, multivariate algorithms are used to process the findings from the patient assessment, giving extra weight and relevance to certain factors deemed more important to the risk outcome. Even though these can be convenient and helpful for teaching and research purposes, there is a risk that

TABLE 3.3 Factors in Assessing Caries Risk/Susceptibility and Categorising Patient's Susceptibility to Caries as High or Low Risk[a]

CARIES RISK/SUSCEPTIBILITY ASSESSMENT	
High Risk	**Low Risk**
Social History	
Socially deprived	Middle class
High caries in siblings	Low caries in siblings
Low knowledge of dental disease	Dentally aware
Irregular attender	Regular attender
Ready availability of snacks	Work does not allow regular snacks
Low dental aspirations	High dental aspirations
Medical History	
Medically compromised	No medical problem
Handicapped	No physical problem
Xerostomia	Normal salivary flow
Long-term cariogenic medicine	No long-term medication
Dietary Habits	
Frequent sugar intake	Infrequent sugar intake
Fluoride Use	
Non-fluoride area	Fluoridation area
No fluoride supplements	Fluoride supplements used
No fluoride toothpaste	Fluoride toothpaste used
Plaque Control	
Infrequent/ineffective cleaning	Frequent/effective cleaning
Poor manual control	Good manual control
Saliva	
Low flow rate	Normal flow rate
Low buffering capacity	High buffering capacity
High *S.mutans* and lactobacillus counts	Low *S.mutans* and lactobacillus counts
Clinical Evidence	
New lesions	No new lesions
Premature extractions	Nil extractions for caries
Anterior caries or restorations	Sound anterior teeth
Multiple restorations	No or few restorations
History of repeated restorations	Restorations inserted years ago
No fissure sealants	Fissure sealed
Multiband orthodontics	No appliances
Partial dentures	

[a]This information can be gathered from a targeted verbal history and clinical examination (Chapter 2, Table 2.1).

the analysis becomes too standardised and the nuances and variations for each patient are not fully appreciated or understood, especially at the general practice primary care level. It is more important for the dentist and the oral healthcare team to tailor the risk assessment for each patient, with the team and patient appreciating and fully understanding the relevance and significance of all the information gathered for that specific individual. With the increase in litigation against dentists, risk/susceptibility assessments that are interpreted and recorded formally in the clinical notes are becoming essential dento-legal requirements, not forgetting the obvious ethical dimension to this best practice. The CRSA will change over time and therefore should be assessed longitudinally, especially when the pattern of disease presentation changes in the same patient. The overall patient management of caries is as dynamic as the disease process itself.

In terms of the numbers of lesions detected during the clinical oral examination, a high caries risk patient is one who presents with or has a history of ≥2 new/progressing/restored carious lesions in the previous 2 years. The patient's caries risk/susceptibility is classified generally into three categories: high, medium or low (or red, amber and green (RAG) traffic lights). Some classifications extend the range to very high and extremely high risk. This, although useful for epidemiological and research purposes, can add an unnecessary layer of complexity, or even ambiguity, for the oral healthcare team in the assessment of patients in primary care general dental practice and in communication with patients. A simpler division into low or high risk/susceptibility is usually more than sufficient to paint the individual risk status for the patient and helps the team, with the patient, to formulate their personalised care plan accordingly. It is of course recognised that there are patient subgroups within the general population who are susceptible to factors (e.g., radiotherapy patients, those with systemic autoimmune conditions) elevating their risk to an extreme level (also classified as high risk with unmodifiable factors), and these may require periodic referral for advice regarding care planning and, indeed, sometimes care in a specialist environment (see Chapter 4, Section 4.2.1).

Longitudinal CRSA should be regarded as a cornerstone for clinical decision-making and disease management but its implementation in everyday practice is not common. There is, however, no particular method with perfect accuracy and no conclusive evidence to support the use of one CRSA tool, model or technology over another. Single predictors, or even prediction models,

TABLE 3.4 **A Simple CRSA Chart**		
Status	**'Yes': High Risk**	**'No': Low Risk**
Lesions: ≥2 new/progressing/restored lesions in the past 2 years? Activity state?		
General Factors		
Diet: Frequent snacks between meals? Anorexia, bulimia? Prolonged nursing/ bottle feeding? Use of sugar-free chewing gum after meals?		
Fluoride: Deficient fluoride exposure (toothpaste/rinse daily, fluoridated water community)?		
Health: Sjögren's syndrome, chemotherapy, radiation to head and neck?		
Medications: Hypo-salivatory medication, polypharmacy?		
Social: Socio-economic status? Parents/siblings with active caries? Symptom-driven attendance?		
Age: Adolescent? Older adult? Orthodontic/prosthetic appliances?		
Oral Factors		
Oral hygiene: Quality? What aids are used?		
Saliva: Stimulated saliva flow <0.7mL/min? pH/buffering capacity? Saliva quality? Clinical Oral Dryness Scale scor?		
Plaque: Readily visible dense plaque deposits; plaque scores? Quality vs. quantity		
Bacterial balance: Levels of *S. mutans, salivary lactobacilli*		

Note: This simple chart is to note down some key findings from the patient's history and examination to help evaluate their caries risk/susceptibility. Some of this information can be gleaned remotely, perhaps by having the patient complete the form online prior to any face-to-face consultation. (Adapted from Domejean-Orliaguet, S., Banerjee, A., Gaucher, C., et al. Minimum Intervention Treatment Plan (MTIP): practical implementation in general dental practice. JMID, 2009;2(2):103–123.

rarely exhibit high sensitivity and specificity values (close to 1.0) at the same time, so using any individual factor individually is not appropriate. Multivariate models tend to display an improved accuracy over those using single predictors. The ability to predict future caries is greater among preschoolers and schoolchildren than later in life, with an accuracy that can exceed 80%. Validated tools for root caries prediction are currently lacking. There is emerging evidence that interventions based on CRSA can increase patient behavioural adherence and reduce the onset of new disease. Further research is needed, in particular on the health-economic impact of CRSA and its value for patients, oral healthcare providers and other stakeholders.

3.4 DIAGNOSING TOOTHWEAR

The detection of toothwear from its causative factors has been discussed in detail in Chapter 2. A targeted verbal history coupled with rigorous examination of the teeth is essential to return a diagnosis of and prognosis for this common multifactorial problem. Differentiating between acceptable, slow-progressing, age-related toothwear and pathological levels of wear can be difficult as this depends on the patient's age, dental history, lifestyle and experience and the rate of progress of the toothwear, which can be difficult to assess clinically unless the patient is reviewed periodically, at least annually in the first instance. Study models can record more gross changes over longer periods of time. Intra-oral digital scans can offer a periodic record of more subtle changes, with the need for suitable fixed reference points as a constant to measure to (see Chapter 9, Section 9.1.3). Wear facets on teeth with staining or dental plaque biofilm present at the time of clinical examination may be indicative of a very slow or arrested rate of progress whereas significant dental sensitivity from such lesions may indicate a more rapid rate of wear, as there would not have been enough time for the upregulated odontoblasts to lay down translucent or tertiary dentine (see Chapter 1, Section 1.1.8).

3.5 DIAGNOSING DENTAL TRAUMA AND DEVELOPMENTAL DEFECTS

Again, as with toothwear, the degree of separation between detection and diagnosis of trauma and developmental defects is negligible as the two processes are linked with the verbal history and the oral/dental examination. These have been discussed in detail in Chapter 2.

3.6 PROGNOSTIC INDICATORS

The clinician should give the patient a verbal and written prognosis of their responsibilities and potential outcomes of preventive care, individual tooth/teeth requiring interventional treatment and/or a prognosis for the management of the overall condition the patient has. At the tooth level, factors affecting the prognosis include:

- Restorability. This depends on the severity of damage incurred to the coronal hard tissues (extent of the carious lesion, amount of tooth structure lost due to trauma, toothwear or developmental defect). Can operative treatment repair and reinstate the tooth structure successfully in the mid- to long term?
- The viability of the pulp.
- The status of the periodontium (alveolar bone levels, periodontal ligament).

In terms of the underlying condition, prognostic factors include:

- The ease with which the aetiological factors can be removed or modified to prevent or slow the progress of the disease and its reoccurrence. As an example, the aetiology of xerostomia caused by head and neck radiation therapy cannot be modified, so dental conditions (e.g., caries) will generally have a poorer prognosis. However, with the judicious use of oral hygiene procedures to a high standard complemented by high concentrations of fluoride, the prognosis might be improved to an acceptable level.
- The overall level of patient/caregiver motivation to manage the condition. If a patient is not particularly concerned or does not wish to take responsibility for maintaining their personal oral health, then the long-term outlook for oral healthcare team-administered treatment will be bleak at best and only short-term repairs can be considered. This, along with the long-term consequences of further tooth destruction,

must be made clear to patients and documented fully in the clinical notes. There are three emotional/behavioural subcategories that may be displayed by patients in this regard:

- A positive attitude and clear self-confidence that improved health can or will be achieved
- A passive attitude that everything will be all right and fixed by the dentist and the team
- A negative attitude characterised by frustration, a tendency to give up and ultimate non-attendance.

The latter subcategory must not be overlooked or underestimated. To be pointed out as 'almost sick' or vulnerable may negatively affect a person's self-confidence and increase feelings of hopelessness. It is therefore important that oral healthcare providers are able to assist those persons by offering empowerment and supporting and facilitating self-efficacy in terms of robust, reinforced advice.

3.7 FORMULATING A RISK-RELATED, PERSONALISED CARE PLAN

3.7.1 Why Is a Personalised Care Plan (PCP) Necessary?

The need to and importance of making individualised, adaptable holistic plans, both simple and complex, and of recording the decisions in the patient's clinical record can be summarised as follows:

- It ensures that the lead clinician reviews the care in the light of all available evidence at the start of treatment and at stages throughout it.
- It is a record for later reference, particularly in complicated cases or after a lapse of time has occurred during the treatment period. This is available mostly for the benefit of the patient, but on occasions, when patients complain, it will have dento-legal importance and may protect the dentist and their team against unjustified complaints. In this context, when the care plan is complex and expensive it is essential to put the advice in the form of a letter to the patient so that they have time to consider it, have time to digest it and its implications and can question it before acceptance or rejection (shared decision-making). This process of two-way communication between the dentist/team and the patient is of critical importance. The vast majority of

all dento-legal litigation pursued in the UK in the past decade was blamed on poor communication and/or understanding between the two parties, lack of management of patients' expectations and an inadequacy in recordkeeping. The UK's General Dental Council now suggests this formalised two-way planning approach as a recommended practice in all cases.

- It avoids the risk of disorderly and ill-advised treatment, which may arise if treatment is undertaken piecemeal or by different members of the oral healthcare team or specialists. The personalised care plan items of treatment must be accompanied by their justification.

Written personalised care plans, however simple, should be made for every patient. They should be tailored specifically to each individual patient's holistic needs, should take all factors into consideration from the detection and diagnostic phases and must have realistic goals and be achievable for the dentist, oral healthcare team and patient. They must also be planned by the dentist and their team to manage patient expectations as regards to the quality and success of any potential outcome of care. They must include all aspects of care, including a non-operative primary preventive care and recall strategy, including the clinical justification for each item of treatment or active surveillance carried out, rather than just being a list of specific surgical procedures carried out by the dentist to treat symptoms of the disease. The traditional 'treatment plan' terminology is dated and clinically inappropriate. All too often, treatment plans are a simplistic shopping list of procedures to be carried out as opposed to outlining with reasons the purpose and justification of each treatment item within a particular phase of care and how they interlink with the responsibilities of the oral healthcare team, clinician and patient to secure a successful outcome: the complete and adaptable *personalised care plan*.

Patients must understand the implications of the treatment and appreciate that their original personalised care plan may deviate from the initial path as treatment progresses. They must also appreciate their own pivotal role in its ultimate success, the time frame for its delivery and its cost (if applicable).

3.7.2 Structuring a Personalised Care Plan

However simple a PCP may be for a particular management episode, it is wise to have an adaptable structure to follow. One such scheme is outlined in Table 3.5 and includes:

- An initial *stabilisation phase* (which may take several appointments to complete depending on the amount/type of work required, including acute phase of pain relief)

TABLE 3.5 Personalised Care Plan Flowchart: Three Basic Phases of Patient Care	
Personalised Care Plan Phases	**Comments**
Stabilisation	Acute pain relief/infection management (see Table 3.6) ↓ Control active disease Primary prevention Extraction of teeth with hopeless prognosis Temporary/transitional/intermediate restorations of cavitated, broken down teeth ↓
Re-assess/active surveillance	Re-assess patient's response to the preventive stabilisation phase, behaviour change adherence, changes in risk/susceptibility, active surveillance of existing lesions, their subsequent needs, aesthetic expectations, motivation, dental examination, costs ↓
Rehabilitation	Reorganising or conforming to existing occlusal scheme (see later); intermediate/definitive restorations/prostheses ↓ Review, re-assess, recall (maintenance, active surveillance)

Note: The three care phases can overlap one another depending on the complexity of the plan. The direction of the patient journey may also reverse/cycle back, depending on the outcomes from each phase of care (see Chapter 10).

TABLE 3.6   Clinical Methods of Providing Acute Infection Management, Including Judicious Use of Antimicrobial Prescribing

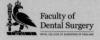

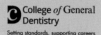

Antimicrobial Prescribing in Dentistry: Good Practice Guidelines

Chairside synopsis for common conditions

Antimicrobial Prescribing in Dentistry: Good Practice Guidelines gives clear, simple and practical guidance on the use of antimicrobials in the management of oral and dental infections: when (and when not) to prescribe, what to prescribe (where indicated), for how long and at what dosage - or when to make an urgent referral. It was developed by the Faculty of General Dental Practice (now College of General Dentistry) and the Faculty of Dental Surgery of the Royal College of Surgeons of England.

Condition	Summary of recommendations*	Where antimicrobial indicated*, 1st choice for adults	See*
Acute periapical infection (dental abscess)	• Drain abscess, remove infected pulp or extract tooth • Antimicrobials as an adjunct to definitive treatment **ONLY if evidence of systemic spread or diffuse swelling** • Clindamycin/cephalosporins/co-amoxiclav **ONLY at the direction of an oral/medical microbiology or infectious diseases specialist**	Phenoxymethylpenicillin 500mg orally four times a day for up to 5 days or Amoxicillin 500mg orally three times a day for up to 5 days	p13
Periodontal abscess	• Drain abscess (ideally by RSD via the pocket) or extract tooth • Antimicrobials as an adjunct to definitive treatment **ONLY if evidence of systemic spread or diffuse swelling**		p58
Necrotising periodontal disease	• Debride under local anaesthetic and OHI • Antimicrobials as an adjunct to local measures **ONLY if evidence of systemic involvement**	Metronidazole 400mg orally three times a day for up to 5 days or Amoxicillin: 500mg orally three times a day for up to 5 days	p49
Pericoronitis	• Debride and irrigate pericoronal space, and drain if localised abscess • Antimicrobials as an adjunct to local measures **ONLY if evidence of systemic spread, severe swelling or trismus**		p35
Acute pulpitis	• Provide definitive treatment of the cause, such as extirpation of the pulp or extraction for a tooth with irreversible pulpitis		p65
Dry socket	• Irrigate with sterile solution to remove debris and consider placing a suitable dressing in the socket which may relieve symptoms	None	p39
Peri-implantitis	• Local management with mechanical debridement and OHI		p59

*Practitioners should refer to *Antimicrobial Prescribing in Dentistry: Good Practice Guidelines* for full wordings, recommendations for other conditions, second choice antimicrobials, dosages for children and hospital patients, consideration of medically compromised patients, and guidance on prophylactic prescribing for the prevention of local and distant site infections

v1.0, November 2022

Source: Reproduced with permission from the Faculty of Dental Surgery and the College of General Dentistry, https://cgdent.uk/antimicrobial-prescribing-in-dentistry/

- *Re-assessment/active surveillance* to reevaluate patient behaviour change adherence, the response to any initial treatment, changes in risk/susceptibility of the patient over time and the future needs and expectations of the patient (which may have changed since presentation)
- A *rehabilitation phase* in which definitive restorations/prostheses can be designed and placed

Other considerations include the type of restorative material to use (see Chapter 7) and the extent of invasiveness of any operative intervention, ranging from non-operative to micro-invasive to minimally invasive where it is paramount to conserve as much viable tooth tissue as possible to extraction (i.e., whether to restore or attempt to arrest a carious lesion in dentine, restore or monitor an erosive toothwear lesion or extract or endodontically treat an infected tooth). These decisions must be made with input from the patient/caregiver (including their own perceived need, aesthetic considerations, number of appointments, costs, dental anxiety [that is, appreciating and managing the patient's expectations] shared decision-making), as this will confer ownership and therefore responsibility to the patient in terms of the success of the final outcome. Second opinions from more experienced specialists in practice or hospital can be helpful, especially for more complex cases, as there is rarely an absolute right or wrong decision made in developing a personalised care plan. Choosing the best option from several for the patient is a skill that comes with further clinical experience and, unfortunately, by making some errors in judgment along the way! It is perhaps intriguing to note that these 'errors of judgment' are rarely cause for formal dento-legal action by patients, as long as the patient has been involved in the planning and decision-making journey and the decisions that helped make them. Good communication and documentation is the key! Always be prepared to *justify* the successful personalised care plan to three parties: the patient, yourself and a lawyer! It is vital to learn from these situations and adapt accordingly one's own evidence base in the future.

Table 4.1 (Chapter 4) gives an example of a care pathway flowchart for patients with dental caries. It is based on five possible management options dependent on the presence or absence of active lesions coupled with the individual's caries risk/susceptibility assessment (the overall caries matrix). Of course, real life is not always that simple and patients' conditions do not always fit into such clear-cut categories, but this concept mapping exercise helps the clinician, their team and the patient understand the options and where the management strategy chosen fits in with respect to the alternatives.

REFERENCE

1. Twetman S, Banerjee A. Caries risk assessment. In: Chapple ILC, Papapanou PN, eds. *Risk Assessment in Oral Health: A Concise Guide for Clinical Application*: Springer; 2020.

Minimum Intervention Oral Care (MIOC) – Clinical Domain 2

Minimum Intervention Oral Care (MIOC) – Clinical Domain 2

MIOC Domain 2 Disease Control and Lesion Prevention 2

MIOC Domain 2: Disease Control and Lesion Prevention

4.1 INTRODUCTION

From Chapter 3 it can be seen that in all cases of caries and toothwear, disease control and lesion prevention are key aspects of the management strategy, often commencing in the stabilisation phase of the personalised care plan but continuing throughout the full course of treatment and beyond to maintain lifelong oral health.

4.1.1 Disease Control

Neither the dentist, as part of the oral healthcare team, nor the patient has the power to *prevent* the caries or toothwear process. These ubiquitous processes occur at the ionic, metabolic and microscopic levels at the tooth surface/biofilm interface and are made pathological by other factors in combination. If these factors are *controlled* or modified by the patient (with help from the oral healthcare team), then the processes can be regulated and homeostasis maintained. The term *primary prevention* is sometimes used in this context.

4.1.2 Lesion Prevention

The term *prevention* has been used commonly to describe disease control, but only the manifestation of the pathological process—the carious lesion or toothwear lesion—can be *prevented* if the disease process/condition is controlled. The term *secondary prevention* has been used in this context to slow down or stop (arrest) incipient, progressing lesions. *Tertiary prevention* is a term used to describe the care offered to the patient in an attempt to control or reduce the negative consequences of current disease, all affecting the pattern of future disease.

4.2 CARIES CONTROL AND LESION PREVENTION

4.2.1 Categorising Caries Activity and Risk/ Susceptibility Status

The caries risk/susceptibility assessment (CRSA) was covered in Chapter 3, Section 3.3. Here we will discuss how to categorise a patient's caries activity and risk/susceptibility status.

Based on the history and examination, the patient may be allocated to one of the following categories in terms of their caries activity/risk/susceptibility status:

- *Caries inactive/controlled/low risk*: No new or actively progressing lesions (including new restorations and/or caries associated with restorations or sealants (CARS)) in the past 2 years. A level of patient-administered control (self-care maintenance) is still required to remain in this stable condition. This is a form of primary prevention.
- *Caries active/modifiable risk factors/moderate risk* (plaque biofilm control, fluoride use and other remineralisation agents, diet control): This status is characterised by the presence of active lesions and a yearly increment of more than two new, progressing or filled lesions in the preceding 2 years. Caries process control may be achieved by changing or modifying risk factors as well as treating the signs of early disease (e.g., remineralising incipient lesions).
- **Caries active/unmodifiable or unidentifiable risk factors/high risk** (dry mouth, medications affecting saliva quality and quantity, head and neck radiotherapy): This category of patients will always be high risk although it may still be possible to control the caries process by optimal moderation of risk factors. This status is characterised by the presence of active lesions and a yearly increment of more than two new, progressing or filled lesions in the preceding 2 years.

The aim is to *help* the patient change or modify their risk factors by personal behaviour change so that at recall, the caries activity status may be deemed to have changed because there are no new active lesions and/or because lesions previously judged as active are now deemed arrested. The correlation between current risk status of the patient and presence of active lesions (and their stage of progress; a *caries risk matrix*) can lead to an assessment being made by the oral healthcare team in conjunction with the patient of the patient's likelihood of suffering from new disease in the future. Table 4.1 shows a flowchart of potential caries management pathways depending on active lesion presence and the patient's caries risk/susceptibility. Note that in all cases, disease control is paramount in preventing further lesion development, but different levels of control can be offered depending on the activity/risk status: *standard* and *active* care (Table 4.2).

4.2.2 Behaviour Change/Modification: The COM-B Model

For lesion prevention and control of a lifestyle-related, non-communicable disease such as dental caries, it is imperative that all members of the oral healthcare team work with the patient and/or caregiver to help the patient modify their existing key oral health behaviours to reduce the likelihood of further disease as well as limiting the severity of already manifest disease. These key oral health behaviours include:

- Regular daily toothbrushing with a fluoride-containing toothpaste at the relevant concentration
- Interdental cleaning where applicable, carried out before general toothbrushing
- Reduction in dietary sugar consumption, frequency and amount
- Regular visits to the dentist/oral healthcare team in person, at least once every 2 years depending on the individual's disease risk/susceptibility assessment (as well as online communications where relevant)
- Refraining from or quitting tobacco use if relevant

One currently accepted behavioural psychology model to elicit the relevant changes in patients' behaviours that can be used by all members of the oral healthcare team is the Capability – Opportunity – Motivation - Behaviour change model (COM-B; see Fig. 4.1).

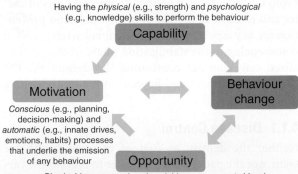

Fig. 4.1 The three interlinked components of the COM-B model required for patient behaviour change/modification. It is suggested that before any change can take place, these conditions need to be met by addressing each individual area; that is, the patient must have the capability to perform the behaviour, be motivated to do so and create or have created for them the opportunity to engage in the behaviour. (Adapted from Newton, J., Asimakopoulou, K. Minimally invasive dentistry: enhancing oral health related behaviour through behaviour change techniques. *Br Dent J.* 2017 Aug 11;223(3):147–150. doi:10.1038/sj.bdj.2017.659.)

TABLE 4.1	Care Pathway Flowchart for Caries Management				
	Active carious lesions			**No/inactive (arrested) lesions**	
IDENTIFY[a] (Chapters 2 and 3)	Cavitated (irreversible)	Non-cavitated (reversible)			
	mICDAS: 3,4 High risk	mICDAS score: 0–2 High risk	mICDAS score: 0–2 Low risk	High risk	Low risk
PREVENT and CONTROL (primary/ secondary prevention; non-invasive/ micro-invasive) (Chapter 4)	**SC + Active care** SDF Sealants High-fluoride toothpastes PMPR Motivation	**SC + Active care Remineralisation:** Fluoride CPP-ACP, fTCP e.g., MI Paste Plus Cervitec + Clinpro Tooth Crème Clinpro 5000 **PMPR Motivation**	**SC + Active care Remineralisation:** Fluoride CPP-ACP, fTCP e.g., Tooth Mousse Clinpro Tooth Crème Clinpro 5000 **PMPR Motivation**	**SC + Active care Remineralisation:** Fluoride CPP-ACP, fTCP e.g., Tooth Mousse Cervitec; MI Paste Plus, Clinpro Tooth Crème Clinpro 5000 **PMPR Motivation**	**SC:** Diet control OHI Fluoride toothpaste Maintenance/ active surveillance
Minimally invasive RESTORE (tertiary prevention) (Chapters 5 and 8)	**Provisional restorations:** e.g., Biodentine, GIC, RM-GIC **Definitive restorations:** e.g., Hybrid GICs, resin composites	**Therapeutic Fissure Sealants/ PRR:** e.g., Fuji Triage Clinpro Sealant Helioseal	**Therapeutic Fissure Sealants:** e.g., Fuji Triage Clinpro Sealant Helioseal	**Preventive Fissure Sealants:** e.g., Fuji Triage Clinpro Sealant Helioseal	
RE-ASSESS (active surveillance) (Chapter 9)	2–6 months	3–6 months	6 months	3–6 months	12–24 months

[a]The left column indicates where in this book those topics are discussed in more detail.

Note: The table shows the interaction of caries susceptibility, the presence or absence of lesions and an emphasis on non-invasive, micro-invasive and minimally invasive operative treatment of individual lesions with suitable recall intervals. The table has been divided into the four MIOC clinical domains (left column) and indicates some examples of products that could be used at the time of publication.

CPP-ACP, Casein phosphopeptide-amorphous calcium phosphate; *fTCP,* functionalised tricalcium phosphate; *GIC,* glass-ionomer cement; *mICDAS,* modified International Caries Detection and Assessment System; *PMPR,* professional mechanical plaque removal; *RM-GIC,* resin-modified glass-ionomer cement; *SC,* standard/self care; *SDF,* silver diamine fluoride; *OHI,* oral hygiene instruction.

When creating *capability* for your patients, the oral healthcare team must document and explain the findings and outcomes of the various examinations they carry out in terms that the patient understands and often supplemented with written or image-based materials. However, it is key that the patient understands, contextualises and remembers the key points. To enable this:

- Tell the patient the important points first (i.e., the points relevant to them personally, the 'primacy effect'), emphasise that information and repeat it.
- Make messaging more understandable. Several dental terms and phrases are taken for granted in our professional capacity but will not be understood by patients. Consider the best form of words to make the message understandable and identify simple ways

TABLE 4.2 Features of Preventive Care Regimens: Standard/self and Active Care	
Standard/self Care (Patient led, oral healthcare team advised, non-invasive, home care, primary prevention) Inactive/controlled, low-risk patient	**Active Care** (Oral healthcare team led, non-invasive/micro-invasive, clinic care, primary and secondary prevention) Active/uncontrolled, medium- to high-risk patient
	Standard/self care plus: **Decontamination** procedures (PMPR, transitional restorations, chlorhexidine)

Plaque biofilm control (toothbrush/interdental brushes
and toothpaste, dental flossing, waterpiks etc.)
Fluoride (various chemical formulae in toothpastes,
water)
Diet modification/control
Continued patient motivation paramount to prevent
onset of disease
Active surveillance (in person, online)
	Remineralisation agents:
	• Fluoride (high-concentration toothpaste, mouthwashes,
	  topical varnishes)
	• Remineralising pastes/solutions (e.g., CPP-ACP, fTCP,
	  SDF, bio-active glasses)
	Managing hyposalivation (medications, saliva
	substitutes)
	Preventive/therapeutic sealant restorations

CPP-ACP, casein phosphopeptides-amorphous calcium phosphate; *fTCP*, functionalised tricalcium phosphate; *PMPR*, professional mechanical plaque removal; *SDF*, silver diamine fluoride.

to explain jargon. Aside from jargon, the words and sentence structures used by the oral healthcare team may be more or less understandable. Short sentences and short words are easier to understand. Avoid long sentences with multiple clauses. Other ways in which sentences can be made more understandable are to use personal statements (e.g., 'I believe…' 'I think…') and to avoid the passive voice.

• Categorise the information in an explicit manner to help with patient recall. You could use diagrams and provide patients with mnemonic devices such as acronyms to help them recall particular points. Even simple categorisation can help to improve recall: for example, 'There are three key points for you to remember…'.

• Use specific statements relevant to the patient rather than general statements. For example, 'I would like you to keep your teeth cleaner' is general; it provides the patient with only limited information about how you want them to change their behaviour. State more explicitly what the patient can do. For example, 'I would like you to do two things to help keep your mouth cleaner. First, I want you to brush your teeth twice a day using the technique I showed you. Clean them for at least 2 minutes each time. Try cleaning each section, bottom right, bottom left and so on for about 30 seconds each. Second, I would like you to floss the gaps between your teeth twice a week, say once on Sunday and once on Wednesday'.

• Send reminders. Contacting the patient to let them know that you are expecting them the next day can

reduce unexpected non-attendance and therefore decrease lost time and opportunity costs.

When *motivating* patients, note that the best behavioural adherence is obtained when positive messages identifying the benefits of change are given in the context of how the patient can achieve those benefits. Ideally the benefits identified should be those that are valued by the patient. Try asking the patient what is important to them about their teeth and mouth and emphasise how they can fulfil those desires through working with you and your team. It is often useful to remind patients that the majority of the care of their teeth is in their own hands—they, after all, look after their teeth every day. As well as this, identifying the patient's susceptibility to disease provides an individualised personal motivation for change.

Creating *opportunity* transforms the desire and motivation for change into pragmatic, personalised action plans. This can be structured using GPS:

• **G**oal setting: These must be SMART (Specific, Measurable, Achievable, Realistic and Timed) and can be cumulative towards an ultimate goal.
• **P**lanning: Encouraging patients to make specific plans of when, where and how particular actions will be executed improves adherence to behaviour change suggestions.
• **S**elf-monitoring: Logging how well patients are achieving the goals they set with the oral healthcare

team provides feedback on performance which can allow the patient to adjust their plans if necessary. Since feedback is most effective if delivered in a timely fashion, encouraging the patient to adopt systems to record and reflect on their own behaviour can be effective (e.g., diet or flossing diaries using pen and paper or apps).

Overall, encourage persistence. The longer the patient continues, the more likely it is that they will form a habit. For infrequent behaviours (such as attending the practice), encourage the patient to link the visit to other significant events that they will recall (e.g., birthdays, holidays etc.). Ultimately, patient behaviour change through these motivational interviewing techniques is pivotal in maintaining good oral health using the minimum intervention oral care delivery approach.

4.2.3 Standard/Self Care: Low-Risk, Caries-Controlled, Disease-Inactive Patient

The standard/self care regimen (non-operative/non-invasive primary preventive therapy) is carried out wholly by the patient or caregiver at home, on the advice of their dental care professional (dentist, oral health educator, dental hygienist, dental therapist). This advice can be given in person at clinical consultations or possibly remotely via online video consultations. The latter encourages sustainability in dentistry as unnecessary patient journeys are kept to a minimum, there is no material waste generated and in-person appointments can be reserved for those in need of direct clinical interventions.

4.2.3.1 Plaque Biofilm Control

Carious lesions form at the tooth surface as a result of the metabolic events in the dental plaque biofilm. Thus plaque biofilm control is the logical cornerstone of non-operative therapy in caries prevention. Teeth should be brushed with a fluoride-containing toothpaste as fluoride interferes with the growth and ecology of the biofilm and retards lesion progression.

The preventive action of tooth brushing can be maximised by following these principles (see also Table 4.3):

- Brushing should start as soon as the first deciduous tooth erupts.
- Brush twice daily: at night before going to bed and at one other time each day.
- Discourage rinsing the mouth with water after brushing. 'Spit, don't rinse' is the correct advice.

- Some evidence exists to show that using electric rotating/oscillating toothbrushes can be more effective in plaque biofilm removal, but this will be patient dependent. Toothbrushes have to be used judiciously with the correct technique, whether manual or electric.
- Children less than 3 years of age should use a toothpaste containing no less than 1000 ppm (parts per million) fluoride.
- Children between 3 and 6 years of age are likely to swallow toothpaste and this may cause fluorosis. To prevent this they should use only a smear of paste (pea-sized amount) on the brush head and not be allowed to eat or lick toothpaste from the tube.
- Currently, it is recommended that over the age of 3 years, family fluoride toothpaste (1350–1500 ppm fluoride) should be used.
- Children need to be helped and supervised by an adult when brushing.
- The occlusal surface of erupting molars should be individually brushed with the brush placed at right angles to the arch.
- Dependent adults should be helped with oral hygiene procedures.

Oral hygiene instruction (OHI) should be generalised for the whole mouth as well as specific to the particular lesion. The patient should be aware of the problem areas and see them in their mouth via a mirror, an image from an intra-oral camera, an augmented reality device and/or a radiograph and be given a clear explanation of the issue. The following may be helpful with respect to toothbrushing:

- The patient should attend each appointment bringing their own toothbrush and toothpaste.
- Check the toothpaste for fluoride content and the brush head to ensure it is not worn.
- Disclose the mouth with a suitable plaque-staining dye so that plaque can be clearly seen by the patient.
- Assess whether the patient (or parent/caregiver) can remove the plaque or whether the technique or brush should be altered. Arthritic patients, for example, may not be able to manipulate the normal handle of a toothbrush, so silicone impression material or cold-cure acrylic may be used to thicken the grip to aid manual dexterity. Rotating or oscillating electric toothbrushes may also be recommended.

TABLE 4.3   General Population and Higher-Risk Disease Control/Lesion Prevention Approaches Categorised by Age

	Up to 3 Years	3–6 Years	7–17 Years	Adults	Older People
General population	• Brush teeth at least twice daily—last thing at night and on one other occasion—with a **smear** of fluoride toothpaste containing at least 1000 ppm fluoride. • Parents/caregivers should brush teeth. • As soon as teeth appear in the mouth, brush them twice each day with a fluoride paste. • Spit out after brushing, do not rinse. • Promote breastfeeding from birth. • Promote healthy diet. • Minimise consumption of sugary food and drinks. • Avoid sugary food and drinks at bedtime. • Maintain good dietary practices. • Use sugar-free versions of medicines. • Breastfeed for around the first 6 months of life. Introduce solids (no added sugar) from around 6 months and continue breastfeeding for the first year. • For parents feeding by bottle: only breastmilk, infant formula or cooled boiled water should be given. Feeding from a bottle should be discouraged from the age of 1 and babies should drink from a free-flow cup from 6 months.	• Brush teeth at least twice daily—last thing at night and on one other occasion—with a **pea-sized** amount of fluoride toothpaste containing at least 1000 ppm fluoride. • Parents/carers should brush and supervise toothbrushing up to 7 years. • As soon as teeth appear in the mouth, brush them effectively twice each day with a fluoride paste. • Spit out after brushing, do not rinse. • 2.2% F - varnish twice yearly. • Promote healthy diet. • Minimise consumption of sugary food and drinks. • Avoid sugary food and drinks at bedtime. • Use sugar-free versions of medicines.	• Brush teeth and the gumline effectively at least twice daily—last thing at night and on one other occasion—with toothpaste containing a standard 1350–1500 ppm fluoride. • Spit out after brushing rather than rinsing with water, to avoid diluting the fluoride concentration. • Promote healthy diet. • Minimise amount and frequency of consumption of sugary food and drinks. • Avoid sugary food and drinks at bedtime. • Avoid tobacco. • Avoid alcohol.	• Brush teeth and the gumline effectively at least twice daily—last thing at night and on one other occasion—with toothpaste containing a standard 1350–1500 ppm fluoride. • Spit out after brushing rather than rinsing with water, to avoid diluting the fluoride concentration. • Minimise amount and frequency of consumption of sugary food and drinks. • Avoid sugary food and drinks at bedtime. • Promote healthy diet. • Avoid tobacco. • Avoid alcohol or drink at safer levels.	• Brush teeth at least twice daily—last thing at night and on one other occasion—with toothpaste containing a standard 1350–1500 ppm fluoride. • Spit out after brushing rather than rinsing with water, to avoid diluting the fluoride concentration. • Minimise amount and frequency of consumption of sugary food and drinks. • Promote healthy diet. • Avoid tobacco. • Avoid alcohol or drink at safer levels.

TABLE 4.3   **General Population and Higher-Risk Disease Control/Lesion Prevention Approaches Categorised by Age—cont'd**

	Up to 3 Years	3–6 Years	7–17 Years	Adults	Older People
Dental caries *(Higher risk)*	2.26% F - varnish twice yearly. Investigate diet and assist adoption of good dietary practice in line with the Eatwell Guide. Liaise with medical practitioner to request that any long-term medication is sugar-free.	2.26% F - varnish twice yearly. Investigate diet and assist adoption of good dietary practice in line with the Eatwell Guide. Liaise with medical practitioner to request that any long-term medication is sugar-free.	2.26% F - varnish twice or more times yearly. Daily fluoride rinse. Higher fluoride toothpaste: 10+ years 2800 ppm 16+ years 2800 ppm or 5000 ppm Dietary analysis and sugar reduction Apply fissure sealants Liaise with medical practitioner to request that any long-term medication is sugar-free.	2.26% F - varnish twice yearly. Daily fluoride rinse (0.05% NaF). Higher-fluoride toothpaste (2800 ppm or 5000 ppm) Dietary analysis and sugar reduction Liaise with medical practitioner to request that any long-term medication is sugar-free.	2.26% F - varnish twice yearly. Daily fluoride rinse (0.05% NaF) Higher-fluoride toothpaste Dietary analysis and sugar reduction Liaise with medical practitioner to request that any long-term medication is sugar-free.

Modified from Office for Health Improvement and Disparities, Department of Health and Social Care, NHS England, and NHS Improvement. *Delivering Better Oral Health v4.* https://www.gov.uk/government/publications/delivering-better-oral-health-an-evidence-based-toolkit-for-prevention

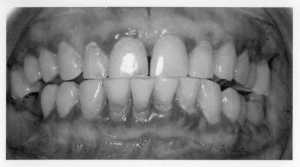

Fig. 4.2 Clinical presentation, anterior view of a patient suffering from desquamative gingivitis. Notice the generalised erythema and ulceration/desquamation of the gingivae. This is making it painful for the patient to disrupt the plaque biofilm at the cervical margins of the teeth using conventional toothbrushing techniques. Thus the biofilm stagnates in these areas, causing acute inflammation and therefore exacerbating the gingival problems. (Courtesy B Dawett.)

- Are there acute mucosal conditions present that might be preventing adequate biofilm control through conventional oral hygiene methods (see Fig. 4.2)?
- Is thorough brushing in the surgery causing gingival bleeding? If so, does the patient realise this indicates gingivitis caused by dental plaque?
- If active lesions are present, is the patient aware of where they are and able to remove the disclosed plaque from the lesions?

Where active proximal lesions are present, either in the enamel or on the root surface, an interdental cleaning aid will be needed. In young patients, lesions are best cleaned with dental floss, whereas interdental brushes are preferred for cleaning larger interdental spaces following gingival recession. The following may be helpful with respect to interdental cleaning, to be carried out prior to general toothbrushing:

- Advice given must be site specific.
- Examining the tape or brush after use may show the plaque that has been removed and this can be a useful motivating factor.
- A special holder for the floss or brush may help the patient.
- Super-floss may be used to clean around bridge pontics or crown margins.
- If the gingivae bleed, the relevance of this should be explained to the patient. If bleeding persists for days after effective cleaning is instituted, this may indicate a cavity or plaque-retentive feature is present that prevents

the patient from adequately disrupting or removing the plaque. A restoration may be needed to restore tooth integrity to allow the surface to be cleaned adequately.

4.2.3.2 Fluoride

Fluoride delays carious lesion progression by being incorporated physico-chemically into the hydroxyapatite lattice structure and by inhibiting carbohydrate metabolism within the plaque bacteria (enolase and phosphoenolpyruvate (PEP)-phosphotransferase system inhibition). Vehicles for fluoride include:

- Water: To date, approximately 15% of the UK population has access to 1 ppm F^- water. UK government legislation is changing, however, so in the future it is hoped that a greater percentage of the population will have access to fluoridated water supplies.
- Toothpaste: Fluoride toothpaste is inexpensive, requires minimal patient cooperation and enhances patients' appreciation of their essential role in caries control. See Table 4.3 for advice on fluoride concentration and toothpaste use.

The choice of vehicle is not crucial, but it must be combined with improvement in oral hygiene. It is important that the patient accepts the mode of treatment and complies with advice (see Table 4.3).

The topic of fluoride is covered further in Section 4.2.4.3.

4.2.3.3 Diet

The evidence that the frequency and amount of sugar consumption is linked to caries is irrefutable. Thus emphasis on diet in caries control would seem logical. Unfortunately, the evidence that it is possible to modify people's diets is lacking! Since the advent of fluoride, the emphasis in caries control has shifted from diet to oral hygiene in conjunction with a fluoride-containing toothpaste. However, this does not preclude the dental care professional from giving dietary advice to all patients. Reducing the amount and frequency of sugary food intake can reduce dental caries and aids in weight control as well as offering general health improvements. All health professionals have a responsibility to give advice on diet in the same way have a responsibility to give advice on smoking cessation (see Chapter 2, Section 2.5.5).

No change in diet is required for the caries-inactive/controlled patient, but the dentist/team should make the patient aware of how an adverse change in diet and/or salivary flow could pose a future problem, especially if oral hygiene efficiency deteriorates. All patients should be aware of the link between saliva, sugar and caries.

All of these aspects of *standard/self care* for controlling disease and preventing lesions require patient responsibility, cooperation and motivation. The oral healthcare team collectively is the adviser and the patients are the executors of their own personalised preventive care plan.

4.2.4 Active Care: High-Risk, Caries-Uncontrolled, Disease-Active Patient

This regimen includes all aspects of standard/self care *plus* those listed in Table 4.2, where the oral healthcare team may have to take on some of the treatment as well as providing an advisory role.

4.2.4.1 Decontamination Procedures

Professional mechanical plaque removal (PMPR) is carried out by members of the oral healthcare team (dentist, dental hygienist, dental therapist) using hand scalers as well as ultrasonic or air-polishing instrumentation to remove gross calculus deposits both supra- and subgingivally, and rotating brushes with prophy paste to mechanically debride particularly thick, tenacious plaque deposits on the tooth surfaces. This will allow the patient to clean more effectively with their toothbrush whilst enabling the clinician to examine the tooth surfaces directly.

Transitional (stabilising) restorations In some cases, early stabilising minimally invasive adhesive restorations (high-viscosity glass-ionomer cements [GICs] or resin-modified [RM] GICs; see Chapters 7 and 8) can be placed to strengthen the remaining tooth structure after removing the caries-infected dentine biomass. This tissue acts as a bacterial reservoir, and its roughened exposed surface in a cavitated lesion along with the accumulating biofilm is difficult for the patient to disrupt effectively with conventional oral hygiene procedures (Fig. 4.3).

4.2.4.2 Antimicrobial Agents

As the dental caries process is the result of a medium- to long-term imbalance in the ecological microbial enrichment of the plaque biofilm, driven by nutrients that encourage acidogenic and acid-tolerant bacteria (the ecological plaque hypothesis), this may justify the inclusion of chemical control into a caries prevention regimen. Such dysbiotic biofilm formation modulators or disruptors could be included in toothpastes, mouthrinses, varnishes or other slow-release vehicles such as slow-dissolving mints or lozenges. Whatever the delivery method, they should be aimed at:

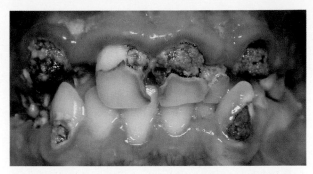

Fig. 4.3 Anterior view of a 24-year-old caries-active/uncontrolled, high-risk patient with rampant caries. The large cavitated lesions are covered with a tenacious plaque biofilm. In such patients, transitional (stabilising) restorations might be necessary to remove the bacterial reservoir and to recontour the smooth tooth restoration surfaces to facilitate improved oral hygiene procedures by the patient (standard/self care).

> **Q4.3:** What might be the possible aetiology of the degree of caries attack found in this patient?

- Minimising dysbiotic plaque formation
- Affecting the proliferation of specific bacteria
- Affecting the development of the extracellular polymeric substance in the biofilm
- Modifying enzymes which control the production of bacterial acids, leading to demineralisation of the underlying tooth surface

There is also a growing literature about the abundance of natural oligopeptide molecules as the first line of innate defence against microbial attack. To date, several experimental laboratory studies have shown that some naturally occurring as well as synthetic antimicrobial peptides can be effective in inhibiting the growth of *Streptococcus mutans*. However, it must be appreciated that there is only an associative link between *S. mutans* and the caries process, not a causative one. Therefore, preventive regimens targeting one bacterial species will not be the answer for caries prevention as a whole.

Chlorhexidine (CHX) rinses There is little clinical evidence for the use of chlorhexidine in the medium- to long-term control of the caries process. CHX (>0.12%) can affect plaque biofilm adherence and bacterial diversity on a short-term basis and can be used after oral surgical procedures when normal oral hygiene procedures would be difficult to perform due to pain, risk of postoperative bleeding and limited access for oral hygiene aids. Due to a high substantivity, its efficacy is related to both concentration and frequency of application. Long-term use may, however, lead to altered taste perception, extrinsic dental staining and possible mucosal irritation, and is therefore not recommended.

Xylitol Several studies have shown a significant decrease in *S. mutans* load after 5 weeks of chewing gum containing xylitol as a sweetener. The minimal effective dose was around 6.5 g per day, divided into at least three chewing periods. Xylitol is safe at this recommended dose; its main side effect, along with other sugar alcohols, is a mild laxative effect at much higher doses. Indeed, more recent systematic reviews and meta-analyses of the literature investigating the use of xylitol-containing sugar-free chewing gums indicate a potential clinical beneficial role for their use in an adjunctive prevention regimen to reduce the incidence of dental caries, especially in children. Manufacturers are aware of the environmental impact of waste gum and littering and are developing biodegradable gums to combat this problem.

4.2.4.3 Remineralisation

Fluoride High-concentration prescription toothpastes can be beneficial to control caries (2800/5000 ppm fluoride) especially for high-risk or highly susceptible patients with unmodifiable factors such as multiple lesions, dry mouth and radiation therapy. This is because it tips the demineralisation–remineralisation balance at the tooth surface in favour of remineralisation and has the following antimicrobial effects on the plaque biofilm:

- Impairs glycolysis and metabolic processes in plaque
- Inactivates metabolic enzymes
- Impairs bacterial membrane permeability to ionic transfer
- Inhibits the synthesis of extracellular polymers

Fluoride mouthwash can be prescribed for patients aged ≥8 years,[1] for daily (0.05% NaF) or weekly (0.2% NaF) use. For patients younger than 8 years, these mouthwashes are not advised because there is a risk of sufficient fluoride concentration in potentially ingested mouthwash to cause fluorosis in the developing dentition. The rinse should be used in addition to twice-daily brushing with toothpaste containing at least 1350 ppm fluoride. Rinses require patient compliance and should be used at a different time to toothbrushing to maximise the topical effect, which relates to frequency of availability. The product should be rinsed around the mouth for

a timed minute. Be aware that some products are astringent and will be uncomfortable for children and painful for those with a dry mouth and thin, friable intra-oral mucosa. A bland, non-alcohol mouthwash should be advised in these cases. The indications for the use of fluoride mouthwash are:

- Patients >8 years with high caries activity.
- Patients with orthodontic appliances, which inevitably encourage plaque accumulation and predispose to carious lesions.
- Patients with a dry mouth (xerostomia).
- Patients developing root caries. In these patients a weekly concentrated mouthwash may be advised for daily use.
- Professionally applied topical fluoride varnishes or fluids (e.g., Duraphat, Clinpro, Elmex Fluid) with concentrations of 22 600 ppm F or 2.2% F. Systematic reviews of research have shown fluoride varnish application by dental care professionals can reduce caries increment in the deciduous dentition by one-third and in the permanent dentition by one-half. These are impressive reductions in caries, but the dental professional should be aware that:
  - To be effective, professional application must be repeated every 3 months for high-risk or highly susceptible children and adults and every 6 months for patients over age 3 and for adults with dry mouth or active caries, and this is inevitably costly.
  - The emphasis switches to the care being provided by the professional rather than by the patient. This is important as it is essential that the patient is motivated and fully appreciates their responsibility in maintaining their oral health. Fluoride is not a panacea for controlling dental disease.
  - The concentration of fluoride is high and this means the varnish is potentially toxic to a small child if swallowed. The maximum dose advised for use in the primary dentition is 0.25 mL (5.65 mg F), in the mixed dentition is 0.4 mL (9.04 mg F) and in the permanent dentition is 0.5 mL (11.3 mg F).
  - The varnish should be applied professionally to isolated, clean, dry teeth. An ideal time to apply varnish is therefore when the teeth are being examined for carious lesions because to detect lesions, the tooth surfaces must be isolated, clean and dry (see Chapter 2, Section 2.5). Once the charting is complete, it takes only seconds to apply varnish to fissures, through contact points, cervical margins

buccally and lingually and the more susceptible exposed root surfaces.

- Apply using a disposable brush, avoiding gingivae. Include occlusal pits and fissures and floss varnish through proximal contact areas. Avoid elective toothbrushing for 4 hours and the consumption of hard, abrasive foodstuffs if possible.

Topical remineralising agents[2,3] Research is ongoing into the development of calcium- and phosphate-rich ionic solutions that can potentially act as a reservoir for these mineralising ions, therefore encouraging new mineral deposition in the right ionic conditions at the exposed tooth surface. These solutions can be incorporated with or without fluoride into toothpastes, mouthrinses, varnishes, chewing gums and topical creams and have the potential to help combat and prevent carious lesions and dental erosion. An elevated concentration of calcium in plaque biofilm fluid also facilitates a higher buildup of fluoride in this reservoir. It has also been demonstrated that there is a symbiotic relationship between calcium and fluoride. CPP-ACP (casein phosphopeptide-amorphous calcium phosphate ($Ca_9(PO_4)_6 + H_2O$)) is one such stabilised calcium phosphate system, produced under the trade name Recaldent™. ACP has a natural predilection to convert to hydroxyapatite (HAP) in wet, ionically favourable environments, and the phosphopeptide chains are thought to help bind these complexes to the tooth or biofilm surfaces and envelop them, thus regulating and directing the ultimate precipitation of the HAP where it is needed (i.e., demineralised surfaces). Combinations of CPP-ACP with fluoride have also been developed as pastes and varnishes and clinical evidence is being gathered as to their overall efficacy in the preventive management of early carious and fluorotic lesions, especially in adults where the mix of fluoride, calcium and phosphate ions has a synergistic effect (Fig. 4.4A–B). Current research evidence tends towards a favourable short-term remineralising effect, but further long-term trials are needed for conclusive clinical evidence.

Other solid calcium- and phosphate-rich formulations include calcium phosphosilicate glass-based dentifrices, functionalised β-tricalcium phosphate, unstabilised amorphous calcium phosphates, methacrylate-functionalised calcium phosphates (Crysta™), nano-hydroxyapatite and calcium sodium phosphosilicate bioactive glass (NovaMin®), which has been combined with sodium fluoride in a toothpaste. Bioactive

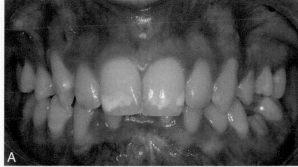

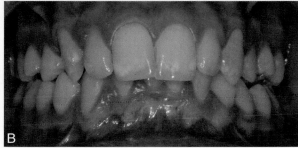

Fig. 4.4 (A) Patient with chalky, matte fluorotic lesions on the labial surfaces of the upper central incisors (see Chapter 2, Table 2.6). (B) One month later, after professional application of topical fluoride/CPP-ACP paste. The lesions are less clinically evident. (Courtesy Dr M Basso.)

Q4.4: How can you clinically distinguish these lesions from incipient white spot carious lesions?

glass particles produce crystalline hydroxycarbonate apatite (HCA) in biological aqueous environments over time, thus encouraging nucleation sites for further remineralisation. Recent in-vitro studies have shown how these particles may also be used to surface precondition white spot lesions using air-abrasion, thus aiding new mineral deposition. However, real-life clinical evidence is lacking on the effectiveness of many of these formulations and more medium- and long-term clinical trial data are required. However, there are three key drawbacks of all such topical remineralising agents that still need to be overcome for effective clinical use:

- Their relative inability to cause mineral deposition in the oral cavity when only exposed to tooth surfaces in fairly low doses over multiple short intervals. The artificial conditions in most in-vitro studies tend to bias towards a more prolonged exposure of higher concentrations of the remineralising agents to susceptible tooth surfaces (or other substrates) to encourage mineral crystal deposition to show that the product biochemistry is technically feasible.

- Such topical solutions to mineral deposition work from the top down on a demineralised tooth surface. That is, the superficial surface closest to the applied agent is remineralised but the depth of the demineralised tissue remains relatively unaffected, with porosities still evident histologically. As the surface porosities become infiltrated with new mineral crystal accretion over time, this reduces the penetration of such ions into the depths of the tissues, thus reducing any beneficial effect.

- The newly mineralised tissue surfaces in the normal oral environment are exposed to attritive, erosive and abrasive wear over time. Therefore the clinical longevity of such surface mineral crystal deposition needs to be better evaluated.

There is also the issue with carrying out and interpreting data from clinical trials on the clinical effectiveness of such topical remineralising systems. The most sought after evidence is produced from data collected from randomised controlled trials across a representative population subset. This will include patients with varying levels of caries susceptibility, from low to high, and other factors. As the outcome measures are subtle to record and any beneficial changes will only become evident over longer periods of time, such trials have to be carried out over prolonged periods with large sample numbers to account for clinical variables and the potential lack of controlled environments *in vivo*. These features make such trials very expensive to set up and carry out. Therefore data from shorter-duration trials with fewer subjects and fewer controls, as are many of those that are published, need to be interpreted with caution. Most conclude that there is limited real-life evidence of the *efficacy* (whether the intervention produces a result under ideal circumstances) and *effectiveness* (whether the intervention produces results under real-world conditions) of many of these remineralisation formulae. However, if datasets focusing of the higher risk/more susceptible populations are analysed, there is often a tailored benefit to these patients. Therefore all such aforementioned regimens should be instigated as part of the preventive caries care pathway, be specific to each patient and be delivered by the oral healthcare team as part of the MIOC delivery framework.

4.2.4.3.1 *Managing Hyposalivation*.

Altered saliva quality and quantity affects up to 20% of the UK population, especially older adults who have an altered physiology due to the ageing process and/or are taking multiple medications with a synergistic deleterious effect on saliva production (polypharmacy); patients suffering from autoimmune conditions (e.g., Sjögren's syndrome), diabetes, Parkinson's disease or Alzheimer's disease, to name but four; patients who have received head and neck radiotherapy to treat malignancies. The fact that saliva has an important protective role in the oral cavity means the detection of dry mouth (xerostomia) signs and symptoms in general dental practice is of paramount importance. It should be based on the clinical findings from a targeted examination of the quality and quantity of saliva present and the use of a suitably straightforward clinical assessment system such as the Challacombe Scale of Clinical Oral Dryness (see Chapter 2, Table 2.5). Controlling the caries process and preventing carious lesions when the mouth is dry can be very difficult for both the oral healthcare team and the patient. A dry mouth is miserable for the patient, with known significant reductions in quality-of-life indices reported extensively in the literature and is a concern for the dentist and their oral healthcare team. The long-term management goals for caries control in these high caries risk patients should be to:

- Optimise oral hygiene.
- Prescribe a high fluoride concentration toothpaste (5000 ppm F).
- Prescribe a non-alcohol containing fluoride mouthwash.
- Apply fluoride varnish to existing lesions every 3 months (see earlier).
- Ask the patient to keep a regular diet sheet or diary and to try to minimise sugar intake where possible.
- Make the patient aware that they need to moisten their mouth frequently and that plain water is safe.
- Re-assess the patient at a minimum of 3 months with members of the oral healthcare team and consider regular online consultations (active surveillance).
- Make the patient aware that saliva can be stimulated by chewing a xylitol-containing sugar-free gum, provided there is sufficient salivary gland activity, or pharmacologically.
- In cases of Sjögren's syndrome or post-radiotherapy of the head and neck, a saliva substitute may be required including proprietary dry-mouth gels.
- Check that any prescribed antifungal agent does not contain sugar.

- Check with the patient's medical practitioner regarding alternatives to medications causing hyposalivation (this may be limited as the medical benefits of the medication will usually outweigh the negative effect of reduced saliva output).

4.2.4.3.2 Preventive Fissure Sealants. This micro-invasive, primary preventive procedure has been included in this section on caries control as it helps to modify local surface factors that affect the onset and progress of caries and its lesions, namely eradicating caries-susceptible deep fissures and pits on posterior occlusal surfaces of high-risk patients. There are two types of fissure sealant materials:

- *Resin-based*: Visible light-cured systems based on methacrylate resin composite chemistry (detailed in Chapter 7, Section 7.2). These resins are only lightly filled to permit a readily flowable consistency, thus creating a void-free infill of deeper pits and fissures. After checking the pre-operative occlusion, the dental practitioner must isolate the teeth, ideally using a rubber dam, to obtain effective moisture control; next, the teeth then must be thoroughly debrided and acid-etched so that the fissure sealant is micro-mechanically retained to the enamel surface and then light-cured (see Chapter 8, Table 8.2). Care must be taken to ensure the sealant is not in direct occlusion as it will wear or chip readily, with the subsequent risk of increasing plaque accumulation in an uncleansable site. Therefore occlusion should be checked before commencing treatment as well as afterwards.
- *Glass-ionomer cement (GIC)-based*: Can be used to chemically bond to the 10% polyacrylic acid-conditioned enamel surface. These materials are more soluble than the resin-based systems, but they do leach fluoride ions which may have a cariostatic effect (Fig. 4.5A–C). They can be beneficial in clinical scenarios where moisture control is sub-optimal (e.g., sealing occlusal surfaces of erupting molars in high caries risk children).

Evidence-based systematic reviews have concluded that there is no clinically significant advantage of one or the other material type, although it appears that the resin-based preventive sealants show an increased longevity in clinical use when careful application steps are adhered to, with optimal moisture control being achieved and with a better overall wear resistance. However, in clinical situations where adequate moisture control is difficult to achieve, GIC-based preventive fissure sealants may still be recommended. Both types of fissure sealant require careful review, inspection and maintenance (active surveillance) to ensure their long-term integrity, dependent upon the longitudinal caries susceptibility assessment for that individual patient. If fissure sealants chip or debond in the short to medium term, they will need refurbishing, repair or replacement (see Chapter 9, Section 9.4).

The detailed clinical procedure of placing a micro-invasive preventive fissure sealant is described in Chapter 8 (Table 8.2). Fissure sealants are indicated:

- In high-risk, caries-active, susceptible adolescents. Fissure sealing all erupting molars may be advisable as a primary preventive measure.
- In high-risk young adults where there is evidence of caries on molar teeth which need restoration. In these cases other susceptible occlusal fissures may be sealed as a precaution.
- In young patients with deep fissure patterns who may otherwise be susceptible due to changes in diet or other local factors (e.g., the mentally or physically disabled with less than optimal oral hygiene, patients undergoing extensive orthodontic treatment, medically compromised patients).
- In patients with cleaned teeth which can be easily isolated using a rubber dam (see Chapters 5 and 8). Saliva contamination during placement may lead to premature complete loss of the resin-based fissure sealant or leakage at the margins of a partially debonded restoration, which might then lead to active caries. In such clinical scenarios, GIC-based fissure sealants may be advised, but with suitable review and monitoring (active surveillance; Fig. 4.5).

4.2.4.3.3 Therapeutic Fissure Sealants. Therapeutic fissure sealants can be used as micro-invasive, secondary preventive therapy on teeth which have undergone early physical damage due to the caries process but are clinically non-cavitated or micro-cavitated. These sealants are most often placed in the pits and fissures of posterior teeth, ideally under isolation by a rubber dam, after the incipient lesions have been debrided thoroughly, perhaps treated with remineralising agents (discussed earlier), but not excavated physically (Fig. 4.6A–F). The sealing action of this micro-invasive tooth surface modification along with suitable maintenance from the patient to regularly disturb the plaque biofilm will cause the early lesion to become inactive or arrested. There is some ambiguity in this terminology as the term

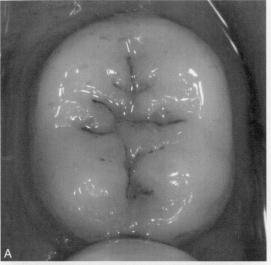

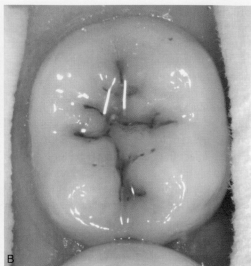

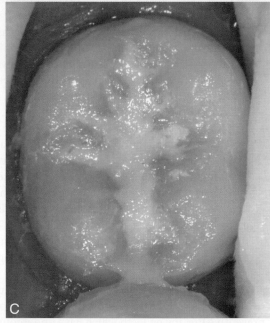

Fig. 4.5 (A) Recently erupted mandibular left second molar in a high caries risk/susceptible patient with difficult moisture control and access. The occlusal surface and fissure pattern is firstly debrided with prophypaste on a rotating bristle brush. (B) A 10% polyacrylic acid conditioner is placed on the occlusal surface to remove the smear layer. Moisture control was achieved with cotton wool roll isolation (see Chapter 5, Section 5.6). (C) After thoroughly washing away the conditioner and blotting the tooth surface dry, the GIC fissure sealant is placed and gross excess is removed. Ideally, the occlusion should be checked with articulating paper before and after the placement of the fissure sealant to ensure the material is not encroaching on the occlusal table, increasing the risk of fracture of the sealant during mastication. (Courtesy I Miletic.)

> **Q4.5:** How long would you expect GIC fissure sealants to last? In the aforementioned case, do you think the fissure sealant on the LL7 will need to be replaced indefinitely?

therapeutic fissure sealant has also been used erroneously by some to describe what are known also as *sealant restorations* (discussed next).

4.2.4.3.4 Sealant Restoration/Preventive Resin Restoration.
Sealant restoration/preventive resin restoration (PRR) is usually carried out as secondary preventive therapy in high caries risk/susceptible patients

presenting with multiple carious lesions at differing stages of progression. These restorations can have diagnostic value in helping to ascertain the histological penetration of lesions where the demineralisation extent is not necessarily evident on a radiograph. They are placed after the minimally invasive excavation of initially cavitated occlusal caries, just beyond the enamel–dentine

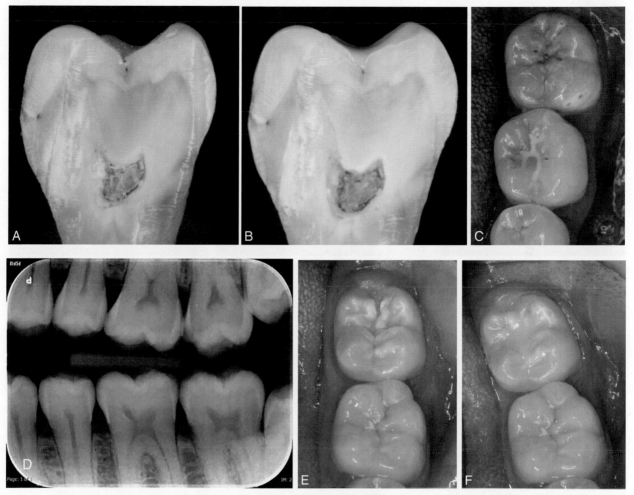

Fig. 4.6 (A) Sectioned tooth with an early occlusal enamel fissure lesion. (B) resin-based fissure sealant placed occlusally after debriding the fissure and acid etching. The fissure pattern is now more cleansable with conventional oral hygiene procedures for the patient ((A, B) *from Dawett B, Young S, Deery C, Banerjee A. Minimally invasive selective caries removal put into practice. Dent Update 2020; 47: 841-847).* (C) LL6 managed with a resin-based fissure sealant whilst the LL7 has been reviewed and maintained with adequate patient oral hygiene, fluoride toothpaste and the application of Tooth Mousse™. (D) the left bitewing radiograph including the two teeth described in image (C) *((C & D) courtesy of P Mylonas).* (E) pre-operative occlusal incipient enamel fissure lesion, LL7, where occlusion should be checked prior to (F) the post-operative placement of resin-based therapeutic fissure sealant after fissure debridement. Note the presence of remnants of preventive fissure sealant on the LL6, placed as the tooth was erupting into occlusion (E & F *courtesy of B Dawett).*

Q4.6C: What classification of fissure sealant is shown in Fig. 4.6C?

Q4.6C and D: What features on clinical and radiographic examination of the LL6 and LL7 would you carefully examine and record on periodical re-assessment/active surveillance?

---

junction (EDJ). In essence, the operator will have undertaken a small enamel–dentine pit-fissure 'biopsy' to determine the extent of carious lesion penetration into the tooth. The sealant restoration restores the small cavity with a suitable adhesive restorative material (adhesive plus resin composite or GIC) followed with an overlying preventive resin-based fissure sealant which extends onto the unrestored fissures on the remaining

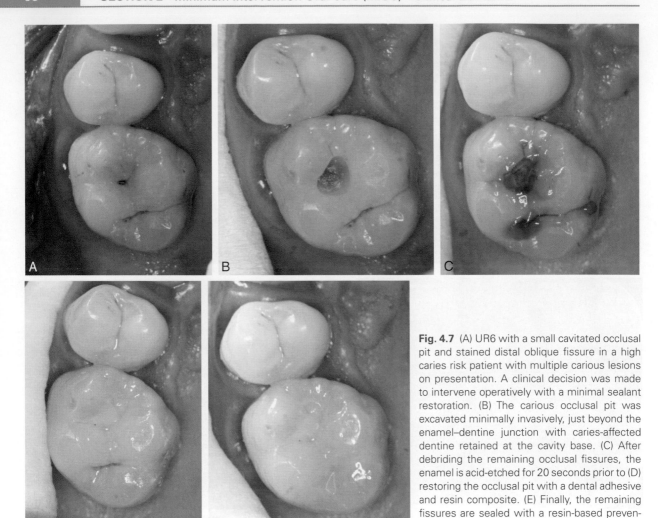

Fig. 4.7 (A) UR6 with a small cavitated occlusal pit and stained distal oblique fissure in a high caries risk patient with multiple carious lesions on presentation. A clinical decision was made to intervene operatively with a minimal sealant restoration. (B) The carious occlusal pit was excavated minimally invasively, just beyond the enamel–dentine junction with caries-affected dentine retained at the cavity base. (C) After debriding the remaining occlusal fissures, the enamel is acid-etched for 20 seconds prior to (D) restoring the occlusal pit with a dental adhesive and resin composite. (E) Finally, the remaining fissures are sealed with a resin-based preventive fissure sealant. (Courtesy B Dawett.)

debrided and acid-etched sound portion of the occlusal surface, placed as a primary preventive measure for the remaining tooth surface (see Fig. 4.7A–E and Chapter 8, Table 8.3).

4.2.4.3.5 Smooth Surface Resin Infiltration.
Resin infiltrants are low-viscosity, light-cured, methacrylate-based materials which are encouraged to penetrate into the subsurface enamel lesion, thus reducing microporosities, affording micro-mechanical support and obstructing the acids, thus hampering further progressive demineralisation. Used as a micro-invasive secondary preventive therapy, resin infiltration treatment for such tooth surfaces, consists of the following clinical steps:

> **Q4.7:** What important clinical step has been omitted in this case?

1. The tooth surface needs to be clean and dry.
2. A rubber dam is applied.
3. If treating a proximal surface, an interdental wedge is placed to gain sufficient separation of the teeth to pass the application foil between adjacent tooth surfaces.
4. The tooth is surface-etched for 2 minutes with 15% hydrochloric acid (HCl).

5. A water-air spray is used for 30 seconds to thoroughly remove the etching liquid.
6. Ethanol (99%) is applied to the tooth for 30 seconds to thoroughly dry the treated surface.
7. The low-viscosity resin infiltrant is applied and the tooth is light-cured for 40 seconds.

Following are some key points to think about when considering the clinical use of micro-invasive, secondary preventive resin infiltration treatment within a personalised care plan for adults or adolescents as part of the MIOC pathway:

- There is some clinical evidence in the published literature that shows the potential for resin infiltration of smooth/proximal surface incipient enamel carious lesions to hamper or even prevent further acid demineralisation and lesion progression.
- Due to the occlusion of these microporosities, alterations can occur in the refractive index of the enamel, thus affecting the light-scattering effect. This in turn can improve the aesthetics of an infiltrated enamel white spot lesion.
- This micro-invasive approach requires lesion and patient review and recall to ensure the patient is adherent to the preventive behaviour change advice given by the oral healthcare team to reduce and maintain low caries risk/susceptibility in the long term (active surveillance; see earlier).
- Resin infiltration is most effective on smooth-surface, active, non-cavitated carious lesions, histologically within enamel or having just breached the EDJ radiographically.
- The depth of resin penetration into a lesion is more dependent upon the size, number and pore volume of the microporosities created within an active lesion, as opposed to the actual clinical application time.
- Once an incipient lesion is infiltrated, topical remineralising agents will have a reduced beneficial effect as the diffusion pathways will have been obliterated by the resin infiltrant. However, topical remineralisation will still have benefit on other tooth surfaces in a high-risk/susceptible patient, so this must be continued.
- If a deeper lesion is not sufficiently infiltrated, the unfilled deeper microporosities may provide diffusion channels for acids to continue demineralisation and further lesion progression. These porosities

might also trap exogenous, dietary stains, thus adversely affecting the overall aesthetics of the tooth surface lesion. Therefore suitable clinical review is required.

4.3 TOOTHWEAR CONTROL AND LESION PREVENTION

4.3.1 Process

The control and prevention of toothwear and its lesions, as part of the team-delivered, person-focused MIOC delivery approach, are intimately linked with managing the aetiological factors of erosion, attrition and abrasion discussed in Chapters 1 and 2. The patient's understanding and motivation are vital to the ultimate successful prevention and control of toothwear (see Table 4.4). The aetiological factors must be identified (targeted history and examination; MIOC domain 1) and behaviour modified subsequently (with positive suggestion/motivational interviewing skills; MIOC domain 2) to modify and minimise the causative factor(s). For example, high intake of carbonated drinks or acidic fruit juices over a prolonged period can be adjusted by suggesting that initially, 1 in 3 drinks could be tap water and then after 1 month, alternate drinks, and so on, thus gradually reducing the primary causative factor.

4.3.2 Lesions

Once structural tooth surface loss has occurred, the tissue damage cannot be reversed. Early, asymptomatic lesions in enamel, or even just into dentine, may be left untreated, especially if the causes have been eradicated. Reviewing and recall of patients with pathological toothwear not requiring immediate operative intervention is discussed in Chapter 9, Section 9.1.3. More extensive tooth loss accompanied by symptoms including sensitivity, aesthetic considerations and functional difficulties can be repaired, depending on the severity, with minimally invasive direct adhesive aesthetic restorations or with indirect extra-coronal restorations (Fig. 4.8A–D). Important factors including the longevity of the protective restorations placed and changes/compensation in the vertical dimension caused by the tooth surface loss have to be taken into account in more complex restorative care planning, the details of which are beyond the scope of this book.

TABLE 4.4   **Age-Related and Higher-Risk Toothwear Control/Lesion Prevention Approaches for the General Population**

	Up to 3 Years	3–6 Years	7–17 Years	Adults	Older People
Toothwear (Higher risk)	Investigate possible risk factors and advise accordingly.	Investigate possible risk factors and advise accordingly.	Investigate possible risk factors (intrinsic/extrinsic). Advise on lowering risk. Support with behaviour change. Consider different toothpaste.	Investigate possible risk factors (intrinsic/extrinsic). Consider general health including reflux. Advise on lowering risk. Support with behaviour change. Consider different toothpaste.	Investigate possible risk factors (intrinsic/extrinsic). Consider general health including reflux. Advise on lowering risk. Support with behaviour change. Consider different toothpaste.

Modified from Office for Health Improvement and Disparities, Department of Health and Social Care, NHS England, and NHS Improvement. *Delivering Better Oral Health v4.* https://www.gov.uk/government/publications/delivering-better-oral-health-an-evidence-based-toolkit-for-prevention

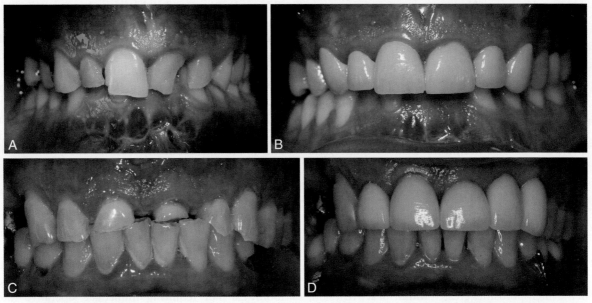

Fig. 4.8 (A) Preoperative anterior view of a patient with erosion-attrition toothwear caused by gastro-oesophageal reflux disease. (B) Anterior view after treatment with metal-ceramic indirect crowns on the UR3 to UL3. (C) A different case showing the anterior pre-operative view of severe attrition-erosive toothwear. (D) The final dental rehabilitation using a combination of crown lengthening periodontal surgery in the maxillary anterior sextant, followed by the provision of indirect porcelain restorations and removable partial dentures. (C and D courtesy of P Mylonas).

Q4.8A: What might the presenting complaints have been?

Q4.8A and B: The long-term tooth loss has caused a loss in occlusal vertical dimension (see Chapter 5, Section 5.13). What clues are present in these images to indicate this process has occurred?

Q4.8A and B: What might have caused the scar on the anterior mandibular mucosae?

Q4.8C: What clinical features can you identify from the anterior view in Fig. 4.8C? What clinical finding might have contributed to the extent of anterior toothwear?

Q4.8D: What restorations have been placed in the maxillary anterior sextant? Why haven't the cavities in the LR45 and LL4 been restored?

4.4   ANSWERS TO SELF-TEST QUESTIONS

Q4.3: What might be the possible aetiology of the degree of caries attack found in this patient?
A: Possibly long-term poor diet and oral hygiene, but this degree of caries attack is very unlikely. The more likely presentation is of recreational drug-induced caries in young adults—possibly methamphetamine or methadone use (a viscous, sugary syrup used by recovering drug addicts).

Q4.4: How can you clinically distinguish these lesions from white spot carious lesions?
A: The site. Discrete carious white spot lesions are usually found closer to the gingival margins and other sites associated with plaque biofilm stagnation due to ineffective oral hygiene procedures. These lesions are present across the incisal third of the labial surface and are not associated with plaque stagnation.

Q4.5: How long would you expect GIC fissure sealants to last? In the aforementioned case, do you think the fissure sealant on the LL7 will need to be replaced indefinitely?
A: Depending on patient factors, realistically probably 2 years or so. The young patient was initially deemed to be high caries risk, so the fissure sealant was clinically justified. However, over time the preventive oral care undertaken by the patient will hopefully change their risk status to low. Indeed, the patient maintained a low-risk status and underwent orthodontic treatment. Therefore the GIC fissure sealant was not replaced when it finally failed.

Q4.6C: What classification of fissure sealant is shown in Fig. 4.6C?
A: Technically, this is a therapeutic fissure sealant as an early enamel lesion is present. This is more evident in the cross-sectioned tooth but would be difficult to detect clinically.

Q4.6C and D: What features on clinical and radiographic examination of the LL6 and LL7 would you carefully examine and record on periodical re-assessment/active surveillance?
A: Careful review of the occlusal shadowing that is present on the lingual extension of the occlusal fissure to check this is not CARS. Use of a sharp dental probe to check the integrity of the margins of the fissure sealant. If the patient is deemed low caries risk/susceptibility, bitewings every 2 years may be indicated to check if any radiolucencies have formed in either the LL6 or LL7. Note that the resin-based fissure sealant is not easily detected

on the radiograph. Serial clinical photographs can be beneficial in the active surveillance of such cases. Review of the efficacy of the patient's oral hygiene regimen and plaque score is required.

Q4.7: What important clinical step has been omitted in this case?
A: There is no rubber dam moisture control. This should be placed where clinically possible. In this case, moisture control was provided with cotton wool rolls and suction with the assistance of the dental nurse to help keep the operating field dry at all times.

Q4.8A: What might the presenting complaints have been?
A: Poor appearance, sharp edges of the incisors cutting/traumatising the tip of the tongue, teeth fracturing and sensitivity.

Q4.8A and B: The long-term tooth loss has caused a loss in occlusal vertical dimension (see Chapter 5, Section 5.13). What clues are present in these images to indicate this process has occurred?
A: Note the step up in the line of the attached gingivae of the mandible subjacent to the lower incisors. This is the classic appearance of the physiological overeruption of these lower incisor teeth leading to *dentoalveolar compensation* that has occurred in an attempt to maintain the vertical relationship between the maxillary and mandibular teeth.

Q4.8A and B: What might have caused the scar on the anterior mandibular mucosae?
A: A postoperative scar after the surgical fixation of a fractured mandible with a bone plate several years ago.

Q4.8C: What clinical features can you identify from the anterior view in Fig. 4.8C? What clinical finding might have contributed to the extent of anterior toothwear?
A: Severe inciso-palatal tooth surface loss in the maxillary anterior sextant that has led to a reduced overbite anteriorly; signs of attrition and erosion; class V buccal cervical cavities in the LR45 and LL4; and plaque stagnation around the gingival margins of the mandibular incisors with concomitant gingivitis. The missing bilateral mandibular posterior teeth may have contributed to an increased occlusal loading on the anterior teeth in function that may have contributed to the extent of tooth surface loss noted.

Continued

4.4   ANSWERS TO SELF-TEST QUESTIONS—cont'd

Q4.8D: What restorations have been placed in the maxillary anterior sextant? Why haven't the cavities in the LR45 and LL4 been restored?

A: A resin composite labial veneer has been placed on the UR3 and porcelain-fused-to-metal indirect crowns on the UR2-UL3. These have gained mechanical retention by surgically moving the position of the periodontium apically in these teeth (crown lengthening). As the patient has adhered to their preventive oral hygiene regimen, an essential prerequisite before any definitive restorative dentistry is carried out, the biofilm control has improved significantly and as the cavities highlighted were not caries active, it was decided between the operator and the patient (shared decision-making) that restorations in these teeth were not currently indicated.

REFERENCES

1. Office for Health Improvement and Disparities, Department of Health and Social Care, NHS England, NHS Improvement. Delivering better oral health: an evidence-based toolkit for prevention. 12 June 2014. Updated 9 November 2021. Accessed 17 September 2023. https://www.gov.uk/government/publications/delivering-better-oral-health-an-evidence-based-toolkit-for-prevention

2. Amaechi, B., 2017. Remineralisation – the buzzword for early MI caries management. Br. Dent. J. 223, 173–182. doi.org/10.1038/sj.bdj.2017.663

3. Philip, N., 2019. State of the art enamel remineralization systems: The next frontier in caries management. Caries Res. 53, 284–295. doi: 10.1159/000493031

Minimum Intervention Oral Care (MIOC) – Clinical Domain 3

SECTION 3

Minimum Intervention Oral Care (MIOC) – Clinical Domain 3

MIOC Domain 3: Minimally Invasive Operative Dentistry

CHAPTER OUTLINE

5.1 CLINICAL MANAGEMENT GUIDELINES

As has already been discussed, all members of the oral healthcare team have a part to play in patient management, comprising the lead dentist (plus other colleagues in the dental practice), dental nurse, dental hygienist, receptionist, laboratory technician and dental therapist. In the UK, registered dental nurses can take further qualifications in teaching, oral health education and radiography and can specialise in other aspects of dentistry including orthodontics, oral surgery, sedation and special care. Dental therapists and dental hygienists in the UK have a developing scope of practice that enables a teamwork environment with dentist colleagues to optimise the patient care delivery journey. A successful oral and dental healthcare practice must utilise the skill sets of all members of the team for its and its patients' benefit.[1,2]

If the dentist wishes to have a specialist's opinion regarding a difficult diagnosis, formulating a more complex personalised care plan or even executing it, they may refer the patient to a registered specialist dentist working in another practice or to a hospital-based consultant specialist in restorative dentistry. These specialists have undergone further postgraduate clinical and academic training and gained qualifications enabling them to be registered as specialists with the General Dental Council (GDC – UK) in their specific trained fields (e.g., endodontics, periodontics, prosthodontics) or have further specialist training in restorative dentistry (hospital consultants). The lead dentist will act as a central hub in the coordinating wheel of patient management, possibly outsourcing different aspects of work to relevant specialist colleagues as spokes of that care delivery wheel. This describes shared care, advocated in the UK National Health Service (NHS).

There is a clear need and benefit to have guidance as to how to deliver minimum intervention oral care (MIOC) and minimally invasive dentistry (MID) to individuals, local regions and country-specific populations. Of course, as all clinicians must appreciate, there is always variation among practitioners as to how to resolve particular clinical challenges, with many, often subjective, factors to be taken into account. To help in such instances, it is useful to have guidelines/standard operating procedures (SOPs) to help oral healthcare teams manage their patients. These cannot be restrictive or prescriptive rules and regulations; they should be a learned summation of the current, collated expert consensus, scientific evidence and clinical evidence, however strong or weak these may be, to be considered along with the individual patient, practitioner and local factors pertaining to each clinical scenario/patient and adapted accordingly. In this way, each patient receives optimal care and the team/practitioner can feel confident in their approach and can also learn from others as well as add to their clinical experience and acumen collectively. The implementation of such consensus guidelines needs to be accompanied with careful communication (shared decision-making) and documentation between the team and patient of decisions made and the reasons as to why (a *personalised care plan* as opposed to a treatment plan, as discussed previously).[3,4]

Many important guideline publications are available for each of the different disciplines in restorative dentistry, including periodontology, prosthodontics and endodontics. These often concentrate on standardising specific operative treatment protocols for more clearly defined clinical situations and outcomes. These are researched and published by expert panels representing learned societies, royal colleges and government bodies in charge of delivering healthcare in society. These groups are sometimes assisted by industry partners to help convene the discussions. It is important, however, that industry partners do not influence the outcomes and that these are kept strictly independent to avoid inappropriate bias towards the use of certain technologies and materials.

The discipline of conservative and MI dentistry in primary care covers a gamut of clinical situations affecting a large, heterogeneous population. Many management variables (technologies, procedures, materials, operator skills, knowledge, experience and a multitude of patient factors including attitudes/behaviour socio-economic status, etc.) all need to be considered when attempting to develop suitable management and treatment guidelines to help practitioners and their teams. Due to this complex interaction of a large number of variables, there is a relative paucity of clear-cut, high-quality research evidence (e.g., randomised controlled clinical trials) to enable such guidance to be absolute, conclusive and applicable to all scenarios.

In conservative and minimally invasive (MI) dentistry including endodontics, there are many national and international learned societies and consensus panels, all providing useful information about the terminology, prevention and management of caries,[5-10] toothwear and management protocols for broken-down teeth. As one example, the European Federation of Conservative Dentistry (EFCD) and the European Organisation for Caries Research (ORCA) have collaborated in an attempt to collate and generate pragmatic, evidence-based expert consensus guidance for primary care practitioners.[11-16] These, along with many other published efforts globally, are trying to help the relevant stakeholders manage patients, improve oral health linked to general health and increase awareness in populations of their role in valuing and taking responsibility for their personal healthcare future.[17-19]

5.2 THE DENTAL SURGERY, CLINIC OR OFFICE

This is the clinical environment where patients are diagnosed and treated. This room has been known traditionally as the 'dental surgery' or 'dental operatory', but a more appropriate modern description might be the 'dental clinic' as much of the more holistic preventive care offered to patients within its four walls will be non-surgical in the first instance. The operator and nurse must work closely together. To be successful, they must build up an understanding of how each other works. The clinic consists of a dental operating chair with an attached or mobile bracket table carrying the rotary instruments and 3-1 air/water syringe (and possibly the light-curing unit and ultrasonic scaler), work surfaces (which should be as clutter-free as possible for compliant infection prevention and control; see later), cupboards for storage and two sinks, one for normal handwashing and another for decontaminating soiled instruments prior to sterilisation (this might be located in a separate decontamination room or zone). Often a surgery will also house an X-ray unit for taking intraoral radiographs and perhaps an operating surgical microscope. Most clinics are designed to accommodate right-handed practitioners in terms of the location of many of the instruments and controls, but of course left-handed designs are available. In larger clinics, there may be space to accommodate a table or desk and comfortable chair where the initial verbal consultation may occur before moving to the dental chair for the clinical examination.

5.2.1 Positioning the Clinician, Patient and Nurse

All three must be positioned for maximum comfort, visibility and access whilst maintaining a healthy posture. Initially, the dentist and patient should be sitting at equal eye level, face to face (Fig. 5.1).

The patient is then reclined in the dental chair into a near horizontal position and the height of the chair is adjusted so that the patient's head is level with the dentist's mid-sternum, whose knees are placed beneath the patient's headrest. The operator/clinician should sit with their back straight and upper arms vertical with elbows bent at right angles. Thighs should be near-parallel to the floor and knees bent at right angles, with feet firmly placed flat on the floor (Fig. 5.2). The use of backless saddle chairs can help the clinician obtain and maintain this posture throughout the working day.

For a right-handed clinician, the dental nurse should sit to the left of the patient, facing the patient, sitting approximately 10 to 15 cm higher than the clinician to aid their direct vision into the oral cavity. The dental nurse's chair may have a foot bar and a swivel backrest that can be moved round to support the nurse when assisting the dentist intra-orally. If the patient's head in the dental chair is represented by a clockface with 12 o'clock between the patient's eyes, the clinician can move between 8 o'clock (to view the lower-right quadrant with direct vision and the patient slightly more upright in the chair) and 1 o'clock, and the nurse from 1 to 4 o'clock positions (Fig. 5.3). These

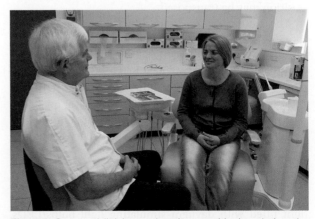

Fig. 5.1 Operator/clinician and patient positioning during the consultation. Note how the clinician is sitting slightly in front of the patient and at the same eye level. This positioning enables the patient to feel more comfortable and relaxed.

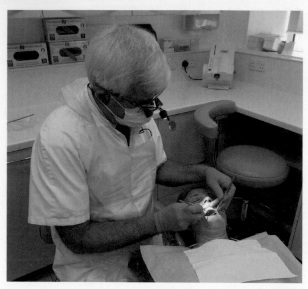

Fig. 5.2 Clinician's operating position with the patient reclined in the dental chair. Note how the clinician's elbows are bent at 90 degrees and the back is straight and shoulders relaxed.

Q5.2: What piece of equipment is the clinician wearing that will aid their posture while examining the patient?

positions may be reversed for the left-handed operator, assuming that the surgery has space and is designed with this in mind. Some dental chairs are designed so that the nurse's suction and operator's bracket table/mobile cart position may be transposed.

The patient can facilitate direct intra-oral vision by moving their head. Assuming there is no medical or physical reason causing a restriction of neck movement (to be checked in the medical history beforehand), the clinician should ask and gently guide the movement, a right head turn to view the upper-left buccal quadrant, tipping head down to view the mandibular dentition and lifting the chin up to help view the maxillary dentition.

5.2.2 Lighting

Good-quality illumination is vital to work in a patient's mouth. This is usually afforded by the overhead chair light fitted with daylight-simulating light bulbs/LEDs. These lights may be focused onto the patient's face and mouth by correct spatial positioning and alignment (some cast a horizontal dark shadow if incorrectly

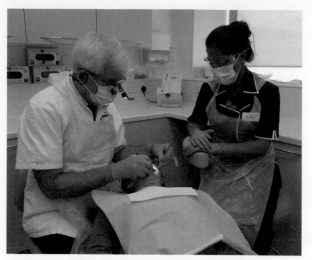

Fig. 5.3 The initial positions of the clinician and dental nurse during the intra-oral examination. See text for details.

focused). They should be aligned to cast their beam of light as directly in line with the operator's line of sight as possible (usually offset by only a few degrees) to reduce the shadows cast intra-orally. The intra-oral mirror should be used to direct light specifically to areas required (e.g., maxillary structures). Light handles must be covered with disposable shields for infection prevention and control purposes. An LED headlight can be worn by the operator, often coupled with magnifying loupes (see Section 5.6), focusing the shadowless light in the direction of the dentist's gaze (Figs. 5.2 and 5.3). Care needs to be taken when working with resin composites, as these can be light-cured prematurely by intense LED outputs or the overhead operating light. An orange filter can be used to prevent this from happening when using the LED headlight, or alternatively the operating light may need to be directed away from the oral cavity when placing the resin composite restorative material.

5.2.3 Zoning

For infection prevention and control purposes, the dental clinic must be divided into zones for clinical notes/clean instruments and dirty instruments. It is important that these zones are designed with practicality in mind as thoroughfare between and through them should be kept to a minimum to prevent cross-contamination between zones. An example in a hospital setting is shown in Fig. 5.4A–C, but variations will obviously be found in different dental practice surgeries. Dirty zones (areas that

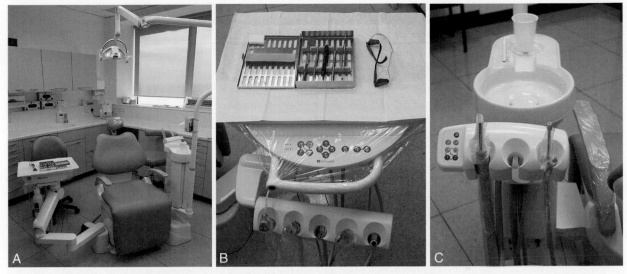

Fig. 5.4 (A) to (C) The infection prevention and control barriers placed when setting up a dental surgery. (A) An overview of the surgery. (B) The bracket table. (C) The spittoon area. Note the use of disposable suction tips and barrier protection on all tubing.

are likely to become contaminated by direct contact, aerosols or splatter during treatment procedures) include:

- Bracket table and handle
- Dental handpiece unit, connectors and switches
- Dental chair headrest
- Light handles/switches
- Chair handle controls
- Suction connectors
- Spittoon

These zones must be cleaned and disinfected appropriately between patients. To aid this process, most of them can be covered with clear plastic wrap (cling film) or plastic sleeves, which are removed, zones cleaned and plastic wrap replaced between patients. With the environmental sustainability in dentistry becoming of ever-increasing importance, it is imperative that industry partners find alternative recyclable materials for this purpose.

5.3 INFECTION PREVENTION AND CONTROL/PERSONAL PROTECTIVE EQUIPMENT

Current UK guidelines[20] require the dentist and nurse to be dressed in short-sleeve tunics or uniforms (bare below the elbow), no neckties that hang loosely from the neck and no jewellery (except wedding bands). Footwear should cover the tops of feet. Standard infection control practise against blood-borne, air-borne and other body fluid–borne pathogens, including nosocomial infections, are outlined in Table 5.1. With regard to protecting the patient, a disposable neck towel should be placed over the patient and suitable eye protection must be worn by the patient while in the reclined position (Fig. 5.5). Of course, the SARS-CoV-2 pandemic of 2020 has highlighted globally the importance of infection prevention and control measures in mitigating the threat of spread of infections to both patients and members of the oral healthcare team, using the hierarchy of controls structure (Fig. 5.6).

5.3.1 Decontamination and Sterilisation Procedures

The days of locating the sterilising unit in the corner of the surgery are numbered and in many countries they are long gone. Separate equipment sterilisation facilities for re-usable equipment are required (either in a decontamination unit or in a segregated area within the surgery) with contaminated entry and clean exit pathways clearly demarcated. This area should be separated into dirty, sterilisation and clean zones. Instruments need to be manually washed and placed in an ultrasonic bath to remove debris. A thermal washer-disinfector is

TABLE 5.1   **Infection Prevention and Control Procedures for the Oral Healthcare Team**

Precautions	Comments
Hand hygiene	Soap/detergent and running hot water; alcohol hand gels before donning and after removing gloves.
Skin dressings	Cuts, abrasions and skin conditions protected with waterproof dressings.
Sharps handling	Used needles and sharps should be disposed by the user into rigid sharps containers. Only resheath needles if using a resheathing device/single-handed technique.
Personal protective equipment	Reusable protective eyewear worn (goggles with side protection or visors over spectacles) if risk of blood/body fluid splashing to the face. Single-use surgical face masks provide a physical barrier to splashes to the mouth/face. They do not protect the wearer from aerosol inhalation (FFP1). Respirator-type masks (FFP2/FFP3) can be used to protect against aerosol inhalation created by aerosol-generating procedures. Single-use gloves: natural rubber latex (non-powdered), nitrile (acrylonitrile)/polychloroprene or Tactylon gloves should be worn (non-allergenic). Contact with natural rubber latex can result in development of latex hypersensitivity: delayed type IV (contact dermatitis, rhinitis, conjunctivitis up to 48 hours after exposure) or, less commonly, immediate type I (asthma, urticaria, laryngeal oedema, anaphylactic shock usually within 30 minutes after exposure). Single-use plastic aprons to prevent contamination of clothing.
Blood/body fluid spillages	Dealt with using hypochlorite granules and appropriate personal protective equipment.
Clinical waste handling	Infectious, hazardous waste disposed of in yellow clinical waste bags.
Instruments	Single-use sharp instruments disposed of in appropriate sharps container. Reusable instruments must undergo decontamination prior to sterilisation (see later).

Note: The use of plastics in single-use instrumentation and personal protective equipment needs to be carefully monitored and regulated due to the negative environmental impact these items have in manufacturing and their disposal. Biologically degradable, ecofriendly alternatives need to/are being developed.

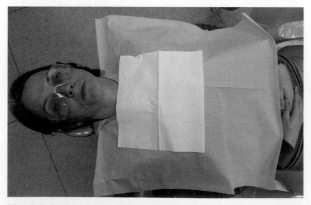

Fig. 5.5 Patient in a reclined position wearing eye protection and a disposable bib and neck towel.

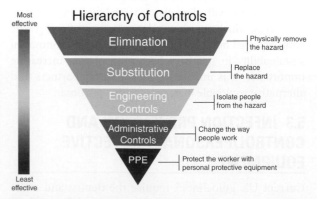

Fig. 5.6 Diagram of the hierarchy of controls used to optimise infection prevention and control measures.

recommended. Dental handpieces require lubrication before and after sterilisation, using manual aerosols or by an air-driven cleaning/lubricating unit.

Once this decontamination cycle is completed, non-vacuum (downward/gravity displacement bench-top steam) or vacuum bench-top steam sterilisation (recommended for wrapped/unwrapped, hollow lumen items) is required before individual instruments are dried (thus preventing long-term corrosion of carbon steel instruments) and finally bagged in sterile packets and stored in the clean zone. Conventional default settings for most steam sterilisers are 134°C to 137°C held for 3 minutes at a pressure of 2.5 bar. In hospitals, central sterilising facilities take on this role and soiled instruments are carefully packaged before transportation to the sterilisation facility.

5.4 PATIENT SAFETY AND RISK MANAGEMENT

During operative dental procedures patient safety is of paramount importance. Accidents may happen, but the risk of these occurring must be minimised or even eradicated at all costs. This is known as *risk management*. In terms of sustaining injury or harm during a dental procedure, the vulnerable areas of the patient include their eyes, airway and exposed soft tissues. The damage can be caused by inappropriate use or maintenance of sharp instruments, burs and small instruments and improper use or handling of dental materials. Table 5.2 outlines the sites, aetiology and types of injury that might be sustained and methods to prevent them from occurring. It is vital that the operator and nurse work as a team, being vigilant at all times to recognise at-risk situations and mitigate them.

5.4.1 Management of Minor Injuries

In all cases of injury, the patient must be informed immediately and the events documented comprehensively in the patient's notes and/or other incident report forms as appropriate.

- *Eyes*: If debris enters the eyes (the patient's or a member of the oral healthcare team), immediate washing in an eye bath with sterile water is essential with follow-up medical care if required.

TABLE 5.2	Potential Patient Injuries Along with Methods to Prevent Them		
Patient	**Aetiology of Injury**	**Type of Injury**	**Prevention**
Eyes	Sharp instruments slipping/burs fracturing, fragments of restoration, aerosolised dental materials/body fluids	Laceration, burn, infection	Protective glasses (with side covers) worn when patient supine
Airway	Small instruments (fractured burs, root canal files), indirect restorations (crowns, inlays), implant components, extracted teeth/fragments	Inhalation or swallowed; lung infection, blockage of upper respiratory tract airway	Rubber dam; safety chains/floss tied to small instruments; gauze squares placed intra-orally to cover back of throat
Soft tissues (lips, mucosae, tongue)	Caustic dental materials (acid etchant, hypochlorite), sharp instruments (including needles), rotary burs, heat, aggressive retraction of soft tissues, compressed air introduced into open wounds; anaesthetised tissues	Burns, lacerations, grazes, surgical emphysema	Rubber dam placed correctly with sufficient seal; proper use/maintenance of handpieces/burs; single-use needles—*do not bend*; avoid directing air jets into broken mucosae, exposed root canals

- *Airway*: If an inhalational blockage occurs, stand the patient bent at the hips and firmly slap the patient's back to help dislodge the object from the oropharynx. Check that the object has not been sucked up the high-volume aspirator (if in use). If the object cannot be accounted for and the patient is not sure whether they have swallowed it, a chest radiograph will be required to help localise the foreign object in the bronchi, lungs, oesophagus or stomach (Fig. 5.7). Follow-up medical attention will be required, especially for the former, as a bronchoscopy may be indicated.
- *Soft tissues*: Haemostasis of cuts and abrasions must be achieved. Cuts to the lips or mucosae may need

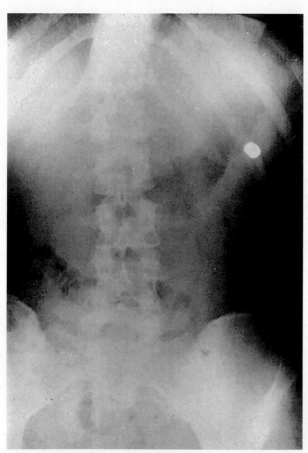

Fig. 5.7 Radiograph showing a gold crown in a patient's stomach. (Courtesy the late Prof A H R Rowe.)

Q5.7: Can you spot the gold crown?

sutures. Caustic sodium hypochlorite burns (caused by a leaking rubber dam during root canal treatment (RCT)) may require medical attention and a suitable dressing to promote healing without scarring. Patients with inferior alveolar nerve anaesthesia should be warned of the persistent numbness for several hours after treatment and to take care in avoiding biting or chewing their lower lip or having hot food or drink in case of burning themselves.

5.5 DENTAL AESTHETICS

The advent in the early 1960s and subsequent continued development of direct and indirect adhesive, tooth-coloured restorative materials have raised patients' expectations with regard to high-quality aesthetic results when it comes to restoring teeth to form and function, especially in the anterior 'aesthetic zone' (classically, UR4–UL4). Indeed, minimally invasive conservative dentistry is at a stage of acceptance now where all operative interventions should be considered *aesthetic*, not *cosmetic*, in nature. An overall aesthetically pleasing dental result depends on the appreciation of numerous complex and interlinked factors including:

Facial/skeletal characteristics:
- Skeletal base relationships between the mandible and maxilla that might affect relative tooth positions
- The overall facial outline shape: round, ovoid, square
- Facial symmetry and proportions, both horizontal and vertical

Oral Soft Tissues:
- Lip line: resting, partial and full smile posture
- Lip morphology: full, thin, vermilion border position
- Lip support
- Soft tissue symmetry

Dental:
- The three-dimensional shape and position of the tooth or teeth
- The surface form and finish of the tooth or teeth (affecting reflectance)
- The morphology of the surrounding periodontal tissues
- The occlusal plane and relationship with adjacent or opposing teeth (symmetry)

- The form of the tooth or teeth, the dental arch in relation to the facial profile and shape
- The inherent shade of the tooth or teeth.

As can be gleaned from the preceding list, numerous complex inter-related factors affect overall dental aesthetics. Many of these factors are not changeable by the practitioner in normal circumstances. If these are not taken into account when care planning, however, it is likely that the final aesthetic outcome will not meet the expectations of the patient or the clinician. It beyond the scope of this textbook to delve into these factors in more detail, so the reader is directed to other expert sources of information, including the series *Essentials of Esthetic Dentistry – Principles and Practice of Esthetic Dentistry* (ed. Wilson NHF, Elsevier, 2014). The actual inherent shade of the tooth (just one of the factors in achieving a satisfactory overall aesthetic outcome) depends upon its histological changes due to aging, toothwear and/or pathology. Extrinsic and intrinsic staining will also play a part in the changes in tooth shade or colour. The dental materials that can offer shades and characteristics that closely match natural tooth aesthetics, shown here in descending order, are:

- Dental porcelains (indirect—made by a dental technician in a laboratory from casts poured from dental impressions and finally cemented in or on the tooth or using CAD/CAM technology)
- Dental resin composites (direct—placed at chairside; and indirect—made in the laboratory)
- Glass-ionomer cements (direct—including conventional, hybrid, resin-modified and polyacid-modified composites)

5.5.1 Colour Perception

The human brain is able to perceive intrinsic physical properties of incident light sensed by the eye. To communicate these, colour scales have been devised. One of the earliest was the system from A H Munsell, which comprised three elements: the dominant wavelength (*hue*), the excitation purity (*chroma*) and its luminous reflectance (*value*) (Table 5.3).

However, the human tooth is structurally heterogeneous and the pulp, dentine, enamel, their interfaces and relative thicknesses along with their changing histological structure all play a part in overall perception of the shade by affecting the interaction between incident light and tooth structure. When attempting to mimic the shade of a tooth, the inherent structure of the restorative material and how it affects the physical characteristics of incident light must also be considered; that is, its reflectance, translucency, opacity and fluorescence. As the Munsell classification does not take these factors into account, another classification was devised by the Commission Internationale de l'Eclairage (CIE): the CIE L* a* b* colour space. This classification applies the amount of red, green and blue colours used; L* measures lightness (0–100, black-white) and CIE a* and b*, the relative hue and chroma (a*, levels of red(+)-green(–); b*, levels of yellow(+)-blue(–)). This system permits quantification and calculation of colour numerically, expressed in units that can be related to visual perception and clinical significance. This scale is used in research studies into colour as well as the electronic shade guides (see later). The properties of the restorative material that can help mimic these interactions include:

- *Refractive index*: Refraction is the change in direction of light when it enters a medium, substrate/tissue of

Property of Light	Comments
Hue (wavelength)	Wavelength of coloured light translated as its actual colour; e.g., red, green, blue, etc. Fig. 5.8 shows the VITA classical shade guide tabs arranged in the four-lettered groups according to hue: A, reddish-brown; B, yellow; C, yellow-grey; and D, reddish-grey.
Chroma (saturation)	Strength/dominance of the colour (hue). Light or dark shade. Fig. 5.8 shows the VITA classical shade tabs arranged with increasing chroma (1–4) in each of the hue (colour) groups (A–D).
Value (greyness)	Luminosity of the colour (the level of black or white; its *greyness*). Figs. 5.9 and 5.10 show the shade tabs arranged in descending order of value. Enamel thickness is the major contributor to the value of a tooth.

TABLE 5.3 Intrinsic Physical Properties of Light Perceivable by The Human Eye According to Munsell Colour Space Classification

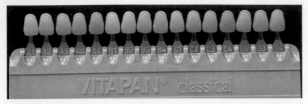

Fig. 5.8 The Vitapan Classical shade guide tabs arranged in four groups (A–D) according to hue (colour), and within each hue a range of increasing chroma (1–4).

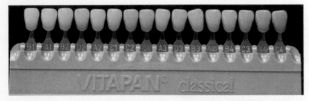

Fig. 5.9 The Vitapan Classical shade guide tabs arranged in order of value (high (whiter) to low (darker)).

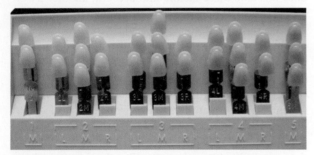

Fig. 5.10 The Vitapan 3D-Master shade guide with value graded from 1 to 5 (light to dark), three chroma choices (2–4) and the individual hue (yellow red).

a different density. Different materials have different refractive indices. The difference between the refractive indices of two materials determines how opaque or translucent one appears when observed from the other. The opacity of a resin composite depends on the difference between the refractive index of the resin composite material and the refractive index of air (refractive index of vacuum/air: 1.0; water, 1.33; enamel, 1.63; dentine, 1.54; cementum, 1.58).

- *Scattering coefficient*: Scattering is the loss of light due to the reversal of its direction. The scattering coefficient varies with the wavelength of the light and the nature of the colourant layer of a resin composite. A resin composite with a greater scattering coefficient (dependent upon the type of polymer matrix, size, type and amount of filler particles; presence of aluminium, zirconium and titanium oxide opacifiers; see Chapter 7, Section 7.2.2.2) will appear more opaque.

- *Absorption coefficient*: Absorption is the taking up of light by a material. The absorption coefficient also depends on the wavelength of light and the nature of the colourant layer of the resin composite. The greater the absorption coefficient, the more opaque and intensely coloured the resin composite will appear.

When restoring a tooth with a direct resin composite primarily for aesthetic considerations, it is advisable to use incremental layering techniques to copy the following structural variations that occur within the tooth.

- In a young tooth, the thicker enamel will affect the value and hue, with the dentine contributing towards the chromatic aspect of its shade.
- As a tooth ages and the enamel thins, the dentine and pulp have more of an influence on the hue, with enamel contributing primarily to the value of the final shade.
- The enamel–dentine junction (EDJ) contributes to the fluorescent characteristics (which can be added in a layering technique using coloured tints and stains).
- The quality of the surface finish and form of the final restoration will affect the reflectivity of incident light; using a flowable, translucent low filler particle content resin composite will assist in producing a smooth, blemish-free surface after careful polishing (see later).

Some manufacturers provide their own shade guide with their layering resin composite system to simplify the choice of dentine and enamel shades, often calibrated to the Vitapan Classical system.

5.5.2 Clinical Tips for Shade Selection

- Avoid brightly coloured neck towels. It is helpful to use a light blue neck cloth. Select the shade before placing the rubber dam as teeth become lighter as they dry out.
- Ask patients to remove bright lipstick or other obstacles, such as hoods or hats, which may affect incident light and shadows.

- Schedule aesthetic restoration appointments early in the morning if at all possible to avoid eye fatigue.
- The light source should be diffuse, not direct. Use natural daylight where possible. Try to avoid conventional fluorescent light sources.
- Fan the shade guide past the patient's mouth and pick the closest tab. Do not stare. Rest your eyes occasionally. After selecting the hue, squinting or half-closing your eyes will aid the determination of the value.
- Cold-sterilise shade guides to prevent damaging them.
- Shade-taking should be carried out after prophylaxis but before tooth isolation and preparation, since dehydration can lighten the natural tooth shade as light is reflected from pore spaces within the enamel as it dries out.
- Select the body shade by examining the centre portion of the tooth (Fig. 5.11). Check with the mouth open and closed (lips parted) for anterior dentition.

- Choose the resin composite shade most closely approximating the centre portion of the shade guide (Fig. 5.11A–D). Custom-made resin composite shade tabs can be constructed from the specific brand of material used by the dentist. Using glass slabs, various thicknesses of each shade of resin composite can be photo-cured and labelled and used subsequently for clinical shade selection.
- Place directly and cure the chosen shade of resin composite on the tooth surface to be restored, using the correct thickness of material (Fig. 5.11). No etch or bond is required. The patient can use a face mirror to help check and agree to the shade of material selected.

As well as the visual shade guides depicted in Figs. 5.8–5.10, there are electronic shade detectors which shine an incident beam of light onto the relevant tooth and then numerically analyse the reflected light. Care has to be taken when assessing particularly translucent

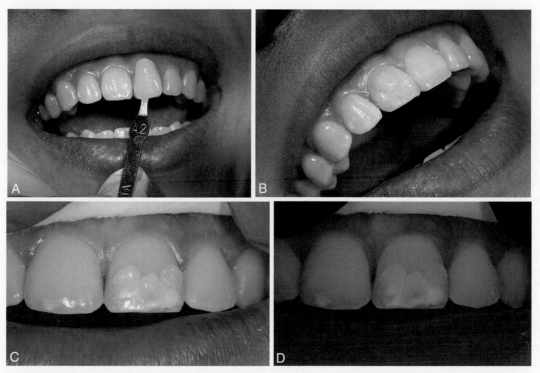

Fig. 5.11 (A) Shade assessment of the UR1 using a shade tab. The shade is assessed from the body of the tab and tooth and then (B) the resin composite is placed on the unetched labial surface of the tooth to make the final assessment, ensuring the tooth is not dehydrated beforehand. (C) Hypoplastic UL1 with different uncured resin composites placed on the hydrated labial tooth surface to assess the colour match directly. (D) UL1 imaged using a polarising filter to remove surface light reflections to aid shade matching with the resin composite. (Courtesy M Thomas.)

incisal edges as these instruments can misreport the translucency as a greyer overall shade since a significant proportion of the light passes through the tooth rather than being reflected back.

5.5.3 MI Management of Tooth Discolouration

The aetiology of tooth discolouration is described in Chapter 1, Section 1.5. A summary of the colour changes affecting teeth is also shown in Table 5.4.

Management principles of tooth discolouration must follow the MIOC delivery framework, following the relevant clinical domains of clinical information gathering (patient history, clinical examination, investigations, risk/susceptibility assessment, diagnosis, prognosis and managing patient expectations), prevention and control (modifying/removing aetiological factors often by the oral healthcare team helping the patient to understand and modify their behaviours appropriately), suitable operative interventions from least to most destructive (micro-invasive → minimally invasive → fully invasive/most destructive) all followed by suitable recall consultation periodicity, to assess patient behaviour response and the outcomes of any treatment provided.

Extrinsic discolouration occurs where higher molecular weight, pigmented molecules are adherent to the tooth surface or just within the enamel surface itself, superficially. This can be managed in vital teeth using:

- Abrasive dentifrices in the first instance, at home by the patient. Some brands will also claim to contain

---

TABLE 5.4	**Variation of Clinical Tooth Discolouration with Some Assigned Causes**
Colour	**Cause**
Extrinsic Colourants	
Brown or black	Tea, coffee, iron
Yellow or brown	Poor oral hygiene, tea
Yellow, brown or black	Tobacco, marijuana
Green, orange, black or brown	Bacteria
Red, purple or brown	Red wine
Intrinsic Colourants	
Grey, brown or black	Pulp death with haemorrhage
Yellow, grey or brown	Pulp necrosis without haemorrhage
Brown, grey or black	Endodontic materials within the tooth
Yellow or brown	Pulpal obliteration/sclerosis
Brown, white lines or spots	Fluorosis: excessive fluoride swallowed during tooth development
Black	Sulphur
Brown or grey	Minocycline taken after tooth formation (adult teeth)
Yellow, brown, grey or blue	Tetracycline taken during tooth development; doxycycline after tooth formation (yellow and brown will bleach out; blue and grey may bleach out)
Pink	Internal resorption
Grey, brown or black	Dental caries
Yellow or brown	Aging
Yellow or brown	Amelogenesis imperfecta
Brown, violet, or yellow brown	Dentinogenesis imperfecta
Brown	Inborn errors of metabolism; e.g., phenylketonuria
Black	Porphyria

From Chapter 3 – Dental bleaching methods. *Minimally Invasive Esthetics,* ed. Banerjee A, Elsevier, 2015.

some form of bleaching chemistry to assist in stain removal. However, as the legal concentration of a common bleaching agent, hydrogen peroxide (H_2O_2), permitted in over-the-counter products on sale to the public in the UK according to the EU Council Directive 2011/84/EU from 31 October 2012 is <0.1%, this will have no effect on removing the discolouration as it is rapidly neutralised on contact with natural salivary peroxidases and catalases. Also, the long-term uncontrolled use of more aggressively abrasive dentifrices in combination with a hard bristle texture toothbrush by patients will often lead to dental abrasion and subsequent loss of enamel, its surface architecture and ultimately aesthetics. Peroxide-containing mouthrinses are freely available to patients but again the concentrations are too low to have any stain-removal effect.

- Micro-abrasion techniques carried out by the clinician, in-surgery. This is a more controlled micro-invasive technique carried out by clinician periodically for superficial extrinsic stains. Using a rubber cup in a slow-speed electric motor handpiece, an acidic abrasive paste (e.g., 37% orthophosphoric acid etch and pumice) can be applied to the affected surfaces and the staining removed locally with insignificant tooth surface wear or damage. This technique may be used in combination with dental bleaching to gain the optimal longer-term beneficial effect. It will only work on superficial extrinsic discolouration.

- Dental bleaching/whitening protocols. To be effective, active hydrogen peroxide concentrations of 0.1% to 6% can only be supplied and administered by registered dental practitioners, for use in nightguard vital bleaching. The delivery agent used in custom-made single or multiple tooth bleaching trays is a maximum 16% carbamide peroxide gel which slowly releases 6% H_2O_2 over a 3- to 5-hour period. A commonly used 'gold standard' concentration, 10% carbamide peroxide, releases 3.5% H_2O_2. This concentration is biologically safe to patients and has no detrimental effects to the soft tissues, enamel histology or pulp or adverse effects to biomaterial adhesion. Temporary post-operative sensitivity may be experienced by some patients. This is usually mild and transient and eases within 24 hours of the bleaching procedure. The patient is taught how to load the tray and use the gel carefully and is

responsible for the ultimate shade change achieved, appreciating that there is likely to be some shade relapse 1 to 2 weeks after the bleaching process is stopped.

Intrinsic discolouration occurs where the pigmented molecules have penetrated deeper into the enamel or within the dentine structure. Indeed, they may reside within the pulp chamber depending on the cause (see Table 5.4). This deeper staining embedded within the structure of the vital tooth can be managed using:

- The nightguard vital bleaching technique described earlier, but for a significantly longer period (months as opposed to weeks). Patients' expectations must be managed in such cases, being informed that the shade change may be more difficult to achieve.
- Chairside, 'in-office' or 'power' bleaching using much higher concentrations of H_2O_2, 15% to 38%. This technique significantly increases the risk of soft tissue damage for both the patient and operator. It requires the judicious use of a rubber dam or other forms of soft tissue isolation and protection for the patient and careful handling by the clinical team. The adjunctive use of light and heat has not been shown in any independent randomised controlled trials to offer any improvement in the longevity or effectiveness of the bleaching outcome. The responsibility for the shade change achieved lies solely with the practitioner and multiple visits will often be required at often significant cost to the patient. From a dento-legal and marketing standpoint, care must be taken not to deceive patients as to the benefits of such practice with mis-appropriated 'before and after' images of cases.

For non-vital, endodontically treated teeth with intrinsic discolouration, different treatment options are available. Table 5.5 summarises the treatment options in order from least to most invasive. In all cases, the MIOC framework must be followed to ensure that the correct treatment option is chosen for the individual patient and that contemporaneous records are kept of all conversations and decisions made. It is vital to work with the patient to manage their expectations. The detailed clinical management protocols listed are described in Chapters 2 and 3 of *Essentials of Esthetic Dentistry– Miminally Invasive Esthetics*. Banerjee A, Millar BJ. eds. Elsevier, 2015.

TABLE 5.5   **Management Options for Treating Discoloured Non-vital, Endodontically Treated Teeth**

Monitor and review	least invasive
Inside/outside bleaching technique with 10% carbamide peroxide	
Internal (walking) bleach technique (concentrated bleaching agent is sealed into the access cavity of a well-sealed, endodontically treated tooth; see Fig. 5.12) 10% carbamide peroxide releases 3.5% hydrogen peroxide Sodium perborate and water releases 7% hydrogen peroxide Sodium perborate and 12% hydrogen peroxide mixed together as a paste releases approximately 25% hydrogen peroxide	
External bleaching	
Chairside bleaching or home/nightguard bleaching or a combination of both Chairside bleaching using heat and a high concentration (30%–38%) of hydrogen peroxide *(highest risk of tooth resorption)*	
Restorative techniques	
Veneers: direct resin composites Veneers: indirect resin composites Veneers: indirect porcelain Crown (partial or full coverage), with or without a post Extraction and prosthetic replacement	Most invasive

Adapted from Chapter 3, *Minimally Invasive Esthetics,* ed. Banerjee A, Elsevier 2015.

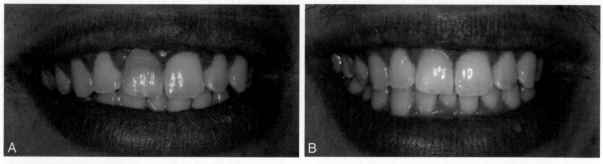

Fig. 5.12 (A) Non-vital, endodontically treated UR1 with intrinsic grey discolouration. (B) Post-operative internal (walking) bleaching has removed the discolouration with a satisfactory aesthetic outcome. (Courtesy D Raju.)

5.6 MAGNIFICATION

Visual magnification to aid careful clinical examination and treatment should be considered an essential requirement in contemporary clinical dental. This can be achieved using *magnifiers*, *dental loupes* and *operating microscopes*. A selection can be seen in Fig. 5.13. In terms of optical physics, there are two fundamental aspects to consider with regard to their clinical application: the *depth of field* (or *focus*) and the *field of view* (or *field width*).

- *Depth of field/focus (DoF)*: Equates to the distance the operator can move towards or away from the object tooth while keeping the view in clear focus. If this range is limited, procedures become tiring as the operator and patient must always remain at a fixed distance from each other with minimal leeway of movement of either person before the view becomes blurred. For a given magnification, the DoF depends on the f-number of the lens (aperture diameter); ↑ f-number (↓ aperture) leads to an ↑ DoF. The higher

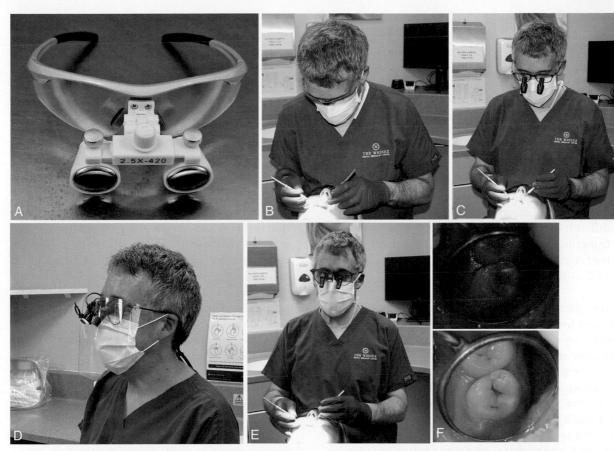

Fig. 5.13 (A) Magnification loupes with a manually adjustable lens block (adjustable interpupillary distance and focal angle) which can be hinged out of the way when not needed. Due to their weight, they require a head cord for retention. (B) Operator's poor posture when not using magnification loupes of any kind. Note the operator's back and neck are bent, shoulders hunched and elbows not at 90 degrees to be able to view the patient's oral cavity. (C) The clinician's fixed interpupillary distance is built in as the lenses are cemented through the prescription/safety spectacle lenses. The magnification optics are closer to the eye, resulting in a greater field width and depth of field, but usually at an increased expense. Note the improvement in musculoskeletal operator posture with a straight back, relaxed shoulders and elbows at 90 degrees. There is still some neck tilt required to view the patient. (D) and (E) These refractive lenses result in minimal neck strain on the operator as they look ahead whilst their field of view is of the reclined patient's teeth. The lenses can weigh as little as 50 g. (F) The clinical mirror view of an inadequately lit maxillary premolar examined without any magnification *(top)*. The same tooth now lit effectively using an LED head-mounted light *(bottom)*. More detail can be observed regarding the state of the mesio-distal fissure. (Courtesy Mackenzie L, Banerjee A. The minimally invasive management of early occlusal caries: a practical guide. *Primary Dent J.* 2014 May;3(2):42–49. doi:10.1308/205016814812143987.)

Q5.13D: Can you spot an important clinical addition to the loupes in Fig. 5.13D?

the magnification of the lens, the less the DoF; an example with the latest refractive lens technology: x3.8 – 80 mm, x5.7 – 55 mm and x7.2 – 40 mm.

- *Field of view (FoV)*: The angular extent of the observable image viewed through fixed-magnification loupes. Normal unaided human binocular vision (with depth perception) permits 140-degree FoV. With increasing magnification, this is greatly reduced; for example, x3 magnification with loupes may only permit a clear, sharp view of the object tooth and one either side (depending on the precise optics of the loupes). This can make introducing dental instruments into the operating field difficult and will require the dentist to look away from the loupe's view to do this. An example of current refractive lenses: x3.8 – 85 mm, x5.7 – 50 mm, x7.2 – 40 mm.

For general restorative dentistry, x2–3.8 magnification is usually satisfactory, but for endodontics and surgery, x4–6 magnification can be used to help detect root canal orifices and fine root canals. Good visual discrimination in dental procedures requires good depth perception, which in turn requires binocular function. To get the most out of the increased magnification, good-quality illumination is also vital. Modern magnification systems come with fitted LED lights that are integrated on the frame above the lenses and can be focused on the same focal plane as the lenses, providing shadow-free, focused, line-of-sight illumination of the operating site, thus improving visual acuity (Fig. 5.13F). These are also more energy efficient and reduce the reliance on the chair overhead light. Orange light filters should be used to prevent premature photo-curing of resin-based materials.

The benefits of clinical magnification plus focused illumination include:

- Improved visual acuity: It is important in modern minimally invasive operative dentistry to be able to see high-resolution detail of the dental and soft tissues. Whether it may be cracks within the tooth structure, carious/demineralised tissues or finding root canal orifices with the pulp chamber, magnification accompanied by suitable illumination will improve visualisation of detail.
- Improved posture/reduced back pain: Without loupes, operators persistently bend or distort their

spine by up to 30 degrees from the natural vertical position leading to long-term postural-related back and neck pain. By using magnification loupes and operating microscopes plus illumination, the clinician is encouraged to sit in an appropriate comfortable position with a straight back and neck, with reduced tension in the shoulders, to optimise the preset depth of focus. Maintaining this ergonomic posture reduces musculoskeletal pain suffered by many clinicians. Refractive lenses can help further by maintaining a completely natural neck posture whilst working (Fig. 5.13E).

- Reduced eye strain: Eye strain is a common condition that arises when your eyes get tired from intense and prolonged use. The symptoms can be unpleasant, resulting in fatigue, sore eyes and headaches at the end of the day. Working in the dental discipline, you are required to concentrate for long periods of time, often causing you to exert effort when focusing on the small details you see on the teeth. Made-to-measure dental loupes reduce eyestrain, magnifying all aspects of the mouth, ensuring eye muscles have no need to strain.
- Improved detection and diagnosis: To provide your patient with the most accurate detection and diagnosis, it is vital that you can view your working field with clear, crisp vision. As dental loupes magnify the visual field to varying degrees (x2–x7.5), operators can easily see details which are not visible to the naked eye, resulting in improved detection, diagnosis and clinical outcomes.

Even though there is an additional expense to purchasing and maintaining dental loupes (including the need for extra batteries for the LED light and the need to charge these) and for those who do not wear spectacles, an increased weight on the bridge of the nose which may be unpleasant for some, it is the author's opinion that using magnification to aid the execution of an effective clinical examination and most intra-oral dental procedures is an essential pre-requisite to practising high-quality minimally invasive operative dentistry. It is important that the skill of using dental loupes is learnt early in the clinical skills laboratory and then transferred to the clinical situation. The physical adjustments made by the operator when using loupes involves practice with a learning curve. The correct use of dental loupes and magnification will also improve the operator's physical posture whilst working, which in turn will reduce the risk of long-term back pain and other posture-related ailments.

5.6.1 Clinical Photography

The use of clinical extra- and intra-oral photography within clinical dentistry provides the opportunity to enhance patient care by allowing oral healthcare professionals to record their clinical findings and reflect on their treatment outcomes (Fig. 5.14A–C). Photographs can be regarded as an essential part of recordkeeping,

particularly in situations where changes in appearance are being considered. The advent of easy-to-use and relatively low-cost equipment enables high-quality images to be obtained in a predictable and reproducible manner. The use of photography therefore has now become a part of everyday dentistry.

The benefits of clinical photography are many, but may be summarised in the following categories:

- *Personalised care planning.* Recording high-quality intra-oral images allows the clinician to plan treatment

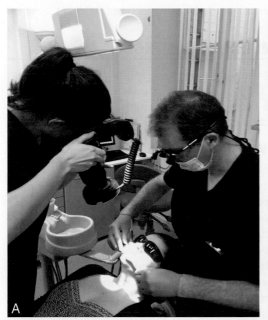
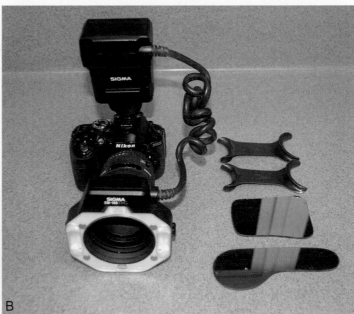
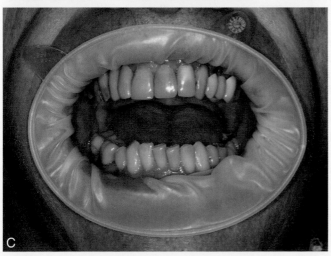

Fig. 5.14 (A) The dental nurse has been trained to take clinical photographs during the initial examination to aid detection, diagnosis, documentation, communication and shared decision-making with the patient and other clinicians where necessary. (Courtesy M Sykes.) (B) A clinical camera kit set up with a suitable ring flash coupled to a macro lens, cheek retractors (held in position by the nurse or patient) and mouth mirrors (occlusal and buccal/lingual). It is important that the mouth mirrors are maintained and stored carefully so as not to scratch them. They should be immersed in hot water a few minutes before use to minimise them steaming up when in use intra-orally. The nurse can also blow a stream of air from the 3-1 air/water syringe over the mirror surface to prevent them from steaming up during use whilst keeping the surface clean and dry. (C) Soft tissue retraction of the lips using the OptraGate (Ivoclar–Vivadent) system. This latex-free option holds itself in position and can be used to protect the lips and extra-oral soft tissues during external dental bleaching techniques as well as for intra-oral photography.

in the absence of the patient and to communicate treatment requirements clearly. Images can also be magnified to assist in detection, diagnosis and monitoring of oral and dental health status.

- *Re-assessment*. A periodic record of restorations/ operative treatment outcomes can provide a useful record of changes that occur over time (see Chapter 9, Section 9.4). This is useful as part of judicious clinical record-keeping and shared decision-making when it comes to deciding whether further interventions are required.
- *Communication*. Images can enhance the communication between the oral healthcare professional and the patient to demonstrate clinical findings and aid discussions regarding prognosis of care plans and the patient's responsibility in their own oral and dental health. Also, with the development of teledentistry, clinical photographs can be used in remote consultations and gaining second opinions from learned colleagues. Images can also be used for peer review and form an important aspect of the reflective practice approach to be carried out by all oral healthcare professionals on a regular basis.
- *Consent*. Images form an integral part of clinical record-keeping and can be included in patient personalised care plans to demonstrate areas where intervention is recommended. They are also useful to act as a reminder as to the initial findings as well as to help manage patient expectations for treatment outcomes or in legal disputes.
- *Education*. Images can be used for education on an individual patient level, in peer review groups for clinicians or, with appropriate consent, to a wider audience.
- *Promotion*. Appropriate, undoctored before and after images of cases where treatment has been carried out within the dental clinic can be used as part of a business marketing plan to promote the skills available within the clinic.

Good equipment and lighting are essential to provide quality images consistently and predictably. In addition to the use of digital SLR cameras, modern mobile phone devices can also produce images of high quality. Care must be taken over the confidentiality of images which are regarded as part of the clinical records and therefore must be consented for appropriately, stored in an encrypted format and used appropriately, keeping in mind the strict adherence to general data protection regulations (GDPR), both in the country where the images originate and globally, thanks to the easy dissemination of images by digital social media. Many commercial intra-oral cameras are also readily available to record static and video images within the oral cavity. The concept of using photography in dentistry has also been enhanced in the use of intra-oral scanners to provide three-dimensional imaging of the structures of the oral cavity. In addition, photography is one aspect of dentistry that can be learned and used by all members of the oral healthcare team and hence can serve to enhance job roles and workplace satisfaction (Fig. 5.14).

5.7 MOISTURE CONTROL

This is the ability to regulate the fluid environment within the oral cavity and around the individual tooth or teeth being operated on. Fluids include water, saliva, gingival exudate, crevicular fluid and blood.

5.7.1 Why?

Moisture control is required:
- To create the optimal conditions required for the proper technical placement of all intra-oral dental restorations. The presence of excessive fluids has a detrimental effect on the adhesion and/or physical properties of all direct plastic restorations, but especially those relying on bonding including the adhesives used to cement indirect restorations.
- To prevent contamination of the restorative procedure, including carious tissue removal, direct pulp capping, RCT and restorative adhesive bonding protocols.
- To improve patient comfort and the visual clarity of the operating field by removing accumulated fluids produced by dental handpiece irrigants, 3-1 air/water syringes and pooled saliva.

5.7.2 Techniques

- *Aspiration*: Fluids can be evacuated using a single-use saliva ejector by the dental nurse, the dentist or even the patient holding the suction device themselves. Plastic tips can be bent into a curved shape to adapt to the contours of the lips and oral cavity, thus accessing the buccal or lingual sulci whilst helping to simultaneously retract these tissues to aid visualisation of the operating field for the clinician and their dental nurse. Wide

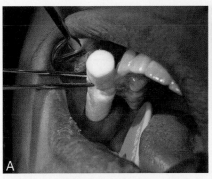
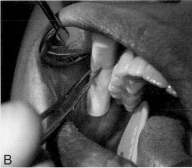
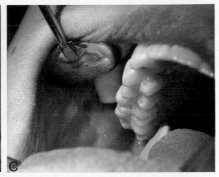

Fig. 5.15 Series of images showing how to successfully place a cotton wool roll into the maxillary right buccal sulcus. Note the way it is rotated into position to ensure it will stay in place. A blue, flanged disposable saliva ejector tip has been placed lingually to help retract the tongue.

and narrow bore suction tips can be used for more precise moisture control and to improve the line of sight for the clinician during clinical intra-oral examination.

- *Cotton wool rolls (cellulose pads)*: These are used to absorb fluids and retract lips or cheeks. They may be placed over salivary duct orifices, upper buccal sulci (parotid ducts) and lingual sulci (submandibular and sublingual ducts; Figs. 5.15 and 5.16). Cotton wool rolls should be rotated into the buccal, labial or lingual sulci to aid their retention. If still dry at the end of treatment, moisten them with a few drops of water

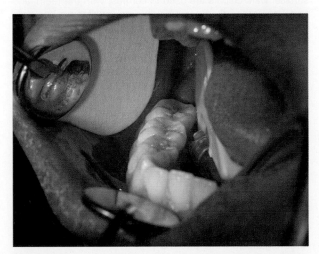

Fig. 5.16 A cellulose pad has been used to absorb moisture from the right parotid duct within the maxillary right buccal sulcus.

from the 3-1 syringe to facilitate their removal and prevent them sticking to the mucosae.

- *Rubber (dental) dam*: This is a thin, preferably latex-free, perforated sheet that isolates a single tooth or groups of teeth, thus allowing the best control of moisture. Its advantages and disadvantages are listed in Table 5.6 and the equipment required along with the techniques to place a rubber dam clinically are shown in Figs. 5.17–5.20.

5.7.3 Rubber (Dental) Dam Placement: Practical Steps

Fig. 5.19 shows how a rubber dam can be placed on a mandibular molar using either a wingless or a winged clamp. Some patients may need local anaesthesia or topical anaesthesia to dull the pain of the clamp on the tooth and periodontium. In some cases plastic soft clamps may be indicated in this regard (Fig. 5.19i). If a matrix band is required to help contour the final restoration proximally, the rubber dam clamp may need to be removed as it will get in the way of the circumferential or sectional matrix system (see later). In this situation, the matrix band will take over the role of the clamp in holding the dam in position while the material is packed into place. Otherwise, planning is required to ensure the clamp is placed on an adjacent tooth to allow space for matrix band placement around the tooth being operated on.

For anterior teeth, there is less need to use clamps as tight contact points are often sufficient to retain the well-adapted dam interdentally; otherwise, a thin strip of rubber dam cut from the peripheral excess or proprietary rubber wedges can be used by 'flossing' them

TABLE 5.6   Advantages and Disadvantages of Placing and Using a Rubber Dam for Intra-oral Moisture Control

Advantages	Disadvantages
Controlled isolation of the teeth from fluids (reducing adverse effects on bonding/physical properties of materials).	More difficult to communicate with the patient.
Reduced bacterial contamination (carious tissue removal, pulp capping, root canal treatment (RCT)).	Some patients dislike the feeling of claustrophobia (may be reduced by relieving the dam away from the nasal passages).
Patient airway protection from accidental inhalation or swallowing instruments (restorations, burs, endodontic files, wedges); orofacial soft tissue protection from chemical agents (acid-etch gel, diluted hypochlorite solution used in RCT).	Attaching the rubber dam to teeth with clamps can cause pain and sometimes post-operative pain for several hours. May rarely need the application of a topical anaesthetic gel on the adjacent gingivae.
Acts as barrier protection from fluid/air-borne pathogen transfer from patient to dentist.	Poorly fitted clamps can cause damage to indirect ceramic restorations (chipping).
Positive psychological experience/improved comfort for some patients. A feeling of detachment/separation from the procedure.	Care needed to check medical history for latex allergies for both patient and dentist. Latex-free dams should be used routinely.
Can aid in tissue retraction, thus improving direct vision; keeps oral mucosae and tongue separate from the operation field.	In inexperienced hands, rubber dam placement can be difficult and time-consuming. Once mastered, this problem is alleviated.
Once in place, the procedure can be completed more efficiently by the oral healthcare team.	

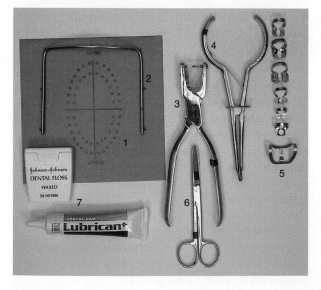

Fig. 5.17 Rubber (dental) dam equipment comprising:

1. A 15 cm square dark green latex-free nitrile sheet (with the position for the perforation holes stamped on using an ink stamp). The nitrile sheet resists tearing and grips the tooth surface. Dark colours are used to contrast with the teeth, and torn fragments, often occurring interproximally, can be easily detected and removed. The sheets can also vary in thickness.

2. Metal rubber dam frame. This holds the free edges away from the face and mouth. The dam is stretched around the tines on the frame itself, keeping it under tension. A trough can be created with the dam stretched around the frame, to help collect any excess water spray during operative procedures.

3. Rubber dam hole punch. This creates a clean-cut perforation of three diameters (corresponding to incisors, premolars and molars).

4. Rubber dam clamp forceps. This is used to place, adjust and remove clamps from teeth.

5. Rubber dam clamps. These metal clips pinch the coronal neck of the tooth holding the dam down against the gingivae. They can be winged or wingless (Fig. 5.19).

6. Scissors to cut excess dam away from the nose and when removing the dam interproximally.

7. Waxed dental floss and a water-based dam lubricant. Both aid the transition of the dam through tight contact points. Floss can act as a ligature, tying the dam down at the gingival margin.

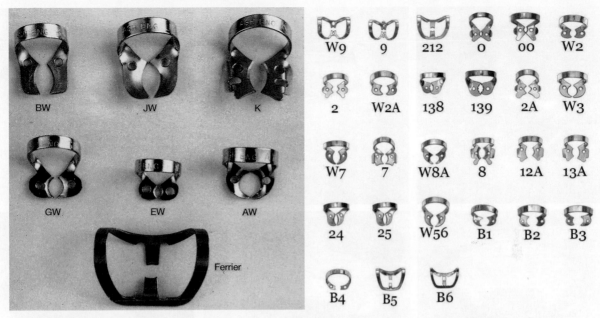

Fig. 5.18 A close-up view of a series of metal rubber dam clamps, with different identification codes, comprising two jaws joined by a curved connecting arm. The two holes accommodate the clamp forceps, which allow the opposing jaws to be separated when placing or removing them over the tooth crown bulbosity. Dentsply Ash codes: BW, JW, K, and AW clamps are molar patterned (AW is more retentive for partially erupted crowns), GW is used for canines and premolars and EW is configured for any other smaller tooth. The K clamp is winged; it has two extensions onto which the dam can be placed prior to inserting the dam and clamp together onto the tooth (useful when isolating just one tooth in the arch). The remaining wingless clamps must be first placed onto the teeth followed by the manual application of the precut dam holes over them. The Ferrier clamp is used for retracting gingivae when isolating anterior teeth, working in the cervical area (care is needed not to traumatise the gingivae and cause blood contamination of the field). A second classification of clamps with different sized jaws indicating their use for left- or right-side teeth.

through the contact points, after the dam is in position (Fig. 5.20). Floss ligatures may also be used for this purpose. If the contact points are too tight initially for even floss to pass through, then interdental pre-wedging with a wooden wedge for a couple of minutes before placing the dam will usually cause enough tooth movement within its periodontal ligament (and that of the adjacent tooth) to allow the dam to pass between. Careful use of the anterior Ferrier clamp is required so as not to traumatise the gingival margins.

Good adaptation of the latex-free/nitrile dam around the cervical aspect of the tooth or teeth to be isolated is critical for its successful placement and moisture control. A poorly adapted dam will allow seepage of water, blood, saliva and crevicular fluid into the operating area (often seen as bubbles appearing at the dam margin within the cavity) that will subsequently compromise any adhesive

restorative procedure or surgical dental procedure being carried out. Good marginal adaptation and seal of the dam around the tooth can be achieved by:

- Cutting clean, well-defined holes in the dam using a suitably sharp rubber dam hole punch. Holes with damaged or frayed margins are more likely to tear and not adapt snugly around the cervical aspect of the tooth and therefore allow seepage of moisture.
- Ensuring the dam margins are inverted against the tooth using a flat plastic instrument (Fig. 5.20D).
- Using a floss ligature around the tooth to hold and adapt the dam margin against the tooth.
- Using a liquid dam or caulking agent to seal the tooth–dam margin. This low-viscosity, resin-based material can be syringed around the interface and

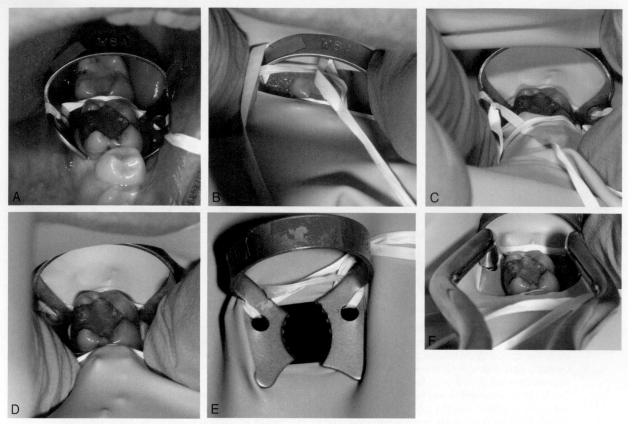

Fig. 5.19 (A) A wingless W8A (JW; Ash Dentsply) clamp placed on the LL6 to isolate the tooth. Clamp forceps were used to open the jaws of the clamp sufficiently to allow it to pass over the bulbosity of the crown. Note the floss tied through both clamp holes. This makes any clamp fragments retrievable if the connector arm fractures under tension when in use. The connector arm is placed distally to prevent the clamp from blocking operator access to the tooth to be treated. (B) The dam is stretched gently by the dentist to widen the lubricated perforation and the free end of the floss is passed through the hole. The dam is then eased over the clamp connector arm. (C) The dam is stretched over the connector arm first and then over the two jaws engaging the cervical bulbosity at the neck of the tooth, buccally and lingually. The nurse can help by keeping the floss taught throughout the procedure. (D) Dental floss is used to work the dam down through the mesial contact of the LL6. (E) A winged molar clamp (13A) with the wings engaged in the lubricated perforation in the dam, outside the mouth. Again, dental floss is tied through both jaw holes to be able to retrieve each part if the connector separates during use. (F) Clamp and rubber dam being secured to the LL6 as one, using the clamp forceps (note the two pairs of holes to engage the forceps in each jaw). The nurse can assist the process by gently retracting the loose rubber dam edges to aid operator vision. Again, the connector arm is placed distal to the tooth being operated upon so as not to block access to instrumentation or operator visibility.

adjacent soft tissues (e.g., gingivae) and then photo-cured to offer soft-tissue protection and a sealed tooth–dam interface. As the liquid dam is slightly flexible when cured, it can be easily and cleanly flicked away, often in one piece, with a suitable hand instrument, prior to finally removing the rubber dam and clamp(s). The liquid dam can also be useful to help support a sectional matrix band and block out impression undercuts (e.g., wide and deep interdental embrasure spaces especially between mobile teeth, or undercuts associated with implant components).

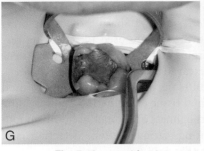
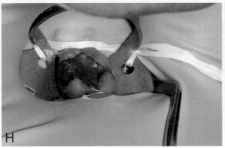
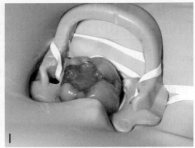

Fig. 5.19—cont'd. (G) and (H) Once firmly in place, the rubber dam forceps are removed and the dam is disengaged from the wings using a flat plastic instrument; the contact areas will be flossed to ensure interdental adaptation of the dam. Tissue paper can be placed between the rubber dam and the patient's face to prevent irritation and the rubber dam frame applied to hold the dam taught whilst in use. (I) A soft resin winged clamp is placed on the LL6 using the same placement protocol as shown in (A–H). This clamp causes less discomfort than a metal clamp on the gingivae, but will only engage effectively on teeth with a greater bulbosity at the cervical margin. They too come in a range of designs and sizes.

Q5.19A: What might this patient complain of once the clamp has been placed?
Q5.19E: Which teeth is this clamp designed ideally to be used on?

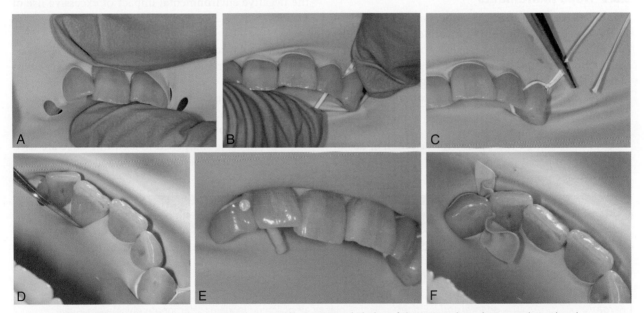

Fig. 5.20 (A) When isolating the maxillary anterior sextant, six holes of the appropriate size are selected and perforated into the dam using the hole punch. The dam around the holes is lubricated and gently stretched over each tooth using one's fingers. (B) Once all the teeth are engaged, dental floss can be used to work the rubber dam interproximally. (C) To hold the rubber dam in place, a dental floss ligature can be tied around the neck of a tooth and the excess removed. (D) A flat plastic instrument is used to invert the rubber dam around the necks of all the teeth both palatally and buccally. (E) Instead of securing the rubber dam with a floss ligature, rubber stabilising wedges can be inserted interproximally by stretching a length of widget, flossing it down through the contact point and then trimming away the excess. (F) In a similar way, if the rubber dam wedge is not available, a small piece of dam could be cut from the corner of the sheet and flossed through the contact point as shown. Sometimes the contact points may be tight enough to retain the dam cervically around the isolated teeth.

5.8 INSTRUMENTATION IN MINIMALLY INVASIVE OPERATIVE DENTISTRY

Instruments are used to examine, clean, cut and help restore teeth. The main types of cutting instruments are either handheld or rotary instruments driven by a handpiece. Other equipment includes fibre-optic lights for illumination, caries detection technologies, light-curing systems used for polymerisation of resin-based materials, new instruments for tooth preparation/carious tissue removal and ultrasonic scalers (Table 5.7). These instruments may be re-used after suitable decontamination and sterilisation procedures, or else are disposable, single-use items. As has been stated previously, plastic disposable items do put a stress on the environment with regards to their manufacture and waste disposal, so alternative biodegradable materials need to be developed and made cost-effective for mass production and use.

5.8.1 Hand Instruments

Manufactured from medical-grade stainless or carbon steel (sometimes with tungsten carbide brazed to the cutting edges for increased longevity of sharpness), the majority of hand instruments are designed with a handle, shank and blade configuration (Fig. 5.21).

Hand instruments can be used for the following purposes:

- Oral examination (mouth mirror, selection of dental probes/explorers, pair of tweezers):

- *Mouth mirrors*: Front or rear surfaced (Fig. 5.22).
- *Dental explorers/probes*: Sharp probes/explorers (straight and Briault) are used for checking restoration margins and the texture of carious dentine to be excavated within a cavity (see later). Rounded ball/blunt periodontal probes are used for periodontal tissue examination and assessing the surface roughness of enamel/occlusal/smooth surfaces during carious lesion detection and examination (Fig. 5.23).
- *Locking tweezers*: To place/remove cotton wool rolls, remove larger pieces of intra-oral debris.

With the implementation of modern infection prevention and control guidelines, disposable examination instruments are now manufactured from plastic to allow single-use only (Fig. 5.24). These need to be manufactured from biodegradable plastics or other ecofriendly natural materials (e.g., bamboo) to reduce the negative environmental impact of excessive use of plastics.

- Periodontal scaling: A selection of *handheld scalers* (Fig. 5.25) to remove supra- and subgingival calculus deposits.
- Carious tissue removal/cavity preparation (excavators, chisels/hatchets/hoes):
  - *Hand excavators*: Instruments with a discoid or ovoid blade sharpened to a cutting edge are used to remove soft carious dentine and soft temporary

TABLE 5.7	Tooth-Cutting/Carious Tissue Removal Technologies, the Substrates Acted on and Their Mechanism of Action	
Mechanism	**Substrate Affected**	**Tooth-cutting Technology**
Mechanical, rotary	*Sound or carious enamel and dentine*	Stainless steel, carbon steel, diamond, tungsten carbide, ceramic and plastic burs[a]
Mechanical, non-rotary	*Sound or carious enamel and dentine*	Hand instruments (excavators, chisels), air-abrasion (alumina/bio-active glass), air polishing (sodium bicarbonate/glycine/bio-active glass)[b], ultrasonics, sono-abrasion
Chemo-mechanical	*Carious dentine*	Caridex and Carisolv gel (amino acid–based; neither available commercially in the UK at the time of publication), Papacarie gel, Brix-3000 (papain-based), experimental pepsin-based solutions/gels
Photo-ablation	*Sound or carious enamel and dentine*	Lasers
Others	*Bacteria*	Photo-active disinfection, ozone

[a]Works only on carious dentine; [b]Primarily used for stain-removal.

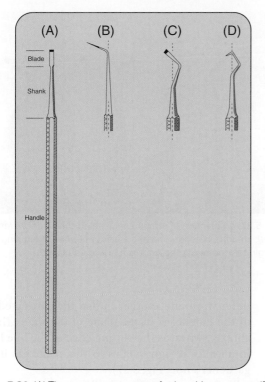

Fig. 5.21 (A) The component parts of a hand instrument. (B) A straight dental probe with a single bend taking the working tip well away from the handle's long axis, thus aiding direct vision. (C) Two bends in a hatchet. (D) Three bends in a Briault probe. Medical-grade stainless steel cutting edges can be resharpened using a sharpening stone with oil lubricant (fine edge) or a dry abrasive disc (coarse edge). Tungsten carbide tips should be sent to the manufacturer for resharpening.

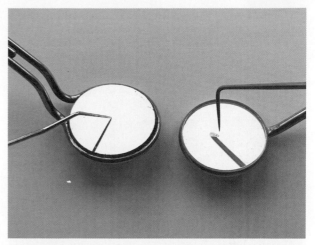

Fig. 5.22 Front- and rear-surface mouth mirrors. The left mirror (front-surface) gives a clearer image than the rear-surface 'double' image *(right)*, but is more prone to scratch damage during injudicious use and sterilisation procedures.

restorations. Can also be used to help shape the occlusal morphology of plastic direct restorative materials (Fig. 5.26).

- *Chisels, hatchets and hoes*: Used to remove unsupported enamel/bevel cavity margins (especially where access for rotary instruments is limited). Hatchets and hoes are similar to chisels in having a straight bevelled cutting edge and are always angled or contra-angled. They

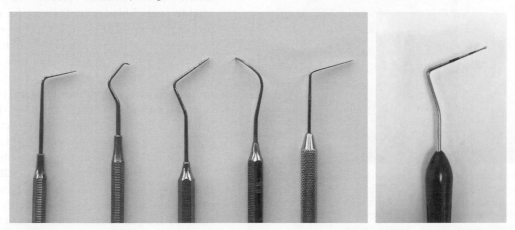

Fig. 5.23 A selection of dental probes *(from left to right)*: straight, Briault, Williams, Nabers, endodontic probe and CPITN.

Q5.23: In which clinical situations might you use each of these probes?

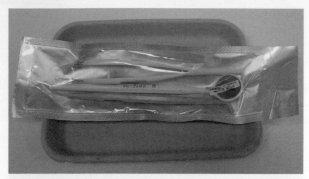

Fig. 5.24 Disposable, single-use plastic examination instruments—mirror, probe, and tweezers—in their sterile packaging.

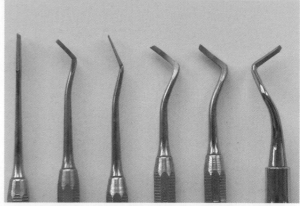

Fig. 5.27 A selection of straight and angled chisels *(from left to right)*: straight, hatchet, hoe and a pair of double-ended gingival margin trimmers. On the right is a tri-angled hatchet.

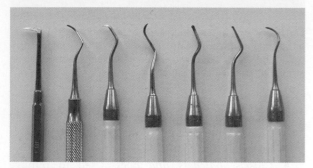

Fig. 5.25 A selection of handheld periodontal scalers (only blade and shank are visible). Note the angulation of the heads and the extent that the cutting blades are offset from the long axis of the handle.

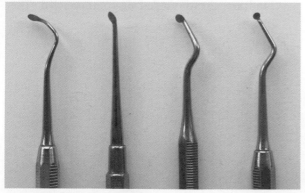

Fig. 5.26 A selection of hand excavators (only blade and shank are visible). Note the different ovoid blade sizes and offset angulations. These instruments will have blades at either end of the handle, oriented in different directions to aid their use when working on either mesial or distal cavities.

Q5.26: What are the advantages of having angulations between the working head and shank of these instruments?

differ from one another in that the cutting edge of the hatchet is in the plane of the *shank* (like an axe), whereas the cutting edge of the hoe lies in an axis at right angles to this plane (as in a gardener's hoe; Fig. 5.27).

- Handling restorative materials (flat plastics, condensers (pluggers), carvers, burnishers, brushes):
  - *Flat plastic instruments*: Used for conveying, placing and shaping plastic materials not requiring heavy pressure. Usually made of stainless steel but for resin composite placement, Teflon-coated, plastic or titanium nitride-coated blades confer a useful non-stick property (Fig. 5.28).
  - *Condensers (pluggers)*: Smooth surface instruments for packing plastic restorative materials into cavities under pressure (eliminating voids; more often used with dental amalgam) (Fig. 5.28).
  - *Carving instruments*: Sharp/semi-sharp blades for helping to carve the shape/contour/occlusal morphology of the final restoration using a cutting or scraping action. Different carver patterns exist (e.g., Ward's, Half-Hollenback) (Fig. 5.28).
  - *Burnishers*: Smooth ball/rounded hand instruments that are useful for finishing the occlusal surfaces of a plastic restoration to ensure the surface is well condensed, eliminate surface irregularities and voids, adapt the restorative material to cavity margins and help create a final sheen to an amalgam restoration (Fig. 5.28).

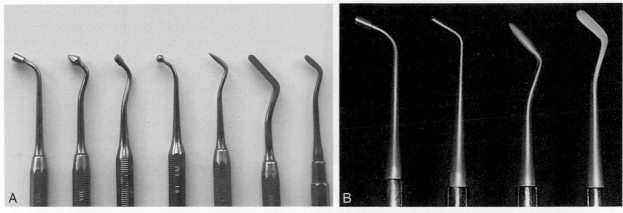

Fig. 5.28 Stainless steel and titanium nitride-coated (non-stick, gold-coloured) instruments for conveying, placing and shaping resin composite materials *(from left to right in both images)*: Guy's pattern condenser (plugger), burnisher (to adapt material to cavity margins), carving instrument (Half-Hollenback pattern), flat plastic (long and short blade).

- *Brushes*: Synthetic bristle brushes that are used for the application of opaques and tints used to characterise resin composite restorations, bonding and silanating agents and for excess cement removal prior to cementation of indirect restorations. They are useful for blending resin composite materials with cavity margins and other incremental layers of material to optimise the final aesthetic result (Fig. 5.29). Note that some brush heads can be cold-sterilised but the brush handles are fully sterilisable and reusable.

5.8.2 Rotary Instruments

Dental burs, stones and cutting and polishing discs and tips are small instruments (essentially, surgical 'drill bits') gripped firmly by a chuck in a handpiece ('dental drill') powered directly by compressed air, a high-speed *air turbine*, or a separate motor, usually electrically driven (the lower-speed *electric motor handpieces*).

- *Air turbine ('high-speed') handpieces*: Clockwise rotary speeds between 250,000 and 500,000 revolutions per minute (rpm) but with relatively low torque, achieved by a small air-driven turbine or rotor mounted in bearings in the head of a contra-angled handpiece. Burs are held via their friction-grip shank, the bur tip shrouded in water spray to act as a coolant and help remove debris and sometimes illuminated with a fibre-optic light (Figs. 5.30 and 5.31). This instrument

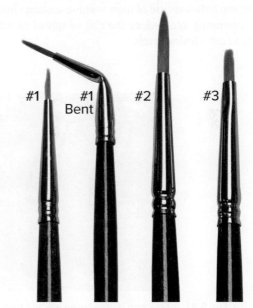

Fig. 5.29 Cosmedent synthetic bristle brushes showing a range of brush head sizes, angulations and filament lengths used to help adapt and shape uncured resin composite increments and surfaces within the cavity during placement, prior to light-curing.

generates an aerosol in use and was highlighted in the SARS-Covid-2 pandemic in 2020 as a possible vector for transmission of viral particles into the atmosphere within a dental surgery. This aerosol generation can be limited significantly by adjusting the water flow

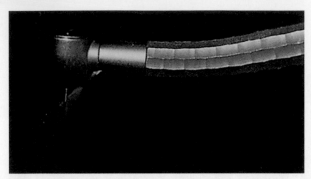

Fig. 5.30 Air turbine handpiece in operation showing the directed water spray over the tip of the bur, the aerosol produced and the fibre-optic light.

through the handpiece and by using rubber dam isolation to prevent the water aerosol mixing with potentially contaminated patient saliva. These actions, along with the judicious use of high-volume suction close to the operating site, reduce the risk of spread of infection to sub-clinical levels.

- *Low-speed electric motor handpieces*: Two-piece system comprising an electric (or sometimes an air-driven) motor coupled to a contra-angled or straight handpiece (rotating clockwise or anticlockwise), with water spray and fibre-optic light; lower speed (conventionally ranging between 5000 and 40,000 rpm) but with higher torque than the air turbine handpiece (Fig. 5.31). These lower rpm/higher torque handpieces can have adjustable speed and torque settings, due to the gearing within the handpiece itself, with reduced or no aerosol generation (speed-reducing/speed-increasing handpieces). The direction of bur rotation can also be changed on some handpieces.
- *Dental burs* (Figs. 5.32 and 5.33), *stones* (Fig. 5.34) and *finishing burs/discs* (Figs. 5.35 and 5.36): Gripped in handpieces by a quick-release clamping chuck (friction-grip diamond grit/tungsten carbide (TC) cutting blades for air turbine handpieces; latch-grip carbon steel/diamond grit/TC/plastic cutting blades for low-speed handpieces).

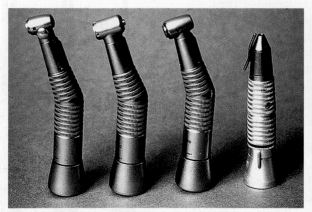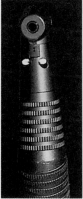

Fig. 5.31 A selection of low-speed electric motor handpieces. From left to right:

1:1 contra-angle handpiece used for most procedures. Latch-grip burs are used. Commonly identified with a blue-coloured band on the shank of the handpiece and a blue dot on the head. Speed in the range 400–40,000 rpm.

1:4 speed-increasing handpiece. Friction-grip burs. Operates at 16,000–160,000 rpm. Commonly identified with a red band. Useful for finishing cavity preparations and for finishing restorations.

7:1 speed-reducing handpiece. Latch-grip burs. Used for drilling pin holes and other procedures where slow speed is indicated. Operates at 550–5500 rpm and is commonly identified with a green band.

Straight handpiece that takes straight burs (may be modified to take latch-grip burs). A 1:1 handpiece is identified with a blue band; speed-reducing is identified with a green band. Used to trim temporary restorations and other similar procedures. Usually used outside the mouth.

A fibre-optic light system built into the head of a contra-angled low-speed handpiece.

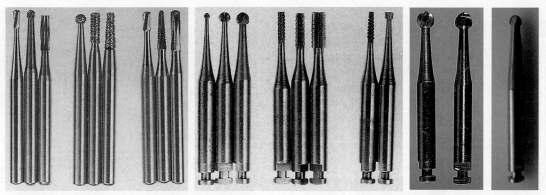

Fig. 5.32 A series of eight sets of burs (first three sets, friction-grip for the air turbine; next five sets, latch-grip for the low-speed handpiece). From left to right:

Friction-grip: tungsten carbide (TC) × 3, diamond grit (round, straight, tapered) and metal-cutting (serrated cross-cut TC blade) burs. TC and diamond used for cutting sound enamel and dentine, removing existing restorations. Diamond burs can be used to cut ceramic.

Latch-grip, carbon steel: three sizes round (rose-head), three sizes straight cross-cut fissure, tapered cross-cut fissure and inverted cone burs (nowadays, rarely used clinically). Burs numbered according to size/diameter of cutting head. Carbon steel heads used for cutting carious dentine but blunt quickly, corrode if not dried after sterilisation, now often used as a single-use bur.

Similar size carbon steel and TC rosehead burs compared. The TC head is a slightly different shape and is attached to the steel shank. Greater longevity and autoclavable.

Developments have included the latch-grip rosehead pattern PKK (polyketone-ketone) plastic bur (far right), for 'self-limiting' carious dentine removal, single-use.

Q5.32: What might be the advantages and disadvantages of single-use disposable burs?

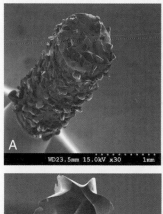

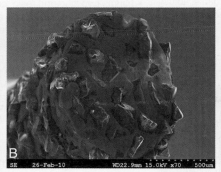

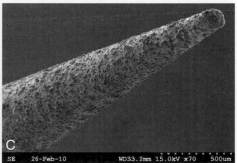

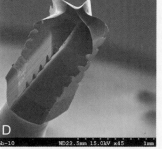

Fig. 5.33 (A) Scanning electron micrograph (30×) of a coarse-grit diamond bur. (B) The same bur as in (A) at 70× magnification showing the random, irregular shapes of the diamond grit. (C) 70× magnification of the yellow stripe diamond resin composite finishing bur with a much smaller grit particle size than the bur in (A) or (B). (D) 45× magnification of a tungsten carbide Beaver bur used for cutting amalgam and gold. Note the sharp notches cut into each flute to increase its cutting efficiency.

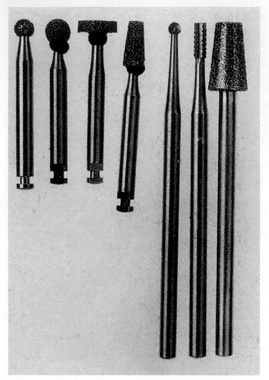

Fig. 5.34 A selection of four dental stones mounted on latch-grip short shanks (abrasive carborundum green stones for adjusting dental amalgam) and three long-shank instruments. Far right is a diamond-coated cone-shaped bur for use in the dental laboratory or rarely at the chairside, for coarse adjustment of indirect restorations and appliances, used at medium speed in a straight handpiece.

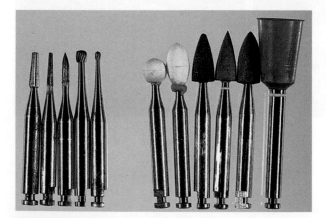

Fig. 5.35 Shaping and finishing burs, stones and points for dental amalgam. From left to right: five plain-cut latch-grip steel shaping burs, two mounted white (alundum) stones, three mounted abrasive rubber points from coarse to fine and a mounted abrasive rubber cup.

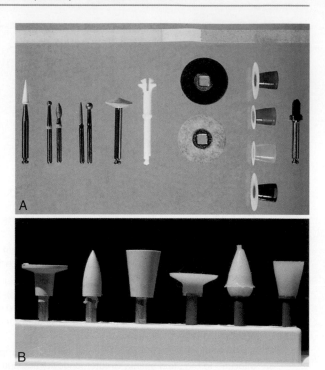

Fig. 5.36 (A) Resin composite finishing burs/discs. Across the top is a proximal plastic finishing strip with a blank area in the middle to facilitate passage through the contact point between the teeth. On the right portion the abrasive is coarse and on the left it is fine. From left to right: a mounted fine white stone, two medium-grit resin composite finishing diamonds (yellow band), two fine-grit resin composite finishing diamonds (red band), a mounted abrasive rubber disc, a mandrel for the two abrasive single-sided flexible discs, which are snap-fit onto the mandrel and four colour-coded flexible abrasive discs (coarse to fine impregnated grit/diamond) mounted on plastic stubs which fit the mandrel on the right of the picture. In (B) is a series of rubber/resin discs, points and cups impregnated with silica grit enabling the finishing of resin composite and glass-ionomer cement restorations.

5.8.3 Using Hand/Rotary Instruments: Clinical Tips

- Rotary instruments do not 'cut' dental hard tissues per se, but mechanically chip, cleave and smash at dental hard tissue ultrastructure. Therefore the resulting prepared surface is often damaged at the microscopic level (Fig. 5.37). This has implications when considering these surfaces' suitability for adhesive bonding (see later).
- Rotary instruments generate heat at the cutting interface (dissipated by the water spray from both

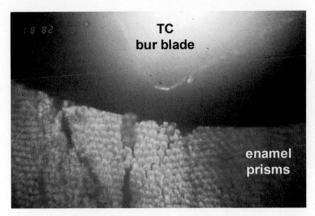

Fig. 5.37 Cracks, clefts and cleaving of prisms (horse-shoe-shaped structures) after enamel has been prepared using a tungsten carbide bur in an air-turbine handpiece. This inherent damage is unavoidable clinically but can be minimised by using only gentle pressure when operating, copious water spray and new, sharp burs in a handpiece with sound bearings, allowing vibration-free rotation. The surface and sub-surface damage will have implications for adhesive bonding as the shrinkage stresses of resin-based adhesive materials exerted on these weakened prisms may open the cracks further, leading to cohesive failure within the enamel structure (field width: 200 µm).

high- and low-speed handpieces), vibration, pressure and noise, all of which are unpleasant stimuli for patients. They offer a reduced tactile feel for the operator compared to hand instruments and therefore cutting is guided visually. As a general rule, hard materials (sound enamel, cast metals and restorations) are cut more efficiently at high speeds and less pressure, whereas softer material (carious dentine) is removed more efficiently at lower speeds and higher torque. In both cases, it is important that the operator does not apply excessive pressure or force when using these instruments as their efficiency and efficacy will be compromised.

- Water spray ejected from tiny nozzles built into the handpieces should be directed to the tip of the rotating bur head (Fig. 5.30). This cools the tooth surface as it is cut, thus preventing excessive frictional heat generation from having a potentially deleterious effect on the pulp. It also helps to flush away debris from the cut tooth surface and the bur head itself. The dental nurse should endeavour to keep the mouth mirror free from spray during rotary instrument use, using the 3-1 air/water syringe and aspiration. This action also reduces the risk of aerosol spread.

- Some handpieces when coupled to the main dental unit enabled with fibre optics have the ability to transmit the fibre-optic light from the head of the handpiece directly onto the bur head (Fig. 5.31). This can greatly improve direct vision for the operator and nurse.

- Air-turbine rotary burs produce less vibration and pressure, unless the bearings are worn. Latch-grip burs have a greater potential to vibrate.

- The cutting action of rotary (and hand) instrumentation causes a *smear layer* to be formed on cut hard tissue surfaces (usually <100 µm thick). This is a tenacious layer of organic, inorganic and bacterial debris which is either removed or incorporated in a modified form into the bond when placing an adhesive restoration (see Chapter 7, Section 7.2.4).

- It is essential that support is available to stabilise the operator's hand when using hand and rotary instrumentation. This can be achieved by resting the free fingers of the operating hand on a firm structure in the patient's mouth (e.g., the adjacent/contralateral/opposing teeth). This improves fine control significantly and reduces risk of iatrogenic damage, especially if the patient moves suddenly and unexpectedly (Figs. 5.38 and 5.39).

- The operator's free hand is used to hold the mouth mirror to provide indirect vision of the maxillary arch, reflect light intra-orally and/or retract soft tissues to aid visibility.

- For the inexperienced operator (and even some experienced ones!) when using rotary instruments, there is a risk of damaging adjacent sound teeth and restorations (operator-induced, *iatrogenic* collateral damage). Therefore there may be a case for protecting the adjacent tooth surface with a matrix band when operating proximally, but this may then interfere with direct vision. Fender wedges can be used to protect adjacent proximal sound tooth surfaces from iatrogenic damage (Fig. 5.40).

- With respect to carious tissue removal, burs are not innately self-limiting and rely on the operator to distinguish between that tissue requiring excavation or not. A single-use polymer bur (Fig. 5.32) only removes tooth structure that is softer than itself (anything harder and it will blunt during use) and so is more self-limiting in use. Hand excavators rely on the tactile feedback offered to the operator to distinguish the tissue requiring excavation and permit finer discrimination between the carious dentine zones

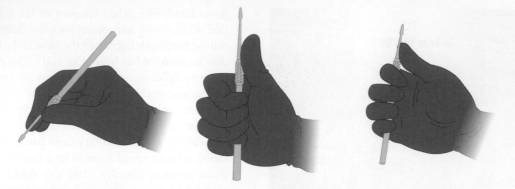

Fig. 5.38 From left to right: pen, palm and finger grip of hand instruments, with clinical examples below. Pen grip: most commonly used, most control for fine movement, enabling finger rests to be sought using the free fingers of the same hand. Palm and finger grip: limited use for more forceful movements in the maxillary arch. Instrument held between thumb (support) and forefinger with handle across palm, clasped by the remaining fingers. Very difficult to gain finger rest support, so these grips are rarely used clinically.

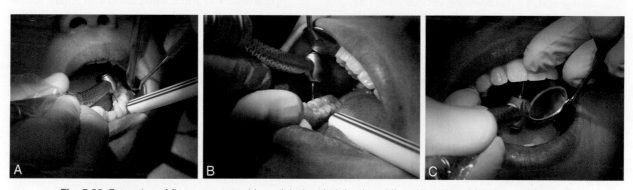

Fig. 5.39 Examples of finger rests used by a right-handed dentist while using a dental handpiece. From left to right: finger rest on the mandibular incisors when operating in the mandibular left quadrant; finger rest on the mandibular right lateral incisor/canine when operating on the mandibular right quadrant; finger rest on the maxillary right canine/premolar region when accessing the maxillary anterior teeth.

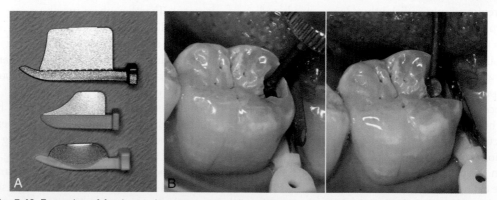

Fig. 5.40 Examples of fender wedges to protect adjacent proximal tooth surfaces during tooth preparation (FenderPrep/FenderWedge/Fenderprime; Directa Upplands Väsby, Sweden) as shown in the clinical images using a rotary bur in a slow-speed electric motor handpiece to gain access to the proximal lesion and a hand excavator to break through the contact area. (From Mackenzie L, Banerjee A. Minimally invasive direct restorations: a practical guide. *Brit Dent J.* 2017 Aug 11;223(3):163-171. doi:10.1038/sj.bdj.2017.661.)

(infected vs. affected vs. sound; see Chapter 1) than rotary instrumentation.

5.8.4 Dental Air-abrasion

- Developed in 1945 by R B Black, air-abrasion is a pseudo-mechanical method for cutting hard dental tissue where the tooth surface is bombarded with high-velocity abrasive particles in air, transferring kinetic energy to the tooth surface, which is then chipped away microscopically, with minimal subsurface damage.
- Adjustable parameters include the type of gas used, its pressure, powder flow rate, operating distance, type/size/morphology of the abrasive particles and diameter of the nozzle tip, all of which affect the efficacy and cutting rate.
- Particles approved by the US Food and Drug Administration (FDA) and/or with CE accreditation for clinical use in the mouth include >27 μm alumina, sodium bicarbonate, glycine and bio-active glass powders.
- Air-abrasion is useful for minimal invasive operative/reparative dentistry with no heat, vibration, pressure, pain or noise generated and for rapid operator-dependent tissue removal when using alumina particles. The extent of surface/subsurface hard tissue damage (cracks/cleft formation) is minimal when compared to rotary instruments, thus making the air-abraded hard surface more histologically suitable for adhesive bonding (Fig. 5.41).
- Preparation with air-abrasion produces rounded cavity line angles that will generate less stress at bonded interfaces during polymerisation shrinkage.
- Studies have demonstrated that air-abrasion with bio-active glass particles is capable of creating a therapeutic bioactive smear layer that encourages remineralisation, preserves the integrity of dentine-bonded interfaces and enhances the bond strength to certain adhesive materials.
- Bio-active glass particles can be used for extrinsic stain removal, desensitisation of exposed cervical dentine, resin composite repair and removal and selective demineralised enamel removal (e.g., preventive resin restorations in high caries risk patients (Fig. 5.42), cleaning residual resin cement deposits after orthodontic bracket removal). In-vitro research also indicates a potential use of bio-active glass powders to aid remineralisation of white spot lesions.

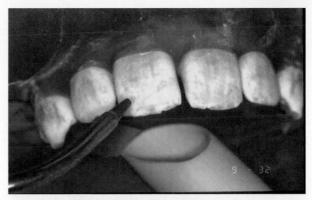

Fig. 5.41 An air-abrasion handpiece being used to prepare the labial enamel surfaces of the upper anterior teeth for direct resin composite veneers. Powder used: dry, 27 μm alumina. Note the blue aspirator tip held close to the operating field to vacuum up the spent powder.

> **Q5.41:** What clinical situations may benefit from using air-abrasion tooth preparation?

- New powders are being investigated for self-limiting carious dentine removal and improving their remineralisation potential.
- Multi-chambered air-abrasion units allow a metered flow of different particles (alumina, bio-active glass, sodium bicarbonate) in a shroud of water, reducing the dust generated by the process and permitting instantaneous initiation and termination of the abrasive stream (Fig. 5.42); a rubber dam is advisable for patient comfort.

5.8.5 Chemo-mechanical Carious Tissue Removal

- Chemo-mechanical carious tissue removal (CMCR) is a gel-based carious dentine tissue removal system that reacts theoretically with caries-infected, bacterially contaminated dentine that has undergone proteolytic breakdown of collagen, causing ultimate irretrievable collapse of the collagen network for easy final removal with 'curetting-action' hand instruments or ceramic/polymer burs used in a speed-reducing electric motor handpiece. This biochemical interaction confers an element of self-limiting caries removal ability.
- CMCR can consist of a 0.1% hypochlorite-based alkaline gel (pH 11) with or without amino acids

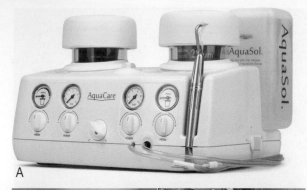

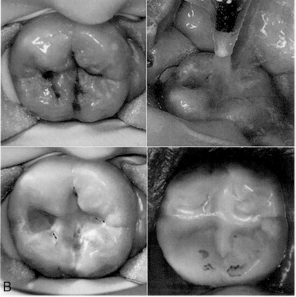

Fig. 5.42 (A) AquaCare Twin – Air Particle Abrasion and Polishing unit. (B) Wet air-abrasion using bio-active glass powder to selectively remove demineralised enamel in an occlusal carious lesion in a high caries risk/susceptible patient (From MacKenzie L and Banerjee A. Minimally invasive direct restorations: a practical guide. *Brit Dent J.* 2017 Aug 11; 223(3):163–171. doi:10.1038/sj.bdj.2017.661.)

Q5.42: What name might be given to the type of restoration placed in Fig. 5.42B?

---

preventing breakdown of sound collagen fibrils, or papain-based enzymatic systems.

• Stainless steel abrasive, non-cutting hand instruments permit more gentle carious dentine removal from cavities (Fig. 5.43). The system requires cavitated lesions for direct access to the carious dentine. Ceramic or polymer burs can also be used to aid excavation.

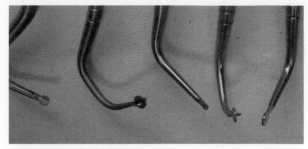

Fig. 5.43 A selection of non-cutting, abrasive hand instruments for use with chemo-mechanical carious tissue removal gels.

• As excavation is concentrated within caries-infected dentine in already deep, cavitated lesions, patients often do not require local anaesthesia (LA). Gentle hand instrumentation pressure (the same force as that exerted during normal toothbrushing or handwriting with a pen) contributes to improved patient comfort when compared to LA injections and the use of the dental drill (Fig. 5.44).

5.8.6 Other Instrumentation Technologies

As can be seen from Table 5.7, there are several clinical operative technologies for cutting teeth and removing caries. Ultrasonic and sonic instrumentation use the principle of probe tip oscillation and micro-cavitation to chip away hard dental tissues. Lasers transfer high energy into the tooth through water causing the photo-ablation of hard tissues. Great control is required by the operator to effectively harness this energy, and the potentially deleterious effects on the remaining enamel, dentine and pulp are under investigation in terms of biological health, residual strength and adhesive bonding capabilities. Other chemical methods include photo-activated disinfection (PAD), introducing tolonium chloride into the cavity which is taken up by the remaining bacteria within the cavity walls and then activated using light of a specific wavelength, thus causing cell lysis and death, as well as ozone (gaseous ozone infused into early lesions causing bacterial death). These technologies currently suffer from a lack of clinical research to validate them for routine evidence-based clinical use.

It is clear that minimally invasive operative cutting technologies must aim to preserve as much naturally repairable tooth structure as possible and at present no perfect instrument exists. Therefore the operator's knowledge of the histology of the dental substrate coupled with their understanding of bio-interactive

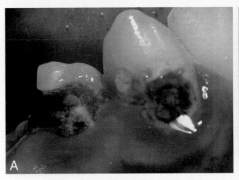
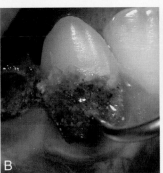
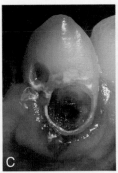
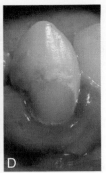

Fig. 5.44 Focus on the buccal cavitated carious lesion (modified International Caries Detection and Assessment System 4/ICCMS extensive) on the LR3. (A) Clear chemo-mechanical carious tissue removal gel sitting in the cavity for 30 seconds prior to mechanical agitation. (B) Gel and carious dentine agitated with a mace tip, abrasive hand instrument using toothbrushing force finger pressure. Note how the contaminated, caries-infected dentine 'emulsifies' into the gel, making it cloudy. A repeat application of gel was required in this case to obtain sufficient carious dentine removal. No local anaesthetic or rubber dam was required. (C) Final cavities before restoration in the LR3. There has been no direct exposure of the pulp, even though caries excavation is deep. Caries-affected dentine (scratchy but sticky/flaky; leathery) has been retained around the gingival margins in this case, along with an intact periphery of enamel (prepared using chisels/gingival margin trimmers (Fig. 5.27). See also Section 5.9. (D) Cavity has been restored provisionally with a glass-ionomer cement (GIC) during the stabilisation phase of this high caries risk patient's personalised care plan (see Chapter 3, Section 3.7).

Q5.44: Can you explain why the decision was made to retain such relatively large quantities of caries-affected dentine, especially at the gingival periphery of this particular lesion?

---

restorative materials and their adhesion chemistry as well as the clinical handling of the restorative materials, instruments, biological tissues and patient as a whole, all must be combined and balanced pragmatically to operatively manage the deeper cavitated carious lesion most effectively. This can be considered the 'golden triangle' of minimally invasive operative dentistry and bio-interactive restoration of teeth.

5.9 "MI" OPERATIVE MANAGEMENT OF THE CAVITATED CARIOUS LESION

5.9.1 Rationale

The critical, underpinning aspects of non-operative primary prevention, micro-invasive secondary prevention and control of disease couple with patient behaviour management, the second clinical domain of the MIOC framework for delivering better oral health, are discussed in detail in Chapters 3 and 4.

There are important factors that will now influence the decision to operatively intervene in a minimally invasive way to treat the cavitated, active carious lesion (MIOC Domain 3; refer to Section 5.1 for published guidelines and Fig. 5.45):

- *Alleviate pain/'protect' the pulp*: Carious tissue removal and a sedative dressing followed by a temporary, provisional or definitive sealed restoration can remove the symptoms of an acute, reversible pulpitis and allow the dentine–pulp complex to react and heal at a cellular level.
- *Restore form, function and appearance*: A large cavitated lesion will weaken the tooth, impeding normal mastication. Smaller, unsightly lesions in the anterior aesthetic zone may require operative intervention, rather than preventive measures alone for reasons of appearance affecting the patient's inclination to smile and ultimately, their self-confidence.
- *Aid patient plaque biofilm control*: Rough/cavitated tooth surfaces may be difficult for the high-risk patient to keep plaque-free (especially in deep occlusal pits and fissures or proximally).

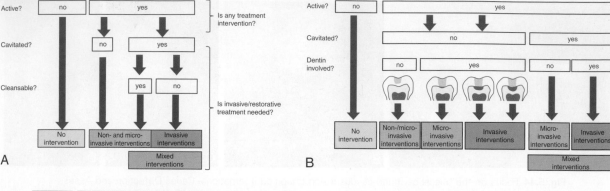

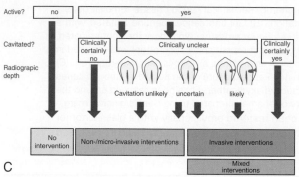

Fig. 5.45 (A) The three most evidence-based clinical factors to be considered when deciding to operatively intervene in the caries process are lesion activity, lesion cavitation and lesion cleansability. (B) These three factors applied to occlusal carious lesions depending on radiographic lesion depth. (C) These three factors applied to proximal lesions depending on radiographic lesion depth. (From Banerjee A, Splieth C, Breschi L, et al. When to intervene in the caries process? A Delphi consensus statement. *Brit Dent J.* 2020;229(7):474-482. doi:10.1038/s41415-020-2220-4.)

- *The patient's caries risk-susceptibility assessment (CRSA)/prediction*: Relatively small, early lesions in a high-risk patient with poor plaque control where repeated primary and secondary micro-invasive preventive management has been unsuccessful may require minimally invasive operative intervention whereas in a lower-risk patient, these same lesions may benefit from non-operative control measures alone (Chapter 4, Section 4.2.3). This is relevant particularly if previous preventive regimens have failed and lesions are progressing actively.

5.9.2 Minimally Invasive Dentistry (MID)

This is the third clinical domain of the overall MIOC framework used to deliver better oral health, followed throughout this book and epitomising good, contemporary evidence-based clinical practice: an approach where the oral healthcare team bases its individualised patient care on early detection of disease, risk/susceptibility assessment, diagnosis and prevention/control of further disease with suitably tailored recall consultation (active surveillance) frequencies (see Chapters 3 and 9).

As has been discussed previously, forms of non-invasive primary dental caries prevention include diet control, optimal oral hygiene protocols allowing the patient to disrupt the plaque biofilm regularly and daily use of fluoride-containing toothpastes and potentially other remineralising agents on at-risk tooth surfaces. Micro-invasive secondary prevention measures would include the placement of sealants and resin infiltration techniques on those tooth surfaces that have undergone incipient demineralisation to arrest the caries process and reverse the tissue damage. Minimally invasive tertiary prevention includes the full operative intervention of more progressed carious lesions, preventing them from causing further irreparable tooth damage.

Three factors interplay in deciding when to intervene operatively:

- Degree of lesion cavitation
- Plaque biofilm stagnation on the lesion surface (cleansability)
- The activity of the lesion (difficult to objectively measure clinically)

These factors are clearly interlinked. The often undermined cavitation of an mICDAS 3 or 4 lesion (moderate/advanced ICCMS lesion) will act as a plaque trap which will be difficult for the patient to routinely clean effectively. The resulting plaque stagnation will create a local environment encouraging biofilm dysbiosis, thus activating the caries process within the undisrupted plaque, as well as in the underlying lesion with progressive, destructive demineralisation and proteolytic breakdown of the tissues. Therefore minimally invasive operative intervention is necessary to prevent the tissue destruction of a developing lesion from worsening (tertiary prevention). Expert consensus guidelines exist to help the practitioner navigate this decision-making process for occlusal and proximal lesions, depending on radiographic lesion depth (Fig. 5.45).

5.9.2.1 Assessing Clinical Cavitation of a Carious Lesion

On directly visible smooth surfaces (buccal/labial, lingual/palatal and proximal when no adjacent tooth is present) and occlusally, clinical cavitation can often be detected with the aid of magnification, good lighting and careful use of a rounded dental explorer to feel across the surface for any catches or roughness on those accessible sites. Plaque and surface debris should be removed prior to the detection of such defects. On proximal surfaces with adjacent teeth contact points present, this becomes a more difficult task. Intra-oral radiographs may help, but the correlation between the presence of cavitation and depth of

radiolucency is not absolute. Lesions into the middle third of dentine and deeper are more likely to be cavitated, but this is not a certainty. Conversely, shallower lesions tend not to be cavitated, but not always. If in doubt and to make the correct decision as to whether to operatively intervene, proximal surfaces of adjacent teeth can be separated using orthodontic separators or wooden wedges placed for a few minutes before the detailed clinical examination using dental magnification ideally. Once removed, direct visual access of the proximal surface(s) may be possible and a further silicone impression of the proximal surfaces could also be taken, if deemed necessary to aid in cavity detection. This technique could be used especially in those higher risk/more caries susceptible patients with multiple lesions present where a decision is required as to which lesion requires operative intervention (Figs. 5.46 and 5.47).

When operative intervention is eventually required for these reasons, the surgical intervention itself should be *minimally invasive*, that is:

1. Limited to the removal of the unrepairable, diseased enamel and dentine only, keeping cavities as small as possible and preserving as much sound and repairable tissue where possible, allowing the dentine–pulp complex to help regenerate and heal the tissues biologically

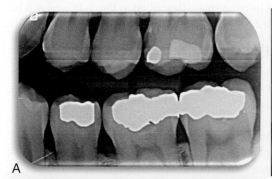
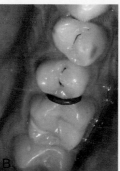
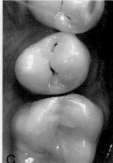
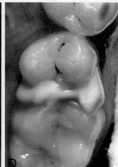
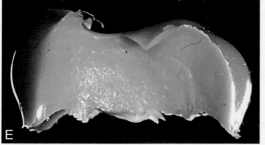

Fig. 5.46 (A) Left bitewing radiograph with a dubious radiolucency mesial UL6; is this carious lesion in a clearly high risk/susceptible patient cavitated? (B) An orthodontic separator is inserted proximally between the UL5 and UL6 and (C) after removal, the interproximal space has been widened with physiological tooth movement within the limits of the periodontal ligament spaces of the two teeth. (D) A quick-setting light-bodied silicone material is syringed into the space and (E) on its removal after setting, the mesial proximal impression surface of the UL6 is clearly smooth and non-cavitated and does not need operative intervention. (Courtesy D Raju.)

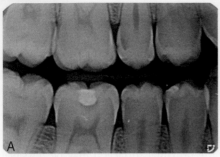
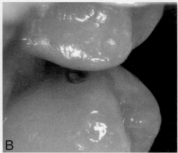
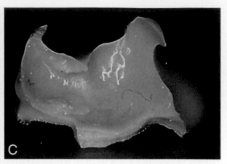

Fig. 5.47 (A) Right bitewing radiograph with a dubious radiolucency distal UR5, extending into the outer third of dentine radiographically; is this carious lesion in a clearly high risk/susceptible patient cavitated? (B) An orthodontic separator is inserted proximally between the UR5 and UR6 and after removal, the interproximal space has been widened with physiological tooth movement within the limits of the periodontal ligament spaces of the two teeth. From the palatal aspect, a small cavity can now be observed directly with a stagnating biofilm present and accessible to a rounded dental explorer. (C) A quick-setting light-bodied silicone material is syringed into the space and on its removal after setting, the distal proximal impression surface of the UR5 is clearly uneven, confirming cavitation that requires operative intervention to improve the surface contour and patient biofilm control in this area. (Courtesy D Raju.)

Q5.47: Can you identify the radiolucency beneath the restoration on the occlusal aspect of the LR6? What might this indicate?

---

2. Physically and chemically modifying and optimising the remaining cavity walls and margins to enable…
3. Restoration of cavities with suitable adhesive, bio-interactive and bio-active materials which will:
   - Confer additional support, infiltrate and strengthen the remaining tooth structure
   - Promote remineralisation and potentially have antibacterial activity
   - Seal off any remaining bacteria from their nutrient supply, thus arresting the lesion within the residual carious tissue retained in the cavity depths
   - Restore appearance, form and function with appropriate long-term maintenance regimens (see Chapter 9, Section 9.4).

For this minimally invasive approach to be successful, integration of the knowledge of tissue histology with the chemistry and handling of dental biomaterials is essential. Also, it is vital that patients understand their responsibility in controlling and preventing further disease progression as discussed in Chapter 4. Remember, 'drilling and filling' teeth does not cure caries! Any dental restoration placed is only ever as good as the operator and their skills in handling the tissues, instruments, materials and placement and the patient then looking after it. In contemporary clinical dental practice, it is imperative that

detailed written records, including operative images, are kept illustrating all of these factors.

The decision-making process during the execution of minimally invasive, selective caries excavation/cavity preparation of the deeper cavitated carious lesion can be divided into the stages described in Fig. 5.48, and will be discussed further in the following subsections.

5.9.3 Enamel Preparation

The aims of gaining and improving access through the enamel when minimally invasively operatively managing a carious lesion are to:

1. Optimise visual/instrumentation access to the full peripheral extent of the deeper carious dentine requiring removal, without removing excessive amounts of enamel in the process.
2. Remove demineralised, weakened (and often unsightly frosty white) carious enamel only.
3. Create a sound peripheral enamel margin to which an adhesive restorative material can bond to and form a seal with.

Fig. 5.49 shows a histological cross section through a cavitated, advanced mICDAS 4 (ICCMS advanced) lesion with unsupported and demineralised enamel and the

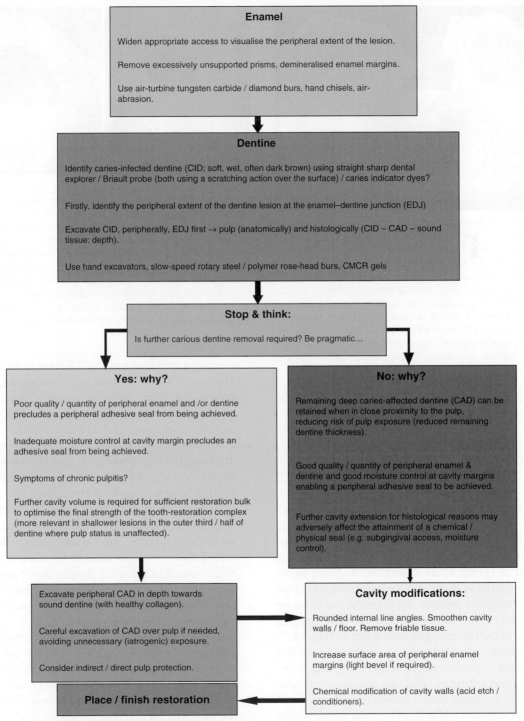

Enamel

Widen appropriate access to visualise the peripheral extent of the lesion.

Remove excessively unsupported prisms, demineralised enamel margins.

Use air-turbine tungsten carbide / diamond burs, hand chisels, air-abrasion.

Dentine

Identify caries-infected dentine (CID; soft, wet, often dark brown) using straight sharp dental explorer / Briault probe (both using a scratching action over the surface) / caries indicator dyes?

Firstly, identify the peripheral extent of the dentine lesion at the enamel–dentine junction (EDJ)

Excavate CID, peripherally, EDJ first → pulp (anatomically) and histologically (CID – CAD – sound tissue: depth).

Use hand excavators, slow-speed rotary steel / polymer rose-head burs, CMCR gels

Stop & think:

Is further carious dentine removal required? Be pragmatic…

Yes: why?

Poor quality / quantity of peripheral enamel and /or dentine precludes a peripheral adhesive seal from being achieved.

Inadequate moisture control at cavity margin precludes an adhesive seal from being achieved.

Symptoms of chronic pulpitis?

Further cavity volume is required for sufficient restoration bulk to optimise the final strength of the tooth-restoration complex (more relevant in shallower lesions in the outer third / half of dentine where pulp status is unaffected).

No: why?

Remaining deep caries-affected dentine (CAD) can be retained when in close proximity to the pulp, reducing risk of pulp exposure (reduced remaining dentine thickness).

Good quality / quantity of peripheral enamel & dentine and good moisture control at cavity margins enabling a peripheral adhesive seal to be achieved.

Further cavity extension for histological reasons may adversely affect the attainment of a chemical / physical seal (e.g. subgingival access, moisture control).

Excavate peripheral CAD in depth towards sound dentine (with healthy collagen).

Careful excavation of CAD over pulp if needed, avoiding unnecessary (iatrogenic) exposure.

Consider indirect / direct pulp protection.

Cavity modifications:

Rounded internal line angles. Smoothen cavity walls / floor. Remove friable tissue.

Increase surface area of peripheral enamel margins (light bevel if required).

Chemical modification of cavity walls (acid etch / conditioners).

Place / finish restoration

Fig. 5.48 Flowchart showing the decision-making process and stages of execution of selective caries removal following minimally invasive principles in the deep, cavitated carious lesion. *CID,* Caries-infected dentine; *CAD,* caries-affected dentine.

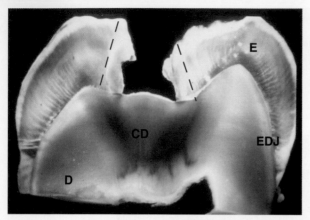

Fig. 5.49 A thin mesio-distal longitudinal section through a cavitated lesion (modified International Caries Detection and Assessment System 4/ICCMS advanced-extensive) viewed in reflected light. Note the demineralised, overhanging enamel bordering the cavity, with the undermining spread of the dentine lesion along the EDJ (see Chapter 1, Section 1.1.6.2). The red dashed lines indicate the extent of enamel removal required to achieve a sound enamel margin with supported prism structure, suitable to affect a seal with an adhesive restorative material while still permitting access to the underlying carious dentine. *E*, Enamel; *D*, dentine; *CD*, carious dentine; *EDJ*, enamel–dentine junction.

> **Q5.49:** What is the name given to the histological appearance of the alternate light and dark stripes evident in the inner third of enamel, arising from the EDJ and radiating towards the tooth surface?

extent of enamel preparation required (red dashed lines). The outer enamel margins may be bevelled lightly to increase the surface area for adhesion. Fig. 5.50 shows the clinical occlusal appearance of such enamel removal using a diamond or TC bur in an air-turbine handpiece before and after preparation. This cutting process must be carried out with only gentle pressure, avoiding the use of coarse grit diamond burs so as not to cause excessive chipping or cracking of the remaining enamel substrate (Fig. 5.37).

Direct visual/instrument access to occlusal, buccal and lingual/palatal carious surfaces is relatively straightforward with good soft tissue retraction and intra-oral lighting. Posterior proximal surface lesions (mesial and distal) can be more awkward and approaches here would include:

- Occlusally, initially accessing just medial to the affected marginal ridge and eventually sacrificing it, thus

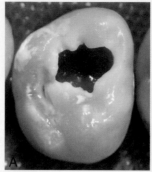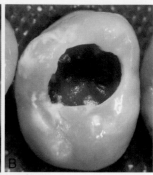

Fig. 5.50 An occlusal cavitated carious lesion in the UR7 (modified International Caries Detection and Assessment System 4/ ICCMS extensive). (A) The lesion on presentation with frosty white demineralised, friable and unsupported enamel at the cavity margin with underlying carious dentine visible. (B) Enamel access has been widened by removal of the weakened peripheral enamel using a diamond bur in an air-turbine handpiece for <5 seconds. The margin has been bevelled lightly. Note that not all the undermined enamel has been removed as the retained tissue is strong enough to help support and be supported by the final tooth-restoration complex.

creating a proximal box (see Chapter 8, Section 8.5). The use of a matrix band on the adjacent tooth to protect the sound adjacent proximal surface, or a proximally placed fender wedge, might be required in some cases (see Figs. 5.51B and 5.55B).

- Occlusally, accessing medial to the marginal ridge, directing the bur towards the proximal lesion, *tunnelling* beneath the marginal ridge and conserving it. This is only successful clinically if the lesion is sufficiently small and it then might be debated as to whether such an operative intervention is appropriate in the first place! There is also a high risk of fracture of the now undermined and weakened marginal ridge enamel in service, following restoration with a suitably flowable adhesive restorative material.
- Buccal/lingual/palatally, especially if the tooth is rotated and has undergone some gingival recession. Tunnelling from these aspects can result in successful management as long as the lesion is not too extensive and effective moisture and cavity margin control can be achieved.
- Directly mesial or distal, if the adjacent tooth is missing and space is present to permit direct visual/instrumentation access.

Anterior proximal lesions are approached conventionally from the lingual/palatal aspect to maintain aesthetics of the natural labial enamel. However, minimally invasive tooth preservation principles would argue that a labial approach might also be appropriate if this led to the least amount of healthy tooth tissue being destroyed. In the modern era of high-quality aesthetic direct adhesive restorative materials, this is an approach that can be encouraged as good operator clinical skills coupled with the placement of such aesthetic materials can achieve a high-quality final aesthetic result (Fig. 5.51).

5.9.4 Carious Dentine Removal

When practising selective carious dentine removal, careful consideration must be given to both the:

- 'Anatomical extent' of the lesion; that is, the lateral extent from the EDJ lesion periphery through to the carious tissue overlying the pulp
- 'Histological depth' of the lesion; that is, the collagen and mineral content of contaminated caries-infected dentine (CID) versus demineralised caries-affected dentine (CAD) versus sound dentine (see Chapter 1, Section 1.1.6.3).

Carious dentine removal must be tailored to the individual lesion, tooth and patient. Following the minimally invasive approach, selective caries removal results in smaller-volume cavities and restorations with the following benefits, ultimately leading to restorations with increased longevity and more importantly, reduced tissue destruction and increased overall tooth-restoration complex longevity:

- Adhesive restorative materials are often easier to handle and place without voids in smaller quantities.
- Moisture control, cavity margin seal and finish can be better controlled.
- The restored crown is often strengthened due to greater retention of natural, repairable tooth structure; consider the tooth-restoration complex as a whole.
- Simpler procedures, improved patient aftercare and long-term maintenance.

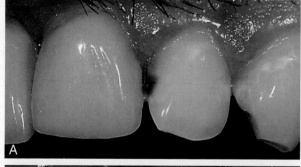
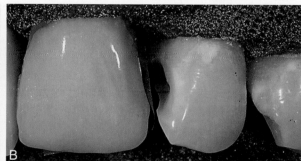
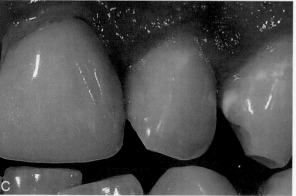

Fig. 5.51 (A) A pre-operative Class III mesial proximal carious lesion in the UL2 that requires operative intervention as it is cavitated, is not easily cleansable by the patient (and therefore at risk of being active) and has poor aesthetics. (B) The lesion has been accessed unconventionally, through the buccal aspect, to reduce the amount of viable tooth tissue loss following minimally invasive principles. Note the presence of an interproximal matrix strip to prevent damage to the adjacent tooth surface. (C) The final resin composite restoration of the UL2 shows the high-quality final aesthetic result. (Courtesy D Raju.)

5.9.4.1 Peripheral Caries Management (EDJ) – (Fig. 5.52)

Prevention of microleakage and subsequent caries associated with restorations and sealants (CARS/secondary or recurrent caries) at the cavity margin depends on the seal formed between the restoration and tooth structure at the periphery of the cavity.

- Histologically, the optimal peripheral seal achieved will be at the interface between the adhesive restorative material and sound enamel > sound dentine > CAD. CID and carious enamel are not suitable substrates for adhesion and should not be retained at the cavity periphery.
- The adhesive seal is created optimally between an adhesive restoration and histologically sound enamel. Even if sound enamel lines the entire periphery of the cavity and moisture control is optimal (e.g., an occlusal cavity or a proximal cavity with a suitably placed rubber dam), ideally the peripheral dentine should be excavated to sound tissue. However, in certain clinical situations, to conserve tooth tissue and perhaps to better manage moisture control, limited quantities of brown-discoloured, slightly leathery but still histologically repairable CAD may be retained at the periphery. This, however, should be removed selectively, down to deeper sound dentine, if there is a risk that the brown tissue discolouration may shine through the final restoration placed, thus jeopardising the aesthetic outcome (especially in the anterior aesthetic zone, classically the mesial surface of the UR4 across to the mesial surface of the UL4). Such a brown peripheral shadow may not only be aesthetically displeasing, but might also be misdiagnosed as secondary caries/CARS at subsequent recall consultation examinations, especially by new clinicians seeing the patient for the first time.
- If minimal or no enamel is present at the EDJ after peripheral caries removal and adequate moisture control cannot be guaranteed (e.g., cervical or proximal lesion, base of a proximal box preparation close to the gingival margin), then sound dentine is a pre-requisite at the EDJ in an attempt to maximise the bond and adhesive seal between the peripheral dentine and final restoration. However, a pragmatic clinical approach is also required alongside the histological analysis and if this means extending the cavity significantly further subgingivally to expose the sound dentine, overall

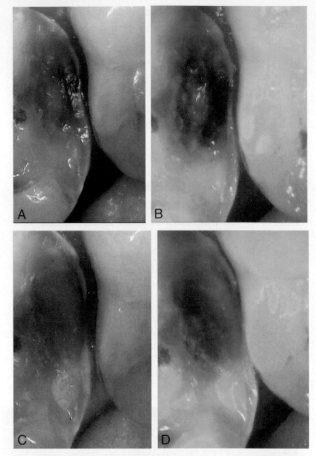

Fig. 5.52 (A) A mesial cavitated carious lesion on an upper molar at presentation with soft, wet caries-affected dentine present overlying the pulp and at the peripheral margin (base of the box). (B) The same lesion on presentation using the fluorescence mode of the Soprolife camera (Acteon) highlighting the more bacterially contaminated dentine in red. (C) The lesion has been excavated using selective caries removal principles, retaining caries-affected dentine (demineralised, leathery) over the pulp but with further excavation towards sound dentine at the enamel–dentine junction (EDJ) at the base of the box. (D) The image in (C) shown more clearly by the fluorescence image showing some decontaminated dentine still present overlying the pulp *(red)* but not present at the EDJ. (From Dawett B, Young S, Deery C, Banerjee A. Minimally invasive selective caries removal put into practice. *Dent Update.* 2020 Nov;47(10):841-847. doi:10.12968/denu.2020.47.10.841.)

consideration must be given to the long-term success rate of the final restoration and ultimately the final restorability of the tooth in question (Fig. 5.44). The patient must be informed and careful records made of the decision outcome and reasoning.

- Distinguishing between caries-infected, affected and sound dentine is a subjective clinical skill and the operator still must use differential tactile feedback (see Table 5.9, Section 5.9.4.3). The brown discolouration of the dentine at the EDJ alone is an indicator neither of its infectivity nor for its removal (unless in the anterior aesthetic zone as mentioned earlier).
- In no clinical situation should caries-infected dentine or grossly demineralised carious enamel be retained at the EDJ. This CID is essentially necrotic and cannot be adhered to, or a suitable seal achieved. It is also too soft to physically support a rigid restoration under occlusal loading.
- Instruments commonly used to excavate carious dentine include hand excavators or steel/polymer rosehead burs in a slow-speed electric motor handpiece. Other technologies might include chemo-mechanical gels (see Table 5.7).

5.9.4.2 Caries Overlying the Pulp

When excavating carious dentine overlying the pulp, consideration must be given to its *proximity* to the pulp (see Section 5.10) and any *symptoms*.

- Where a peripheral seal can be achieved (enamel margins intact) and pulp symptoms are not present or are indicative of a reversible pulpitis only,

leathery, demineralised caries-affected dentine may be retained overlying the pulp, thus reducing the risk of pulp exposure in deep cavities. Clinical evidence shows that affected dentine provides better indirect pulp protection than any artificial restorative material in this situation. The evidence from clinical studies also indicates that pulp exposures in such a clinical scenario tend to lead to a significant increase in ultimate pulp death over a 5- to 10-year period. Therefore pulp exposures should be avoided if possible.

- When using minimally invasive, selective carious dentine removal principles in deep carious lesions, consideration must also be given to the radiographic appearance of the tooth-restoration complex, especially when reviewing over a period of time. Fig. 5.53 shows the radiographic appearance of a Class I, occlusal tooth-restoration complex where resin composite has been used to seal in caries-affected dentine and restore the form, function and aesthetics of the tooth. The radiolucent shadow of the retained caries-affected dentine is clearly visible. The tooth still elicits positive pulp sensibility tests to at least the publication date of this book!
- If the dentine lesion has only penetrated up to the middle third/halfway through the dentine radiographically, thanks to tertiary dentine being laid down at the dentine–pulp border, excavation to

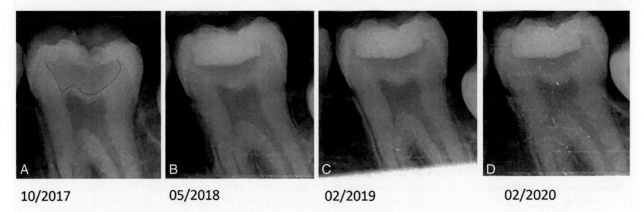

10/2017   05/2018   02/2019   02/2020

Fig. 5.53 (A) A radiograph showing a deep occlusal carious lesion in a lower-left second mandibular molar tooth. The extent of the radiolucency has been demarcated with a red line and is very close to the pulp chamber. (B) to (D) The same tooth-restoration complex after minimally invasive, selective caries removal, retaining caries-affected dentine over the pulp and then restoring the cavity with resin composite. The radiolucent shadow of the residual caries-affected dentine can be clearly observed in the subsequent follow-up radiographs. The tooth still elicits positive pulp sensibility tests. (From Dawett B, Young S, Deery C, Banerjee A. Minimally invasive selective caries removal put into practice. Dent Update. 2020; Nov. 47(10):841-847. doi:10.12968/denu.2020.47.10.841.)

sound dentine may be achievable at the cavity base without the risk of pulp exposure, to improve the adhesive bond and seal (especially if enamel margins are not intact). As pulp proximity is not an issue in this scenario, the restoration bulk/volume of the cavity becomes more clinically significant. Most direct plastic restorative materials are mechanically weaker in thin sections. For improved tooth-restoration complex longevity, an adequate bulk volume of material is required, supported by surrounding tooth structure. If the lesion is distant from the pulp, these material factors become a priority when deciding the extent of tissue preparation required.

- Where chronic pulp symptoms persist along with radiographic changes at the root apex, caries excavation

needs to be complete, exposing the pulp chamber and its necrotic contents as necessary, with a view to commencing a pulpotomy or endodontic treatment.

Table 5.8 summarises the interlinked factors affecting the decision to remove or retain carious dentine. It must be understood that there is no absolute correct or incorrect amount of caries that should be excavated, but whatever decision is made by the operator, it should be made for *pragmatic*, *justifiable* and *documented* reasons. Different quantities of caries can be removed or retained in different parts of the same cavity. Fig. 5.54 highlights this variation in carious dentine removal, showing three depths of potential excavation endpoint, depending on the combined outcome of the factors discussed in Table 5.8.

TABLE 5.8	Interrelating Factors Affecting Decision of How Much Carious Dentine to Remove
Factors Affecting Amount of Carious Dentine Removed	**Comments**
Patient's caries risk/ susceptibility	High-risk, uncontrolled caries progression, unsuccessful non-operative prevention regimens: lesions may be excavated to sound dentine where possible (avoiding pulp exposure). Important for operator and patient to appreciate and record the poorer prognosis of the tooth-restoration complex due to the lack of patient adherence to preventive strategies (see Chapter 9).
Patient/oral factors	Limited oral opening, physical/mental disabilities can affect visual/instrument access directly or indirectly. Broken down, rotated or partially erupted teeth can hinder rubber dam placement. Sedation or general anaesthesia may be required.
Pulp sensibility	Chronic symptoms of an irreversible pulpitis will mean pulp extirpation after complete caries removal to sound dentine.
Pulp proximity	If no or limited acute pulpitis symptoms, in deep lesions close to the pulp (inner third of dentine radiographically), caries-affected dentine retained over the pulp to allow remineralisation from dentine–pulp complex; indirect pulp capping/ protection. Pulp preservation and protection take precedent in deep lesions. In shallower lesions, distant from the pulp, material factors take precedent as adequate bulk volume of direct plastic materials is required to improve the long-term viability of the tooth-restoration complex. Thus excavation to sound tissues may be recommended in such instances.
Remaining coronal tooth structure	Sufficient supragingival tooth structure must remain to support the tooth-restoration complex long term. Excavation to sound dentine should not compromise the physical or adhesive properties of the restorative material (e.g., deep peripheral excavation to sound dentine resulting in a cavity margin >2 mm subgingivally, compromising moisture control and marginal adaptation).
Material factors	Retention mechanisms: mechanical, micro-/nano-mechanical, chemical adhesion. An adverse oral environment can affect the set and physical properties of some materials (e.g., glass-ionomer cements in xerostomia).

Note: The table compares infected vs. affected vs. sound dentine. Read also Section 5.1.

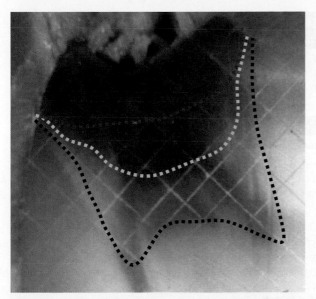

Fig. 5.54 A cavitated carious dentine lesion (modified International Caries Detection and Assessment System 4; ICCMS extensive lesion) showing the brown colour gradation from the superficial caries-infected dentine subjacent to the enamel–dentine junction (EDJ) through to the deeper levels of caries-affected dentine, including the translucent zone and sound dentine. Three depths have been indicated for potential caries excavation endpoints: complete caries removal to sound dentine at the EDJ and over the pulp *(dark blue line)*; minimally invasive selective caries removal retaining stained caries-affected dentine at the EDJ and over the pulp (leathery in texture, sticky and scratchy to the sharp dental explorer dragged across the dentine surface; *light green line*); and minimally invasive excavation with a significant bulk of retained infected/affected dentine over the pulp *(red line)*. Note how all potential cavity excavation endpoints start and finish on sound enamel, thus providing a sealed margin at the periphery. None of these endpoints are right or wrong, but it is essential that the substrate histology at each level is appreciated to enable a successful adhesive restoration to be placed.

Q5.54: Which of the three depths do you think would be best to stop carious dentine removal in the lesion in Fig. 5.54?

5.9.4.3 Discriminating Between the Histological Zones of Carious Dentine

The clinical discrimination of caries-infected, caries-affected and sound dentine is a subjective skill gained using a combination of an understanding of caries histology with clinical experience. These boundaries between the histological zones are not clearly defined; the histological and bacterial changes occur throughout the whole lesion as a continuum from superficial to deeper layers, with different rates of progression within the individual lesion itself. Table 5.9 summarises the techniques available, both clinical and through research development, to help enable the operator to distinguish these important 'histological' layers. From the table it can be seen that none are truly objective, with interpretation required to decide the excavation endpoint and linked to the factors discussed in Table 5.8.

5.9.4.4 'Stepwise Excavation' and Atraumatic Restorative Technique

Stepwise excavation and atraumatic restorative treatment (ART) are the original and more modern application, respectively, of the minimally invasive, biological, selective caries removal approach to managing deep, cavitated carious lesions. Both use simple hand instrumentation (spoon excavators) to remove the necrotic, superficial layer of caries-infected dentine up to and sometimes including some leathery caries-affected dentine as required (Fig. 5.55). The two steps of the original stepwise excavation procedure included the placement of a setting calcium hydroxide 'lining' and a temporary zinc polycarboxylate cement restoration. Between 6 and 9 months later, this provisional restoration was completely removed, exposing the remaining, now arrested caries-affected dentine (darker, harder and dryer) and newly deposited tertiary dentine at the pulp–dentine border. This residual stained dentine was then removed using a steel rosehead bur in a low-speed handpiece and a final amalgam restoration was placed.

The single-step ART restores the cavity with chemically adhesive, high-viscosity glass-ionomer cement (GIC), forming a better adaptive seal to the remaining tooth structure (see Chapter 7, Section 7.3) after the use of specially designed hand instrument cavity openers and excavators to gain access to and remove the caries-infected dentine without the need for rotary instrumentation. Subsequently, this provisional restoration does not require complete replacement as in the original stepwise excavation procedure, as the arrested caries-affected dentine is sealed off from its nutrient

TABLE 5.9   Clinical and Research Methods to Help Discriminate Clinically Between Infected, Affected and Sound Dentine

Discriminating Methods		Caries-infected Dentine (*contaminated*)	Caries-affected Dentine (*demineralised*)	Sound Dentine
Clinical	**Visual examination**	Often a colour gradient from (Fig. 5.54):		
		dark brown→	pale brown/translucent→	yellow/white
		Difficult to judge clinically/OK when examining a sectioned lesion (research).		
	Tactile sensation across the surface	Soft/wet/sticky feel with a sharp dental explorer (straight or Briault probe)	Slightly sticky/flaky and scratchy feel; leathery	Scratchy feel to a sharp dental explorer
	Caries detector dyes	'Fusayama' dyes: based on propylene-glycol, collagen-based stain. Attempts to discriminate infected versus affected dentine, but research has shown these dyes stain deeper collagen and permeate through natural tissue porosities, into affected/sound dentine zones, often leading to cavity overpreparation.		
	Fluorescence	Fluorescence-aided caries excavation technology (see (Fig. 5.52); autofluorescence; optical light scattering, quantitative light-induced fluorescence, optical coherence tomography: all can be adjunctive aids for assisting lesion detection but not necessarily discriminatory for the lesion zones.		
In-vitro research	**Bacterial dyes**	Dyes under research development reacting to bacterial redox by-products, using their concentration gradient drop from infected through affected to sound dentine. Has potential to be zone selective.		
	Biochemical markers	Matrix metalloproteinases, ester groups and advanced glycosylation end-product (AGE) proteins seem to be concentrated more in caries-infected dentine; potential for these histological 'biomarkers' to be labelled with dyes to assist with discriminating lesion zones in the future?		

Note: These zones do not have distinct boundaries but have a gradient of histological/bacterial/biochemical changes through the lesion from the enamel–dentine junction to the pulp (see Chapter 1, Section 1.1.6).

supply and can be healed by the dentine-pulp complex cellular reaction. However, occlusal refurbishment of the GIC may be necessary after a few years, depending on the clinical extent of wear and partial dissolution. This can be accomplished by cutting back the exposed worn GIC surface by up to 2 mm in depth and bonding a layer of resin composite onto the freshly exposed, mature GIC; an *adhesive layered*, *laminate* or '*sandwich*' *restoration* (see Chapters 7 and 8). Indeed, systematic reviews of partial/incomplete minimally invasive caries removal clinical studies have highlighted the one-step procedure with no second re-entry step, that seals in residual affected dentine, resulting in significantly less

pulp exposures than the original two-step stepwise excavation procedure. This was the result of an increase in pulp exposures in the second re-entry procedure where deeper, histologically arrested dentine was removed (forcibly and unnecessarily), too close to the pulp.

Both stepwise excavation and ART follow the underpinning principles of minimally invasive selective carious dentine removal. As this is now an accepted contemporary rationale for operative caries management, these terminologies are gradually becoming redundant as current adhesive dental biomaterials are more capable of sealing in and potentially rehabilitating diseased tissue.

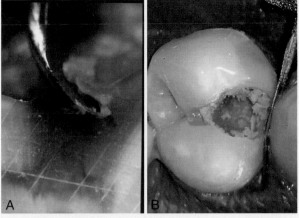

Fig. 5.55 (A) Hand excavator 'scooping' up necrotic, soft caries-infected dentine (CID) once the enamel access has been widened (reference grid lines on the plane cut dentine surface were placed for experimental measuring purposes). (B) An occluso-proximal cavity that has been hand excavated, removing the soft, wet and flaky CID. Note the presence of the fender wedge to prevent iatrogenic damage to the adjacent tooth surface as the contact area is broken using a hand excavator and rotary instrumentation. (Courtesy D Raju.)

5.9.5 CAVITY MODIFICATIONS

Once carious dentine removal has been achieved, the practitioner needs to stop, think and decide which restorative material to use and then modify the remaining cavity accordingly, if required (Fig. 5.56, Table 5.10). These modifications may be necessary to improve the retentive properties of the cavity or to optimise the material properties(e.g., bulk/margin strength or fracture resistance).

- *Retention*: The property of a cavity that resists displacement of the restoration in the path of its insertion.
- *Support*: The property of a cavity that prevents displacement or fracture of the restoration in any other direction, including internal dislodgement within the cavity itself (historically termed *resistance form*). This feature relates to the morphology of cavity walls/floors and rounded internal line angles.

5.10 PULP PROTECTION

5.10.1 Rationale

The final and most important consideration along with any cavity modifications, prior to placing the restoration, is the long-term maintenance of pulp sensibility. This is linked to pulp *signs and symptoms* and *cavity proximity* to the pulp. Assuming the symptoms and signs of pulp sensibility indicate a histologically viable pulp (see Chapter 3, Section 3.2), the pulp tissues may require protection from:

- Bacteria/toxins
- Chemicals leaching from the restorative materials (e.g., unconverted resin monomers from resin composite restoratives, acid etchant)

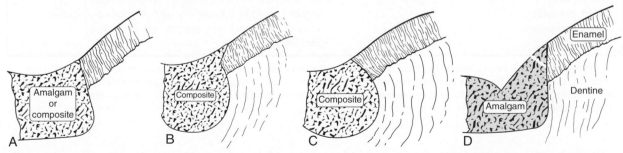

Fig. 5.56 Diagrams outlining the different restoration margin angles and cavo-surface angles suited to different restorative materials. (A) Amalgam and resin composite margins require bulk for strength so that 90-degree restoration margin angles and cavo-surface angles will ensure sufficient intrinsic strength of both the restoration margin and cavity edge. (B) Resin composites adhere to and support enamel to a degree, so light bevelling of the enamel surface can increase the surface area for adhesive bonding while also removing any potentially unsupported enamel prisms at the cavity edge (C). (D) If the amalgam margin angle is too acute, the amalgam margin may be sufficiently weakened for marginal fracture to occur under occlusal loading. Note the internal rounded line angles in all the cavities depicted. It is always important to check the occlusal record before restoring a tooth to try to ensure these margins are not placed under direct occlusal load where possible.

TABLE 5.10   Potential Cavity Modifications Required After Caries Removal and Their Purpose[a]

Restorative Material	Cavity Modification		Purpose
Resin composite/GIC	*Macro*	*Enamel margin bevel (short or long)*	Removes grossly unsupported prisms. Increases surface area for bond/seal. Provides a sound enamel surface to facilitate optimal adhesive bonding (Figs. 5.49, 5.50 and 5.56B).
Resin composite	*Micro*	*Acid etch (37% orthophosphoric acid)*	Enamel: removes smear layer, demineralises prism boundaries creating micromechanical undercuts for adhesive penetration. Dentine: removes smear layer, open dentine tubule orifices, demineralises superficial dentine exposing collagen network, increases surface area for adhesive penetration around exposed collagen and into patent dentine tubules.
GIC	*Micro*	*Dentine conditioner*	10% polyacrylic/citric acid, modifies or removes smear layer, optimising dentine surface for chemical adhesion (Ca^{2+}).
All	*Macro*	*Rounded internal line angles/ smooth cavity surfaces*	Reduces both internal stresses and risk of crack propagation within the body of the restoration (Figs. 5.56–5.60).
Dental amalgam	*Macro*	*Cavity undercuts, grooves, slots, flat surfaces*	Cavities with wider bases than orifices are required for retention of amalgam (undercuts). Slots and grooves cut into cavity walls or floor help prevent further displacement of the restoration (Figs. 5.58 and 5.59). Flat cavity surfaces with rounded internal line angles help improve internal cavity support (Fig. 5.60).
All	*Macro*	*Pulp chamber in endodontically treated teeth*	Pulp chamber is used to add restoration bulk, retentive features and increased surface area for adhesion for the coronal restoration.
Dental amalgam	*Macro*	*Nayyar core*	Packing the coronally flared 2–3 mm of endodontically treated root canals to improve core retention.
Indirect cast gold, porcelain, resin composite restorations	*Macro*	*Long marginal taper*	Divergent tapered laterally opposing cavity walls (7–10 degrees) used to aid insertion and to improve retentive features of indirect restorations (see Chapter 6, Section 6.5).

[a]The modifications have been classified as *macro* (those created using a bur or hand instrument) or *micro* (those created using chemicals). Dentine pins have been omitted as there are no justifiable clinical indications for their use in contemporary minimally invasive dentistry. See Chapter 7 for a description of the material science and Chapter 8 for practical step-by-step guides. *GIC*, Glass-ionomer cement.

- Thermal and/or electrical stimulation via conductance through the overlying restoration

If the floor of the cavity is close to the pulp but the pulp chamber has not been breached during MI carious tissue removal, then this protection can be afforded by a process termed *indirect pulp capping/protection (IPC)*. If a small breach, or *pulp exposure*, has occurred (usually no wider than the tip of a Williams periodontal probe), created either iatrogenically or due to the caries process, a *direct pulp cap (DPC)* may be placed in an attempt to maintain pulp sensibility, but the patient must be warned that this is not guaranteed, especially when this is a consequence of a deep carious lesion (Fig. 5.61).

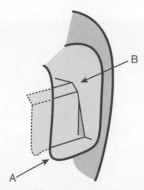

Fig. 5.57 Diagram indicating the internal bevelling/rounding off of the internal line angles between adjacent internal cavity surfaces *(A and B)*. This reduces the risk of crack propagation within the restorative material.

5.10.2 Terminology

Historically, two terms are used synonymously in the dental literature to describe this form of material-based pulp protection where an exposure has not occurred: *cavity lining* and *structural base*. These terms were coined when dental amalgam was the only material of choice to restore cavities long term and it was thought the pulp required an 'insulating' layer between it and the metal-based restoration. The excessively large, undercut cavities designed for dental amalgam could be artificially reduced in size by placing zinc oxide-based plastic materials as 'structural bases' on to which was packed a reduced volume of amalgam. In the contemporary era of

minimally invasive operative dentistry, these terms are no longer relevant or applicable.

5.10.3 Materials

Materials used for both IPC and DPC should ideally:

- Be bacteriocidal (able to kill bacteria) and bacteriostatic (prevent them from multiplying)
- Be mildly irritant to the pulp to stimulate a cellular response with tertiary dentine bridge formation (usually via pH changes)
- Be adhesive to affect a bond and seal
- Not dissolve away over time
- Be easily applied and strong in thin sections
- Be able to ionically infiltrate into the remaining dentine overlying the pulp, thus strengthening/reinforcing it
- Be biocompatible with the pulp and the overlying restorative material

Clinical dental materials used for IPC/DPC (see Chapter 7) include:

- Glass-ionomer cements (GICs)
- Dentine bonding agents and adhesives
- Setting calcium hydroxide
- Tricalcium silicate cements (e.g., Biodentine)

The first two materials fulfil the majority of the criteria of an ideal IPC mentioned earlier. When using

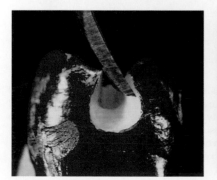
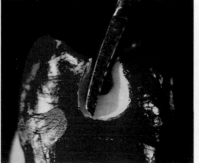
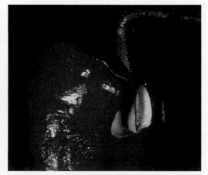

Fig. 5.58 A proximal box cavity prepared with retentive undercuts (a wider base and a narrower occlusal opening) to prevent displacement of the restoration (amalgam) occlusally, from its path of insertion.

Q5.58: Which hand instrument is being used in Fig. 5.58?

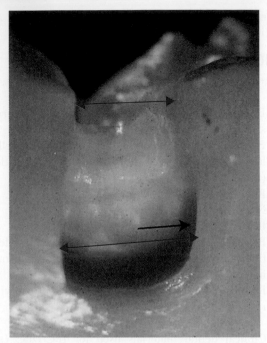

Fig. 5.59 A proximal box cavity prepared with occlusal under-cuts (wider base, narrow occlusal opening; *red arrows*) to prevent displacement of the restoration (amalgam) from its path of insertion occlusally. Note the rounded internal line angles. The black arrow shows the placement of a groove at the junction between the buccal wall of the box and the pulpal wall, thus providing stability (resistance) to proximal displacement.

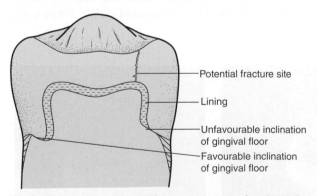

Fig. 5.60 Potential problems of the morphology of cavity walls and floor, requiring modification. Rounded internal line angles reduce the risk of crack propagation and eventual restoration fracture of rigid materials (e.g., amalgam). Use of a rose-head bur to remove carious dentine tends to create the cavity floor morphology on the left, but care must be taken to remove any very prominent unsupported enamel lip at the periphery. The floor morphology on the right offers limited support to the final restoration and should be avoided.

Potential fracture site

Lining

Unfavourable inclination of gingival floor

Favourable inclination of gingival floor

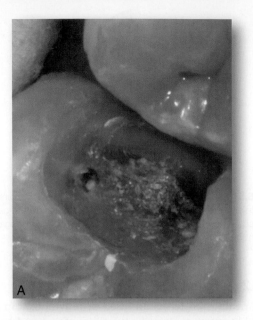

A

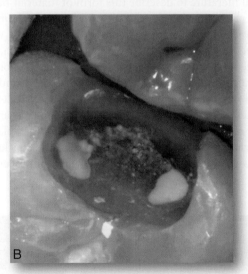

B

Fig. 5.61 (A) Caries excavated from a proximal lesion in a vital tooth with residual caries-affected dentine evident on the pulpal aspect of the cavity. Note the spot of blood exuding from a small carious exposure through the pulp horn. (B) Setting calcium hydroxide has been placed as a direct pulp cap/protection. (Courtesy of L Mackenzie.)

Q5.61: After placing the direct pulp cap as shown, what are the next steps in the restoration of this cavity?

these adhesive materials as the final restorative solution, it can be argued that a separate thin layer of pulp protection is not necessary as the properties are 'built into' the bulk restorative material itself. Setting calcium hydroxide cements have been used for many years as pulp protection beneath dental amalgam restorations but in recent times, more sparingly. The author cannot suggest any positive indications for its use beneath adhesive restorations, as an IPC, in contemporary clinical practice. GICs and resin-based cements are being used in bonded amalgam restorations, so again, the use of calcium hydroxide is ever more limited in this regard. As a DPC, the alkaline pH of setting calcium hydroxide still has a use as an inflammatory stimulant for pulp odontoblasts to produce tertiary dentine and thus help to biologically close the exposure. Unset mineralised trioxide aggregate (MTA) is primarily calcium oxide in the form of tricalcium silicate, dicalcium silicate and tricalcium aluminate, with bismuth oxide added for radio-opacity. Several studies have indicated its potential use as a DPC as it increases the concentration of available calcium hydroxide, the primary reaction product between MTA and water, as well as providing a seal. However, its high solubility, long setting time (up to 3 hours) and expense are disadvantages. Both setting calcium hydroxide cements and MTA need a protective covering prior to placing the final restoration. This is conventionally a GIC/resin-modified (RM)-GIC material (Chapter 7, Section 7.4). A faster-setting (9–12 minutes) calcium

trisilicate restorative cement, Biodentine, incorporates these pulp protection properties within its bulk restorative properties (see Chapter 7, Section 7.7).

Interestingly, clinical evidence now shows that retained caries-affected dentine overlying an acutely inflamed but viable pulp provides the optimum qualities of indirect biological pulp protection as long as the overlying adhesive restoration affords an adequate seal and the patient can maintain adequate oral hygiene and other preventive measures.

5.11 DENTAL MATRICES

Cavities created with missing proximal walls provide a technical problem when it comes to placing a direct plastic restoration, as there is nothing to contain the restorative material within the cavity or to prevent poor marginal adaptation during placement (ledges, overhangs, surface contour and contact point formation). This clinical problem can be overcome with the judicious use and placement of dental matrix bands (see also Chapter 8).

Two types of dental matrix bands are available for clinical use:

- *Circumferential* matrix bands with retainers (e.g., reusable Siqveland and Tofflemire; disposable AutoMatrix and Omni-matrix [Fig. 5.62A]) or without retainers (e.g., copper rings, AutoMatrix or SuperMat matrices [Fig. 5.62B])

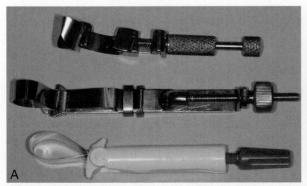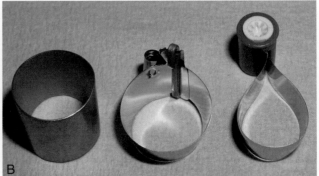

Fig. 5.62 (A) Three examples of circumferential metal matrix bands with retainers: Tofflemire retainer with precured matrix band *(top)*; Siqveland retainer with matrix band *(middle)*; Omni-matrix disposable system *(bottom)*. (B) Three examples of circumferential matrices without retainers: copper ring, AutoMatrix and SuperMat systems.

- *Sectional* matrix bands that are placed on a single proximal surface (e.g., Palodent, Composi-Tight, V-Ring, QuickMat amongst others).

Traditional dental matrix systems consist of two components:

- *Single-use matrix band*: Thin metal or clear plastic band of varying widths and gauges (30–50 μm) used to form the missing wall of the cavity. More rigid and wider bands are used posteriorly (metal) and narrower pliable, transparent plastic bands are used anteriorly (for resin composites, to enable some light transmission proximally when photo-curing resin-based materials).
- *Retainer*: A device used to tighten and hold matrix bands in place proximally. These can be sterilised and used again. Sectional matrix systems have oval or round ring retainers with curved tines to adapt the matrix to the proximal tooth contour (Fig. 5.63).

5.11.1 Clinical Tips

- Cervical margin adaptation of the matrix band to the tooth is essential to prevent ledges or overhangs of excess restorative material, often achieved using wooden or plastic wedges in the interproximal space placed either buccally or lingual/palatally as is convenient. Liquid dam may also be used to stabilise a sectional matrix band in position, helping with this cervical adaptation to the natural tooth surface.
- Tight interdental contact points may need to be opened slightly by causing differential movement of

the adjacent teeth within their periodontal ligament spaces. This is accomplished by pre-wedging using wooden wedges or orthodontic separators for a few minutes prior to placing the band.

- Sectional matrices may be of benefit in situations where teeth are rotated or tilted, thus making the placement of circumferential bands more difficult.
- Sectional bands are importantly more adaptable to create anatomically contoured proximal surfaces and contact areas.
- Circumferential bands can be more painful for the patient to endure than equivalent sectional bands.
- Clear plastic matrix bands and wedges can be used when placing resin composite restorations to permit light penetration to the depths of the proximal cavity when curing the material.
- Rubber dam clamps may have to be removed prior to placing matrix bands, although some designs now allow space for the matrix band retainers.
- Anteriorly, if contact areas are tight and the flexible, clear plastic matrix band refuses to pass through in an incisal direction, the end of the clear matrix band can be cut at an angle to a point and then passed cervically beneath the contact and lifted incisally through it.
- Cervical metal or transparent matrices can be used to develop the surface contour of buccal cervical restorations in anterior and posterior teeth. They can be flexible and adaptable by the clinician to the ideal anatomical surface contour required. Tapering margins allow subgingival placement with little or no excess outflow of material during adaptation (Fig. 5.64).

5.11.2 Silicone Matrices, Stents and Splints

Contemporary aesthetic Class IV buildups of anterior teeth (those cavities or fractures involving the proximal and incisal edges of anterior teeth) are commonly restored using direct resin composite restorations in the first instance. This will depend on (1) the size of the defect to be restored, (2) the quality and quantity of the tooth structure remaining for the restorative material to adhere to and be supported by and (3) the occlusion.

If a set of original study casts are available of the sound tooth or teeth that have been damaged subsequently, a lingual/palatal addition-cured silicone putty, directly hand-adapted mould of that original cast model can be made. This should include the lingual/palatal

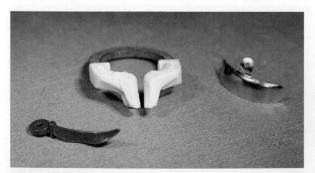

Fig. 5.63 A pre-curved and contoured single-use sectional metal matrix band *(right)* with a plastic gingivally contoured wedge *(left)* and the oval ring retainer with curved tines *(middle)* to adapt the band to the approximal surface of the tooth. The retainer can be sterilised.

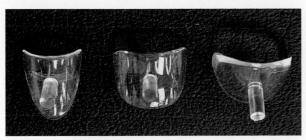

Fig. 5.64 Examples of different configurations of cervical matrices to help contour buccal cervical smooth surface restorations (Class V). Transparent matrices will allow photo-curing through them if required, prior to their removal from the restoration surface. Shown here is the Hawe Transparent Cervical Matrix system.

surfaces of the tooth in question and at least two adjacent sound teeth on either side (to help with locating the set putty mould in the mouth), proximal embrasure contours between the teeth and incorporating/overlapping the incisal edges, just encroaching onto the labial surface. Once set, this flexible lingual/palatal mould can be removed from the study model and located intra-orally to provide the morphologically natural palatal outline of the now damaged tooth. This is used, with finger pressure, to support the first increments of resin composite placed to form the appropriate lingual/palatal contoured surface, proximal and incisal extension of the restoration. Once the resin composite is photo-cured, the mould can be removed and the restoration built up normally (see later).

If pre-operative study models of the intact teeth are not available, then full arch impressions of both the maxillary and mandibular dentition can be taken in suitably fitting stock trays. Plaster models of the teeth could then be cast in a dental laboratory (either on site or sent to a commercial dental laboratory with appropriate instructions for the dental technician to follow). The dental technician can then build up the defects with wax in the laboratory to the specific contour and occlusion required. Either a silicone matrix or a clear, acrylic, rigid, blow-down laboratory splint incorporating the artificially restored tooth/teeth can be manufactured. The clinician can then use this silicone matrix/pre-fabricated clear splint to rebuild the damaged tooth/teeth to the correct morphology and contour (Fig. 5.65A–C). With advances in digital dentistry workflows, intra-oral scans could replace the need for impressions. These scans can be sent wirelessly to the dental technician who could digitally build up the defect(s) and 3D-print the splint in the laboratory, ready for the clinician to use.

Sectional silicone matrices can also be used as an objective guide to the amount of coronal tooth reduction carried out when preparing a tooth for an indirect full-coverage coronal restoration or crown. A silicone putty mould is taken of the tooth to be prepared and the adjacent teeth, encompassing the whole tooth, prior to treatment starting. Once set, the putty impression in trimmed to remove any gingival excess and is then cut with a blade, through the centre of the tooth in a bucco-lingual/palatal direction. Once the coronal reduction has taken place, this sectioned putty matrix is replaced onto the tooth and a space should now be evident where the tooth reduction has taken place. From this, the operator can accurately visualise the extent of coronal tooth reduction on the buccal, occlusal and lingual/palatal surfaces and adjust this as required (Fig. 5.65D).

5.11.3 'Stamp' Matrix Technique

This is an occlusal matrix technique that allows the practitioner to duplicate the natural morphology of posterior teeth, where the intact occlusal surface morphology is present prior to any operative intervention. This in turn means the final restoration will conform to the patient's existing occlusal scheme and should not need occlusal adjustment after placement and curing/setting.

Essentially, the steps to create and use the pattern or 'stamp' of the intact occlusal surface are as follows (see Fig. 5.66A–I):

- After rubber dam placement, a separating medium is painted onto the tooth surface (e.g., soap or other proprietary separating medium).
- Low viscosity utility light-cured resin or hard-setting liquid dam material is flowed over the intact occlusal surface of the tooth, just overlapping the buccal or lingual/palatal cusps that are to be spared during cavity preparation, to aid accurate relocation of the stamp back onto the tooth later.
- A bur or microbrush handle is inserted into the material and then light-cured in place, to act as a handle to hold and position the stamp. The stamp is then removed from the tooth.
- The cavity is prepared according to minimally invasive principles, either occlusal or proximo-occlusal as indicated.

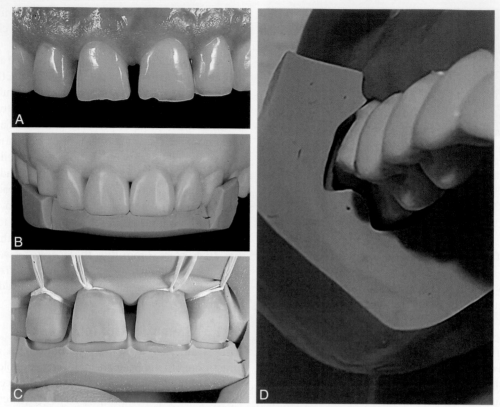

Fig. 5.65 (A) Clinical view of a maxillary anterior sextant with incisal toothwear and diastemas. (B) A study cast has been poured from an impression of the teeth and the technician has built up the teeth on the model in wax to their final shape, building up the incisal edges, diastemas and labial contour. A silicone palatal matrix/mould/stent has then been created from lab putty and trimmed accordingly. (C) After the resin composite shade has been clinically recorded, a rubber dam has been placed with floss retention/adaptation cervically and the palatal putty matrix has been located. The outline for the additional resin composite can now be clearly seen and accurate adaptation of the material is straightforward. (Courtesy A Chandrapal.) (D) A sectioned silicone putty matrix used as a tissue-reduction index when assessing the final indirect crown preparation. The putty matrix was taken as an impression of the original tooth before it was reduced for a full-coverage indirect crown.

- A proximal matrix band is placed and wedged accordingly as required and the proximal box(es) can then be restored with direct plastic flowable materials (e.g., resin composite, RM-GIC, etc.) in the standard way.
- The final occlusal increment of uncured restorative material is placed and the proximal matrix band(s) removed.
- PTFE (Teflon) tape is placed to cover the unset material (Fig. 5.66G).
- The occlusal stamp is then relocated on the tooth using the cuspal overlap to act as a guide for correct replacement. Using the bur/brush handle, firm finger pressure is applied, thus re-creating the natural original occlusal surface anatomy of the tooth.
- The stamp and Teflon tape are removed, any excess material is removed with a suitable hand instrument, the proximal surfaces are flossed accordingly and the restorative material (e.g., resin composite) is then finally light-cured.
- The occlusion can then be checked using articulating paper and the restoration finished accordingly.

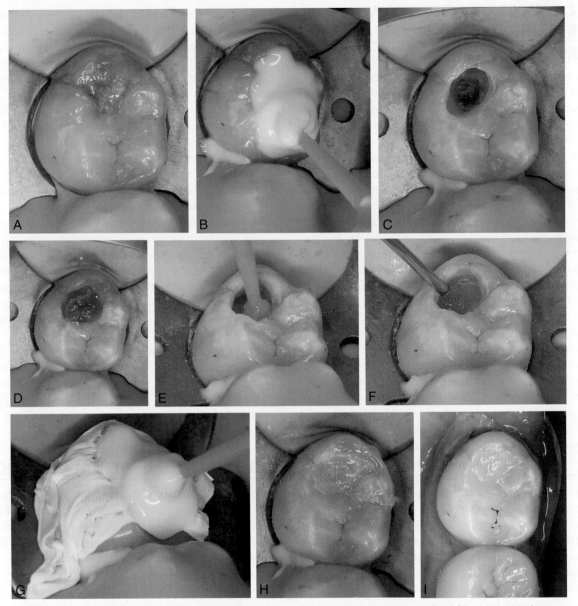

Fig. 5.66 Restoring a carious LR7 with resin composite using the stamp technique. (A) The LR7 on presentation in a high caries risk adolescent patient, with an occlusal, non-cavitated carious lesion evident with symptoms of acute pulpitis (modified International Caries Detection and Assessment System 2; ICCMS late initial/early moderate lesion). (B) Utility LC block-out resin is flowed into the previously debrided occlusal surface to pick up the occlusal surface anatomy detail and light-cured. Then a microbrush is incorporated into further cured layers to act as the stamp handle. (C) Minimally invasive carious dentine excavation is carried out on the LR7, creating a Class I occlusal cavity ready for restoration. (D) A 37% orthophosphoric acid etch is placed on the enamel for 20 seconds and then dentine for 15 seconds. (E) After washing off the acid etch and drying, dentine bonding agent is agitated onto the cavity walls and floor. (F) After photo-curing, the bulk-fill resin composite is syringed into the cavity. (G) Once the cavity is completely filled, PTFE (Teflon) tape is placed over the final uncured resin composite increment and the occlusal stamp is replaced. (H) The occlusal morphology imprinted into the resin composite. After removing the Teflon tape, any excess material can be removed prior to the final photo-cure. (I) The final restoration of the LR7 without the need for any occlusal adjustment. (Courtesy of Dr Ali Salehi of France.)

5.12 TEMPORARY/PROVISIONAL RESTORATIONS

5.12.1 Definitions

A *temporary restoration* is one that is placed for short-term use (usually days or weeks) often between appointments in a course of ongoing definitive treatment (e.g., caries stabilisation, multi-visit root canal treatment, simple fixed prosthodontics).

A *provisional (intermediate) restoration* is one that is placed for a short- or medium-term duration (weeks to months) where diagnostic value is gained from placing the restoration (e.g., complex fixed prosthodontic treatment when reorganising a patient's occlusion or adjusting the vertical dimension of the patient's occlusion (see later); stabilising caries to negate symptoms whilst non-operative preventive behaviours are reinforced and patient behavioural adherence is assessed; active surveillance/phased care).

A *definitive restoration* ideally should be the final restoration placed, with the correct materials, aesthetics, function and finish. Avoid using the term *permanent restoration* as nothing we do as clinical operative interventions are ever permanent! The medium- to long-term management of such definitive tooth-restoration complexes is discussed in Chapter 9.

The dental biomaterial science of temporary restorations (GIC, zinc oxide-eugenol and zinc polycarboxylates) is covered in Chapter 7, Section 7.6. Eugenol-containing temporary restorations should be avoided in cavities where the definitive restoration to be placed is a resin composite as the eugenol can adversely affect the resins' polymerisation chemistry.

Thanks to developments in dental biomaterials, there is now overlap in the properties of materials that could be used for both provisional and definitive restorations. Therefore the definitions of provisional and definitive restorations may become blurred clinically, especially when considering the management of carious lesions.

5.12.2 Clinical Tips

- Care must be taken when placing intermediate restorations to replicate the occlusion and marginal adaptation of the final restoration (e.g., a temporary crown or stabilising direct restorations). This is especially relevant at margins close to the gingivae. If there is poor adaptation of the temporary restoration in this area, there is a risk that the plaque

biofilm will stagnate due to poor oral hygiene in the short term, causing the gingivae to become acutely inflamed (acute gingivitis) and be prone to bleeding. This will ultimately compromise the clinical placement of the definitive restoration at potentially the next visit.

- Zinc oxide–based materials have a relatively poor appearance, so in the anterior aesthetic zone, GIC-based materials might be considered.

- Patients must be made fully aware of the reason and function of the temporary, intermediate or provisional restoration and that it will need replacing as part of the definitive treatment.

- Adequate time must be allocated in the clinical appointment to place temporary restorations. Poor-quality marginal adaptation of temporary indirect crowns, for example, can lead to further marginal staining, plaque accumulation and gingival inflammation/bleeding which in turn makes the cementation of the definitive crown more complicated to manage.

- Frustratingly, if provisional restorations have optimal aesthetics and function, patients may not wish to have them replaced with their definitive counterparts! It is essential that all personalised care plans and conversations are documented carefully in the patient's notes.

5.13 PRINCIPLES OF DENTAL OCCLUSION

To successfully restore dental function in the long term, an understanding of human dental occlusion is of primary importance. This subject is complex and many textbooks exist discussing these complexities and their clinical relevance. The occlusal contacts between the maxillary and mandibular dentition are affected by the skeletal base relationship (condylar head vs. slope of the articular eminence, glenoid fossa), development of the maxilla and mandible and direct factors affecting the development, position and shape of the teeth themselves. Analysis of occlusion is critical in both the *conformative* and *reorganised* approaches to managing dental care.

5.13.1 Definitions

The *conformative approach* to planning and placing restorations ensures the pre-existing occlusal relationships are not altered in any of the three planes (antero-posterior, vertical and horizontal). It is essential therefore to analyse aspects of the occlusion both statically and dynamically prior to commencing so that the final restorations fit into the existing occlusal scheme. This approach most often applies when placing single or multiple plastic, direct restorations or single-unit indirect restorations.

The *reorganised approach* involves changes in the dimensions of occlusion and is often undertaken when rehabilitating major occlusal discrepancies caused by tilting or overeruption of teeth, resulting in premature occlusal interference contacts and/or distortion of the occlusal planes causing reduced interdental space into which to place definitive restorations. Here again considerable planning with the use of provisional restorations is required to calculate the tolerances of

changing the occlusal scheme. This approach is usually indicated in complex prosthodontic cases often involving the use of multiple indirect restorations (crowns, bridges, dentures or implants) and is beyond the scope of this textbook.

5.13.2 Terminology

The terminology used commonly and recorded positions of occlusal analysis are described in Table 5.11.

5.13.3 Occlusal Registration Techniques

The various static and dynamic relationships of the patient's occlusion should be analysed before starting any restorative procedure in the conformative approach to dental care provision, as well as checking again after the restoration(s) has been completed. Many different

---

TABLE 5.11 Occlusal Relationships, Their Definitions and Relevance to Restorative Dentistry

Occlusal Relationship	Definition	Diagram/Comments
Intercuspal position (ICP) **Static**	The occlusal relationship where there is maximum cusp interdigitation between the maxillary and mandibular teeth.	Not always clinically reproducible and can be affected by occlusal interferences.
Occlusal vertical dimension (OVD) **Static**	The vertical relationship between the maxilla and mandible with the teeth in the ICP	Can be reduced by toothwear, missing teeth. Can be compensated biologically by overeruption of teeth/dento-alveolar compensation.
Rest position (RP) **Static**	The vertical relationship between the maxilla and mandible when resting comfortably in an upright position with relaxed facial musculature.	Achieved after swallowing or yawning. Teeth usually slightly apart.
Freeway space (FS) **Static**	The vertical dimension difference between RP and ICP (can range between 0 and 4 mm).	Adaptive in the dentate patient. Essential consideration for the restoration of the edentate individual with complete dentures.
Overjet (OJ) **Static**	The horizontal distance between the maxillary and mandibular incisal edges in the ICP.	

Continued

TABLE 5.11   Occlusal Relationships, Their Definitions and Relevance to Restorative Dentistry—cont'd

Occlusal Relationship	Definition	Diagram/Comments
Overbite (OB) **Static**	The vertical distance between the maxillary and mandibular incisal edges in the ICP. No vertical overlap can lead to an edge–edge incisal relationship or an anterior open bite.	
Retruded contact position (RCP) **Dynamic**	The most retruded position of the mandible when there is initial cusp contact (described as the relationship where the condylar heads are rearmost within their glenoid fossae and rotate about their terminal hinge axis or *centric relation*).	A clinically reproducible and registerable position used in the dental rehabilitation of the edentulous patient as well as in the reorganised approach in the dentate patient.
Lateral excursions **Dynamic**	Occlusal relationship between the teeth when the mandible is shifted horizontally to the right or left. Working side: the side to which the mandible has moved. Non-working side: the side away from which the mandible has moved.	Horizontal movement guided by working side: 1. Palatal/labial surface guidance of canines/incisors 2. Cuspal inclines of premolars/molars 3. A combination of both (group function) Horizontal movement may also be guided by non-working side contacts and condylar head–glenoid fossae relationships.
Protrusion **Dynamic**	The anterior or forward movement of the mandible with teeth in occlusion.	Usually guided by the palatal contour of the maxillary incisors. Leads to a posterior open bite (Christensen's phenomenon).

clinical techniques are available for checking direct occlusal contact relationships in the patient's mouth:

- *Articulating paper*: Ranges from 40 to 200 μm in thickness. Different colours show up contact areas between cusp inclines and fossae on occlusion (Fig. 5.67).
- *Shimstock*: Articulating foil (8 μm) for the fine occlusal adjustment of indirect coronal restorations.
- *Clinical observation*: To assess dental contacts around the arch prior to removing an old or damaged restoration and to ensure these are replicated with the new restoration, especially in the partially dentate.

5.13.4 Clinical Tips

- Occlusion must be checked both *before* and *after* placement of any restoration affecting the occlusal

or guide plane surfaces of teeth. Different colour articulating paper can be used in this regard. This is essential in the conformative approach to dental care provision.
- Occlusal surfaces should be dried with cotton wool rolls (Fig. 5.67A).
- Occlusion must be checked dynamically as well as statically. Patients must be asked to 'grind' their teeth side to side and back to front to check that the guidance paths are free from interferences.
- Even though some authorities classify the buccal cusps of the mandibular teeth and palatal cusps of the maxillary dentition as *functional cusps*, it must be realised that all cusps, ridges and fossae have an important role to play in a harmonious dynamic occlusion.

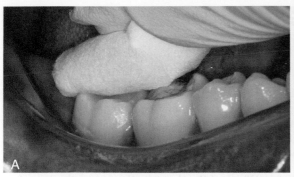
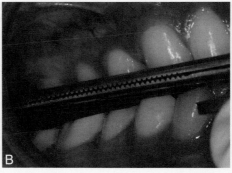
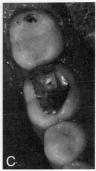

Fig. 5.67 (A) Occlusal surfaces of the LR quadrant being dried with a cotton wool roll. (B) Articulating paper held in forceps placed on occlusal surfaces. The patient is asked to bite together in the intercuspal position and slide the teeth left and right. (C) Heavy occlusal cusp–fossa contact shown on the distal occlusal aspect of the LR7. The red mark indicates indirect pulp capping, with lateral excursions shown in black. This can now be removed selectively with a rotary instrument.

Q5.67A: Why is it important to dry the teeth prior to using dental articulating paper?

Q5.67B: What mandibular movements should the patient be encouraged to make when checking the occlusion using articulating paper?

5.14 ANSWERS TO SELF-TEST QUESTIONS

Q5.2: What piece of equipment is the clinician wearing that will aid their posture while examining the patient?
A: Dental magnification loupes with a fixed visual working length ensures the dentist maintains an optimal posture. See Section 5.7.

Q5.7: Can you spot the gold crown?
A: It is present on the upper right-hand side of the radiograph—the the discrete radio-opacity.

Q5.13D: Can you spot an important clinical addition to the loupes in Fig. 5.13D?
A: There is a clear plastic face shield/visor adapted for use with the loupes to protect the operator from aerosols generated during operative procedures without affecting the vision through the loupes themselves.

Q5.19A: What might this patient complain of once the clamp has been placed?
A: Note the blanching of the mesiolingual papilla/gingiva. This could well be painful for the patient during and soon after placement of the dam. Usually this initial discomfort eases after a few minutes.

Q5.19E: Which teeth is this clamp designed to be used on?
A: Note the broader jaw of the clamp. This should be placed on the buccal surface of a molar tooth. The narrower dimension of the other jaw is adapted for the palatal

surface ideally of an upper posterior tooth. Therefore, if ideally and correctly positioned with the connector distally positioned, this clamp is optimally designed for use on the URQ. That does not mean it cannot be used for other teeth, however, depending on the variability in coronal shape and morphology of human teeth.

Q5.23: In which clinical situations might you use each of these probes?
A: Straight probe: clinical examination of restoration margins and exposed carious dentine; Briault probe: proximal surfaces, internal cavity walls; Williams probe: periodontal pocket assessment, clinical exam of tooth surfaces; Naber's probe: periodontal furcation measurement; CPITN probe: periodontal assessment, clinical examination of tooth surfaces.

Q5.26: What are the advantages of having angulations between the working head and shank of these instruments?
A: To enable the operator to access all aspects of a cavity, undercut or undermined areas as well as off-setting the handle to allow better direct visual access to instrumentation.

Q5.32: What might be the advantages and disadvantages of single-use, disposable burs?
A: Advantages: improved infection control, no maintenance required. Disadvantages: potential long-term cost, possible concerns about quality control over the precision in manufacture, availability of all types of bur.

Continued

5.14 ANSWERS TO SELF-TEST QUESTIONS—cont'd

Q5.41: What clinical situations may benefit from using air-abrasion tooth preparation?
A: Minimally invasive dentistry procedures: diagnosing and treating carious fissures in high-risk patients with unmodifiable risk factors, tooth preparation for direct labial composite veneers, all tooth surface pretreatment prior to adhesive bonding, stain removal/refreshing surfaces of old composites, potential selective enamel/dentine caries removal (with bioactive glass particles; in development).

Q5.42: What name might be given to the type of restoration placed in Fig. 5.42B?
A: Class I occlusal restoration, therapeutic sealant restoration, preventive resin restoration.

Q5.44: Can you explain why the decision was made to retain such relatively large quantities of caries-affected dentine, especially at the gingival periphery of this particular lesion?
A: This was a conscious decision as an intact enamel periphery was present to create an adhesive seal. If the carious dentine was removed at the EDJ (as normal) this would result in a cavity margin that would be located on root dentine at least 3 to 4 mm subgingivally, with no enamel present. Moisture control would then be impossible, no seal achievable, and the tooth/cavity would be unrestorable. By retaining this affected dentine, the tooth (dentine-pulp complex) has been given the opportunity to heal itself, with suitable input from the patient as regards to oral hygiene and dietary concerns.

Q5.47: Can you identify the radiolucency beneath the restoration on the occlusal aspect of the LR6? What might this indicate?
A: The differential diagnosis of the radiolucency beneath the restoration on the LR6 will of course also be dependent upon your clinical examination and signs and symptoms from the patient's history. If the restoration has poor-quality margins, with accompanying biofilm stagnation in a high caries risk/susceptible patient as this, the radiolucency might be indicative of progressing caries associated with restorations and sealants (CARS, secondary caries). This may be associated with symptoms of acute pulpitis, but not always. However, the radiolucency might also be caused by the retention of relatively demineralised caries-affected dentine during selective caries removal, the placement of a radiolucent pulp protection material or excess pooling of dental adhesive during the dentine bonding procedure.

Some biointeractive restorative materials can also affect the underlying dentine (e.g., Biodentine, creating a possible radiolucent effect on a radiograph).

Q5.49: What is the name given to the histological appearance of the alternating light and dark stripes evident in the inner third of enamel, arising from the EDJ and radiating towards the tooth surface?
A: Hunter–Schreger bands.

Q5.54: Which of the three depths do you think would be best to stop carious dentine removal in the above lesion?
A: Probably the second level (light green line) on caries-affected dentine where the collagen has partial structure to enable some form of dentine bonding to take place and the periphery histological status will allow a seal to be achieved, while not encroaching on the pulp and risking exposure. The red line would result in a restoration with minimum bulk for strength and supported by a softer layer of underlying dentine. Such a thin but rigid restoration may be more prone to fracture under occlusal loading (imagine walking on a thin sheet of glass placed on a soft mattress; what would happen?).

Q5.58: Which hand instrument is shown in Fig. 5.58?
A: Gingival margin trimmer.

Q5.61: After placing the direct pulp cap as shown, what are the next steps in the restoration of this cavity?
A: The setting calcium hydroxide should be protected with a layer of GIC/RM-GIC. Then the adhesive restorative procedure—etch, bond and placement of a resin composite restoration—can be carried out.

Q5.67A: Why is it important to dry the teeth prior to using dental articulating paper?
A: To allow the ink from the paper to adhere to and mark the teeth in discrete areas of tooth–tooth contact.

Q5.67B: What mandibular movements should the patient be encouraged to make when checking the occlusion using articulating paper?
A: Vertical intercuspal position (patient should bite up and down) and lateral excursions (patient should be asked to grind their teeth side to side to assess the cuspal inclines guiding the occlusion in these directions).

REFERENCES

1. General Dental Council. Scope of Practice. https://www.gdc-uk.org/docs/default-source/scope-of-practice/scope-of-practice.pdf

2. Young S, Dawett B, Gallie A, Banerjee A, Deery C. Minimum intervention oral care delivery for children – developing the oral healthcare team. *Dent Update.* 2022 May;49(5):424–430. doi:10.12968/denu.2022.49.5.424.

3. British Dental Journal first minimum intervention-themed issue, 2017, vol 223,3: https://www.nature.com/bdj/volumes/223/issues/3

4. British Dental Journal second minimum intervention-themed issue, 2020, vol 229, 7: https://www.nature.com/bdj/volumes/229/issues/7

5. Schwendicke F, Frencken JE, Bjorndal L, et al. Managing caries lesions: consensus recommendations on carious tissue removal. *Adv Dent Res.* 2016;28:58–67.

6. Innes NPT, Frencken JE, Bjorndal L, et al. Managing caries lesions: consensus recommendations on terminology. *Adv Dent Res.* 2016;28:49–57.

7. Machiulskiene V, Campus G, Carvalho J, et al. Terminology of Dental Caries and Dental Caries Management: Consensus Report of a Workshop Organized by ORCA and Cariology Research Group of IADR. *Caries Res.* 2020;54:7–14. doi:10.1159/000503309.

8. Banerjee A, Frencken JE, Schwendicke F, Innes NPT. Contemporary operative caries management: consensus recommendations on minimally invasive caries removal. *Brit Dent J.* 2017;223:215–222.

9. European Society of Endodontology (ESE) developed by Duncan HF, Galler KM, et al. European Society of Endodontology position statement: Management of deep caries and the exposed pulp. *Int Endod J.* 2019;52(7):923–934. doi:10.1111/iej.13080.

10. Brit Dent J. Toothwear-themed issue: Volume 224, Issue 5, March 2018.

11. Schwendicke F, Splieth C, Breschi L et al. When to intervene in the caries process? An expert Delphi consensus statement. *Clin Oral Invest.* 2019: 23: 3691–3703.

12. Banerjee A et al., *Brit Dent J.* 2020; 229: 474–482.

13. Splieth CH, Banerjee A, Bottenberg P et al. How to intervene in the caries process in children? A joint ORCA and EFCD expert Delphi consensus statement. *Caries Res.* 2020; 54: 297-305. https://doi.org/10.1159/000507692.

14. Splieth CH, Kanzow P, Wiegand A, Schmoeckel J, Jablonski-Momeni A. How to intervene in the caries process: proximal caries in adolescents and adults - a systematic review and meta-analysis. *Clin Oral Invest.* 2020: online https://doi.org/10.1007/s00784-020-03201-y.

15. Schwendicke F, Splieth CH, Bottenberg P et al. How to intervene in the caries process in adults? An EFCD-ORCA-DGZ expert Delphi consensus statement. *Clin Oral Invest.* 2020; 24(9): 3315–3321.

16. Paris S, Banerjee A, Bottenberg P et al. How to intervene in the caries process in older adults? A joint ORCA and EFCD expert Delphi consensus statement. *Caries Res.* 2020; 54: 459–465. https://doi.org/10.1159/000510843

17. Askar H, Krois J, Göstemeyer G, et al. Secondary caries: What is it, and how can it be controlled, detected and managed? *Clin Oral Invest.* 2020;24:1869–1876. doi:10.1007/s00784-020-03268-7.

18. Costa RL, Bendo CB, Daher A, et al. A curriculum for behaviour and oral healthcare management for dentally anxious children – recommendations from the Children Experiencing Dental Anxiety: Collaboration on Research and Education (CEDACORE). *Int J Paed Dent.* 2020;30(5):556–569.

19. Martignon S, Pitts NB, Goffin G, et al. CariesCare Practice Guide: Consensus on Evidence into Practice. *Brit Dent J.* 2019;227:353–362.

20. HTM01-05: https://www.england.nhs.uk/publication/decontamination-in-primary-care-dental-practices-htm-01-05/

6

MIOC Domain 3: MI Operative Management of the Badly Broken Down Tooth

6.1 CAUSES OF BROKEN DOWN TEETH

This textbook has described and discussed the common causes of broken down teeth: dental caries, tooth wear and trauma. In addition, long-term failure of parts or all of the existing tooth-restoration complex can be significant and may require further operative intervention for its successful management (see Chapter 9, Section 9.4). Many intra-coronal defects can be repaired with direct adhesive restorations, as discussed in Chapters 5 and 9. However, the situation can be complicated by the loss of significant portions of existing restoration or tooth structure, such as cusps and buccal/lingual walls, which influence the restorative procedures used in an attempt to maintain tooth longevity as well as pulp viability. For direct restorations to succeed clinically, they require healthy dental tissues to aid support, retention and ideally provide an element of protection from excessive occlusal loads. With diminishing amounts of remaining tooth structure to work with, greater thought and care are required to manage and prepare the remaining viable hard tissues to support and retain the larger restoration.

The *core restoration* describes the often large direct plastic restoration used to build up the clinically broken down crown. It is retained and supported by the remaining tooth structure wherever possible (sometimes including the pulp chamber itself as well as posts inserted within root canals of endodontically treated teeth). These large restorations often require further overlying protection to secure their clinical longevity by means of *indirect onlays, partial coverage crowns or full coverage crowns*.

6.2 CLINICAL ASSESSMENT OF BROKEN DOWN TEETH

Before carrying out a detailed clinical examination of the individual tooth and the related oral cavity, it is always important to *justify* your clinical decisions, both for operative and non-operative preventive interventions, as part of the MIOC framework.

6.2.1 Why Restore the Broken Down (or any) Tooth?

As discussed in Chapter 5, Section 5.9, the five key reasons for minimally invasive (MI) operative intervention are:

- To repair hard tissue damage and cavitation caused by the active, progressing caries or toothwear process (where non-operative prevention has failed repeatedly)
- To remove plaque stagnation areas within cavities and defects which will increase the risk of caries activity due to the lack of effective plaque removal by the patient
- To help manage acute pulpitic pain caused by active caries by removing the bacterial biomass and sealing the defect, thus protecting the pulp

- To restore the tooth to maintain structure and function in the dental arch
- Aesthetics

6.2.2 Is the Broken Down Tooth Restorable Clinically?

This is a very important question to answer pragmatically for the patient sitting in the dental chair at the time of consultation. It is important to manage patient expectations in this regard, as often the operative treatment required is technically complex, takes time over multiple appointments and may be expensive. Critical issues to discuss will include:

- The longevity and functionality of the final restoration; the patient has to appreciate the cost versus the clinical benefit of the treatment proposed along with any significant risks of short-, medium-, or long-term failure.
- They also have to appreciate their personal role in maintaining high-quality oral hygiene to ensure the best prognosis of any restoration placed.

Factors that must be considered when deciding whether to restore a broken down tooth are outlined in Table 6.1. These principles must of course be applied to any teeth being restored, but they are highlighted again in this chapter. The operator's clinical skill and level of training must also be considered in this regard and suitable specialist referrals must be made as required.

The clinical oral and dental assessment follows the MIOC guidance outlined and discussed in Chapters 2 and 3. After obtaining a comprehensive patient history and clinical examination of the whole mouth, certain tooth-related factors should be determined:

- Periapical radiographs should be taken to help ascertain the periapical status; the presence, absence and quality of root canal treatment (RCT); the extent of coronal tissue damage relative to the pulp chamber; and the root/canal morphology and periodontal status/alveolar bone levels.
- Pulp sensibility should be assessed.

TABLE 6.1 General Clinical Factors to Consider to Help Decide Whether a Broken Down Tooth Is Restorable

Factors	Favourable	Less Favourable
Pulp	Vital pulp with adequate RDT to incorporate tooth preparation.	Symptoms present, PA pathology (RCT will be required; isolation/access cavity compromised?)
RCT status	Good-quality sealed RCT, assessed radiographically with PA resolution evident. Straight canals and broad roots facilitate post placement.	Symptomatic, recurrence of PA pathology, re-RCT required? Thin roots and curved canals prevent post placement.
Tooth structure	Adequate bulk remaining; e.g., cusps Adequate distribution of coronal tissues; no cracks or defects	Inadequate quantities available once tooth preparation has occurred leads to weakness, fracture
Existing restoration status	Only requires refurbishment or repair (see Chapter 9, Section 9.4)	Active caries present, leaking margins, subgingival extension
Periodontal status	Pocket depths 3–4 mm, minimal recession, >50% bone level from PA radiographs	Active periodontal disease, LOA, <50% bone levels, grades II–III mobility
Occlusion	Protected canine-guided lateral excursions; no interferences	Reduced OVD minimises space for restoration
Dental arch tooth position	Fully/partially dentate with even tooth distribution, minimal tilting/rotation	Tooth bears full occlusal load in a quadrant, drifted/tilted/rotated
Aesthetics	Posterior dentition, previously restored dentition	High smile line in anterior aesthetic zone, recession risk due to thin gingival tissues, subgingival restoration margins and poor contour; complex shade matching
Patient factors – preventive status	Well-motivated, responsible patient; efficacious oral hygiene control (or can be motivated as such)	Refuses responsibility/unable to maintain oral health, poor diet, oral hygiene, no fluoride use

LOA, Loss of attachment; *OVD*, occlusal vertical dimension; *PA*, periapical; *RCT*, root canal treatment; *RDT*, remaining dentine thickness.

- An occlusal analysis should be conducted to ascertain the loading, guidance or interferences that may be related to the tooth in question, in all axes of movement, both static and dynamic.
- An occlusal vertical dimension (OVD) assessment should be conducted to ensure there is enough inter-occlusal space to successfully place a new restoration. Tilting/overeruption of the tooth or opposing teeth may reduce the space available in which to place a secure restoration with adequate strength, thus forcing treatment down the more complex reorganised approach to dental rehabilitation (see Chapter 5, Section 5.13).

When considering the tooth to be restored, further factors to consider would include:

- *The amount and/or distribution of the remaining viable tooth structure.* In posterior teeth, the presence of solid cusps directly or diagonally opposite one another can help support and even retain the core restoration with relative undercuts (see later). Thin, weaker retained buccal or lingual/palatal walls, on the other hand, would be less amenable to preparation for the retention of dental amalgam and more prone to fracture. In these situations, the retained, weaker cusps and walls may be reduced in height vertically and the core material overlaid to offer some occlusal loading pressure relief

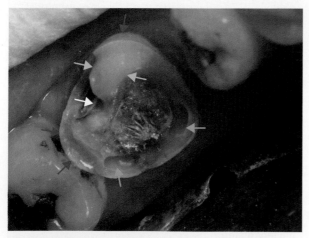

Fig. 6.1 A heavily broken down LL6 which has been prepared macromechanically to receive an amalgam core restoration. The blue arrows indicate the relative undercut prepared around the vertically reduced mesiobuccal cusp, which will be overlaid with amalgam. The green arrows point to two slots that have been prepared in healthy dentine to aid retention of the amalgam. The purple arrows highlight the prepared distal-buccal shoulder to support the amalgam restoration margin. The amalgam placement procedure is covered in detail in Chapter 8, Section 8.9. (Courtesy G Palmer.)

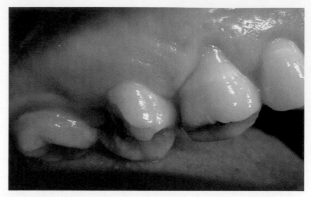

Fig. 6.2 A clinical image of the UR5, 6, 7, and 8, showing a traumatic distal shear fracture of the still-vital UR7 terminating subgingivally on the root surface.

> **Q6.2** What practical difficulties might be encountered when trying to restore the tooth shown in Fig. 6.2?

during function (Fig. 6.1). When placing adhesive resin composite cores, care must be taken to limit shrinkage stresses at the tooth restoration interface using incremental techniques or bulk-fill materials and when considering the axial tooth preparation that might be required for the indirect crown to be fitted.

- *The subgingival extent of the coronal damage.* When fragments of tooth-restoration complex have been lost in function, the fractures that occur often follow natural internal histological tissue planes, leading to shear fractures that can terminate on the root surface, sometimes millimetres subgingivally (Fig. 6.2). This makes their restoration difficult in terms of preparing the subsequent base cavity form to support the core restoration as well as gaining direct access and moisture control, thus adversely affecting the successful medium- to long-term restorability of the tooth.
- *Using the pulp and/or root canal spaces.* If the tooth has undergone successful RCT, there is the potential to prepare the straighter coronal section of a root canal for a post which can then help retain the core restoration (Fig. 6.3A–G). Restorative core material can fill the pulp chamber and even the first 2 to 3 mm of root canal space, close to the orifice, thus gaining another form of macromechanical retention. This type of restoration, originally using dental amalgam, is known as a *Nayyar core* (see Chapter 7, Section 7.5 and Chapter 8, Section 8.10). With the development of modern, high-quality adhesive dental restorative materials to aid core retention, *elective* RCT of a vital tooth for core retention is not normally indicated.

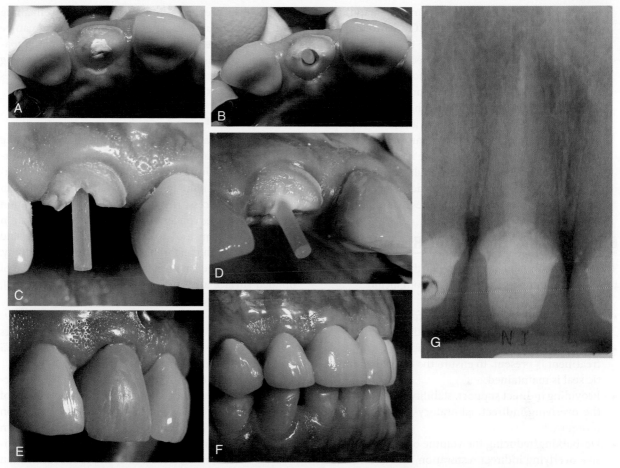

Fig. 6.3 (A) Fractured UR1. The crown fractured through the pulp chamber during mastication. The remaining root was endodontically treated and a temporary restoration placed in the access cavity. The fracture margins are just at the gingival margin or supragingival. The remaining enamel and dentine are sound. (B) and (C) show the root canal post space having been created using increasing sizes of Gates Glidden burs. A fibre-reinforced direct post has been placed into the post space. Its length has been adjusted to ensure it is short of the incisal edge position of the final restoration. (D) A fibre-reinforced post has been cemented into the canal space using a resin cement and the excess has been removed before final photo-curing. (E) Direct provisional resin composite restoration built up incrementally around the fibre post. (F) Definitive indirect ceramic cast restoration on the UR1 in occlusion. (G) Final periapical radiograph showing the fibre-reinforced post in place with 4 mm of root canal filling material (gutta percha) still present at the apical end of the root canal. Note the similar radiodensity of the fibre post compared to the surrounding dentine.

Q6.3 Look at Fig. 6.3.
 i. What other restorative materials could be used to fill the endodontic access cavity shown in Fig. 6.3A?
 ii. Look at Fig. 6.3B. Why should the post diameter not exceed one-third of the root diameter?
 iii. Why should the post extend to 1 to 2 mm below the incisal edge/occlusal surface of the definitive restoration in Fig. 6.3C?
 iv. Look at Fig. 6.3D. Can you suggest any alternative materials used to cement a root canal post?

 v. What is the C-factor of the provisional restoration shown in Fig. 6.3E?
 vi. Look at Fig. 6.3G. Why should the post length within the root canal exceed the length of the final restoration it supports?

- *The direct core restorative material.* The traditional restorative material used for core restorations, especially on posterior teeth, is dental amalgam due to its higher compressive strength and wear resistance under occlusal loading. Contemporary resin composites and now hybrid glass-ionomer cements (GICs) have improved strength and wear resistance over their predecessors, and as they will often be protected with an indirect crown, these are now becoming more popular as core materials for larger posterior restorations (Fig. 6.3E). Their adhesive retention reduces the amount of tooth preparation required, making them an attractive proposition where remaining tooth structure is at a premium. However, moisture control and the relative complexity of their placement technique in multiple increments in cavities that are not always easy to access operatively or keep dry, can limit their success rates in this regard.

6.3 INTRA-CORONAL CORE RESTORATION

The key functions of the direct plastic core restoration used to build up the broken down tooth include:

- Reconstituting the structure, the function and possibly the aesthetics of the crown of the tooth.
- Maintaining pulp sensibility, or where a root canal treatment is present, to ensure the coronal endodontic seal is maintained.
- Providing indirect support, stability and retention for the overlying indirect, laboratory-made restoration, if required.
- De-bulking/reducing the volume of the more expensive overlying indirect restoration. This will be more relevant when precious metals are used.

The direct core restoration is in the form of a plastic restorative material (usually dental amalgam or resin composite, but some modern high-viscosity GICs have also been developed for this purpose). However, in some cases, depending on the distribution and quantity of the remaining tooth structure and the size and shape of the existing cavity, an indirect/cast inlay/onlay or partial crown restoration may be placed instead of the plastic core buildup. Materials used for this type of restoration would include indirect resin composite, precious and nonprecious metal alloys or ceramics.

6.3.1 Direct Core Retention

The retention mechanisms used for different plastic restorative materials have been highlighted in Chapter 5, Table 5.10. *Macro-mechanical* cavity modifications to aid restoration retention will include the provision of diametrically opposing hard tissue undercuts where possible,

without over-preparing and weakening the remaining tooth structure unnecessarily. Opposing surfaces can be made more plane parallel with marginal shoulder preparations to stabilise the final restoration, and stabilising slots and grooves can be placed within healthy tissues where possible (see Fig. 6.1).

6.3.2 C-Factor

Adhesive materials will be placed with suitable bonding systems (see Chapter 8, Table 8.12). Incremental layering techniques must be used for conventional resin composite materials, although bulk-fill resin composites can simplify this process. This minimises the polymerisation shrinkage stresses concentrating at the tooth restoration interface that can lead to potential tooth flexure and even cracks, with concomitant symptoms of sensitivity. However, in large, open cavities with a reduced ratio of bonded surface area to free surface area (the C-factor), the shrinkage stresses will be less problematic.

- An occlusal cavity with a ratio of 5 bonded surfaces to 1 unbonded surface has the highest C-factor of 5 (5:1), thus maximising the interfacial stresses.
- A labial resin composite veneer has the lowest C-factor of 1 (one bonded to one free surface, both of similar surface areas). In this case, the shrinkage (on average between 1.5% and 2.5% vol for many modern resin composites) will be dissipated within the restoration and not concentrated at the tooth restoration interface (see Fig. 6.3D–E).

To date, independent published evidence is building to validate the use of bulk-fill resin composites, which only need one large increment of material to fill a larger cavity, as a core restorative material (see Chapter 7, Section 7.2.2). This class of resin composite is popular amongst clinicians due to its simplicity of use, and these materials seem to offer good medium-term success. High-viscosity, hybrid GICs and their derivatives have been used as core materials, but as a general rule these materials are not routinely recommended for this purpose unless at least two opposing walls of tooth tissue are present. Their only moderate compressive strength and wear resistance, when compared to dental amalgam and resin composites, also make them less appropriate for use as long-lasting restorations exposed to extensive occlusal functional loading in posterior teeth.

In the restoration of non-vital, endodontically treated teeth, the cementation of a post into the root canal space is indicated if the amount of residual tooth structure is insufficient to support a core made of a plastic material (dental amalgam or resin composite). Ideally, the root:

- Must have sufficient bulk (diameter) in which to widen the prepared root canal space to support the post
- Must have a length of straight root canal longer than the height of the final restoration it will support
- Should have at least one-third of its length supported by surrounding healthy alveolar bone

Root canal posts require removal of the root canal filling material (often gutta percha) within the coronal two-thirds of a straight canal. The procedure usually commences with a small rose head bur in a slow-speed handpiece and then continuing with a specially designed steel Gates Glidden bur. This consists of a noncutting point on the end, which melts the gutta percha, and then a bulbous cutting tip with a narrow shank behind that allows the root-filling material to be spun out of the canal space, all in one action. The coronal root canal space then needs to be increased in size to accommodate a post. This is achieved with a special twist drill (often supplied with the post kit) mounted in the slow-speed handpiece, shaped to match the size of post selected. The maximum width of the post is normally equal to one-third the diameter of the remaining root, assessed from the periapical radiograph. There should be at least 4 mm of residual root canal filling material remaining at the root apex to ensure the existing apical endodontic seal is not disturbed. All these dimensions can be assessed from the preoperative periapical radiograph (see Fig. 6.3).

6.4 CLINICAL OPERATIVE TIPS

- The ability to achieve successful moisture control is critical to the ultimate long-term restorability of the broken down tooth. Clamping the individual tooth for rubber dam placement may not be possible due to the scarcity of supragingival tooth structure. A split-dam technique may be required, with the dam anchored to adjacent teeth and the use of circumferential floss ligatures around the broken down tooth, to adapt the dam to the tooth to be restored (see Chapter 5, Section 5.7.3). A liquid dam may also be useful in this regard.
- In some cases, the use of cotton wool rolls and/or judicious suction may be all that is possible in this regard (see Chapter 5, Section 5.7.2).

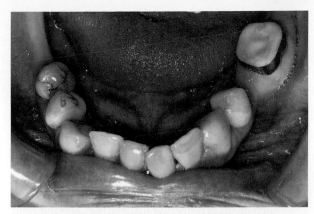

Fig. 6.4 A stainless steel orthodontic band placed around the LL6, supporting a large coronal restoration following endodontic treatment and prior to provision of an indirect full-coverage restoration. Note how the band has been adapted well to the contour of the molar and burnished into the furcation defect buccally.

> **Q6.4** What clinical clues in the patient shown in Fig. 6.4 might help you gain an insight into the patient's caries risk, prior to when the image was taken?

- Historically, a suitably adapted copper ring or, if available, an orthodontic band can be used to circumferentially support the core restoration buildup, and retained whilst the restorative material sets in function before its removal at a subsequent visit (see Fig. 6.4).
- Attempt to make internal cavity walls as plane parallel or slightly undercut as required without the concomitant loss of unnecessary sound tooth structure. Opposing walls help the stability of the core restoration within the cavity (see Fig. 6.1).
- Careful use of slots, grooves and pits can help the retention of large core restorations (see Fig. 6.1).
- *Matrixing:* Various designs of circumferential matrix exist from copper/orthodontic bands to self-tightening and supporting auto-matrix systems (see Chapter 5, Section 5.11). These are most useful for aiding the buildup of multiple missing walls of large cavities. Problems commonly arise when there is little peripheral tooth structure to support the peripheral shape of the band and on tightening, the band collapses over, especially where cusps and walls are missing, resulting in open proximal contacts and poor final restoration morphology.

Clinical techniques to overcome this loss of restoration morphology and contact points include:

- Trimming/shaping the outline of the matrix band to help proximal placement through tight contact points, adaptation and contour of the restoration.
- Using a ball burnisher hand instrument (Chapter 5, Fig. 5.28) to burnish the matrix band. Once the band is in place, tighten and wedge the band proximally to adapt it to the cervical margin of the tooth.
- Tightening and wedging the band proximally, filling the depth of the proximal boxes with initial small increments of restorative material (e.g., flowable resin composite). Once this is done, loosen the matrix a little to adjust its position and allow burnishing adaptation at the contact point followed by further increments of material. This 'adaptive matrixing' permits close adaptation at the cavity floor and adequate contouring of the proximal restoration anatomy.
- Initially restoring the accessible cusps, lingual/palatal–buccal/labial walls without the aid of a matrix band. Once they have been restored, place the matrix band conventionally (circumferential or, more ideally, sectional), then wedge and restore the proximal areas to the correct contact point and proximal morphology. The newly built-up sections will support the matrix band more effectively.

- The clinical procedure to place a fibre-reinforced post and build up a resin composite core is outlined in Chapter 8, Table 8.11. Endodontically treated teeth may need endodontic retreatments in the future and to accomplish this, bonded fibre posts can be removed, but using considerable care. Their removal is achieved by drilling down through the middle of the post, avoiding any additional removal of peripheral root or coronal dentine. In contrast, removal of a non-adhesively cemented metal-based post may be relatively easy, using an ultrasonic scaler to break down the cement lute at the post–dentine interface. Unfortunately, a chemically adhesively cemented metal post will be nearly impossible to remove without damaging the remaining root dentine.

6.5 DESIGN PRINCIPLES FOR INDIRECT RESTORATIONS

This section aims to *outline* the common design features required for the successful placement of indirect laboratory or chair-side made restorations used to reconstruct the crowns of broken down teeth. It does not cover the details of specific individual step-by-step restoration preparations, materials or operative techniques involved in the clinical and laboratory manufacturing processes. This information is covered in alternative prosthodontic texts.

Indirect restorations are classified as those that are fabricated outside the mouth, either by dentists making temporary crowns from putty indices, by technicians in a dental laboratory or from a clinical CAD/CAM processing unit from digitally scanned intra-oral records, and then cemented into place clinically by the operator (Table 6.2). They may be appropriate in the following clinical situations:

- To protect a broken down, weakened tooth from further fracture or to hold together parts of a cracked tooth (cusps, walls)
- To restore an already broken tooth or a tooth that has been severely worn down
- To cover, support and protect a tooth with an extensive core restoration from large occlusal loads when there is little tooth structure remaining

TABLE 6.2 **Indirect Restoration Types and the Materials used to Manufacture them**	
Indirect Restoration Type	**Materials**
Inlay	Gold type I alloy, ceramic, laboratory composite
Onlay	Gold types II and III alloy, composite, ceramic
Partial coverage crown (e.g., three-quarter crown)	Gold type III alloy
Full-coverage crown (full gold crown, metal ceramic crown/porcelain-fused-to-metal crown, all-ceramic crown)	Gold type III alloy, palladium alloy, base metal alloys (nickel, chromium), ceramic, stainless steel (paediatric crowns)
Precision attachments	Gold types III and IV alloy, palladium or base metal alloy (nickel, chromium)
Temporary crowns	Acrylate resin/acrylic based

Note: The intrinsic properties of the materials, often needing to be optimal in thin sections, will include a combination of suitable compressive, shear and tensile strengths to combat occlusal loading, wear resistance (ideally comparable to enamel) and aesthetics.

- To retain a bridge, whose *pontic(s)* replaces the missing tooth/teeth and *abutment(s)* anchors the prosthesis to the adjacent tooth/teeth
- To cover severely misshapen or discoloured teeth where direct restorative methods would not be clinically or practically viable
- To restore dental implant abutments and to act as precision attachments for removable prostheses

For children, an indirect crown may be used on the primary dentition to:

- Save a tooth that has been so damaged by caries that it can no longer support a restoration but requires maintenance in the dental arch for functional and developmental reasons (e.g., the Hall technique in the primary dentition)
- Protect the teeth of a child at high risk for caries, especially when a child and/or carer has difficulty maintaining daily oral hygiene
- Decrease the frequency of sedation and general anaesthesia for children unable, because of age, behaviour or medical history, to fully cooperate with the requirements of proper dental care and maintenance.

In such cases, a paediatric dentist is likely to recommend a stainless steel crown.

6.5.1 Design Features

Retention is the property of a restoration/cavity that prevents its displacement from the cavity in its direction of placement/insertion. Prior to the use of chemical adhesives, this property was reliant on macro-mechanical tooth preparation features including undercuts (only for direct plastic restorations), slots and grooves, which potentially weakened and sacrificed quantities of sound tooth structure (see Chapter 5, Section 5.9.5).

Resistance form is the property of a restoration/cavity that prevents its displacement in any other direction.

These traditional terms are dated now and indeed their use was always rather more theoretical than practical. Their relevance is much reduced in contemporary minimally invasive operative dentistry since the advent and development of effective dental adhesives. However, basic mechanical, operative principles are still relevant and important when designing preparations suited for indirect restorations of all types of material:

- *Occlusal/axial reduction:* This should be sufficient to accommodate the appropriate thickness of restorative material used for the indirect restoration. Gold alloy crowns require the least tooth preparation as they have adequate strength and rigidity in thin sections (0.7 mm). Indirect resin composites and all-ceramic restorations require a greater bulk (up to 2 mm) to achieve this. Newer ceramic formulations allow thinner veneers with adequate strength and aesthetics, thus making tooth preparation more minimally invasive.
- *Axial wall taper (Fig. 6.6A–B):* For indirect restorations that have been manufactured and cast or cured outside the mouth, perfectly parallel walls would be ideal, but in clinical practice these are impossible to achieve without introducing an element of undercut. Instead, a slightly divergent axial taper is recommended of 7 to 10 degrees. Even this level of taper is difficult to achieve/perceive with the naked eye in the oral cavity; therefore 15 degrees is often the minimum achieved in practice. Any undercut in the axial surface preparation (as with classic amalgam cavities, see Section 5.9.5, Figs. 5.58 and 5.59) is contraindicated as it will be impossible to make or seat the restoration.
- *Surface area and finish:* Maximising the surface area between the indirect restoration and tooth will aid cementation and therefore retention. The microscopic roughened surface produced by fine dental diamond or tungsten carbon finishing burs will increase the surface area for adhesive bonding without introducing major flaws or cracks in the tooth tissue (see Chapter 5, Sections 5.8.2 and 5.8.3).
- *Preparation margin – position (*Fig. 6.5A–C) To maximise the axial wall length and surface area, it is desirable to place the finishing margin of the full coverage crown close to, but just, supragingivally. This will aid oral hygiene procedures for the patient and allow simpler impression-taking procedures for the operator. Care must be taken during tooth preparation not to traumatise the gingival tissues or to encroach on the biologic width of the gingival attachment complex (the region between the alveolar bone crest and junctional epithelial attachment), for fear of accelerating irreversible periodontal tissue damage and recession caused by biofilm accumulation. Patients must be advised regarding optimal oral hygiene procedures to prevent plaque biofilm stagnation at all restoration margins. Indeed, if a patient shows evidence of not being able to maintain effective oral hygiene in such areas in the preventive phase of MIOC, this should act as a warning and as a potential contraindication to restoration placement (see Table 6.1).

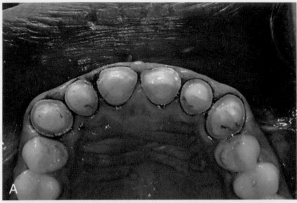

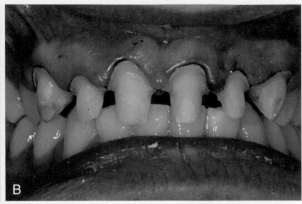

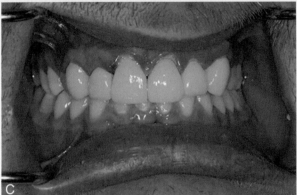

Fig. 6.5 (A) A maxillary anterior occlusal view of full-coverage indirect crown preparations, UR3 to UL3. Note the just supragingival location of the rounded shoulder finishing margins of the tapered axial walls. (B) The labial view of the same tooth preparations where the rounded shoulder finishing margins are more clearly demarcated as are their circumferential positions supragingival to the surrounding gingival papillae. The relative tapering of the axial walls can be clearly seen on the upper central incisor teeth. Sufficient occlusal height reduction of the teeth allows (C) the final ceramic restorations to be cemented using a resin-based luting cement. (Courtesy of Dr Ryan Olley.)

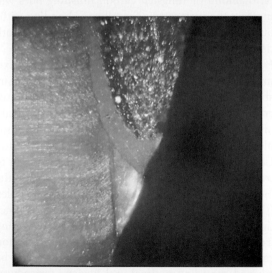

Fig. 6.6 A photomicrograph (field width 2 mm) showing a section through the margin interface of a thin ceramic indirect restoration luted to a tooth. The dentine is on the left of the image and the ceramic restoration is on the upper right. Between it and the dentine and the small triangle of retained enamel is the resin-based luting cement. The profile of the axial finishing margin on the tooth is a chamfer.

Q6.5 Look at Fig. 6.5.

i. What are the advantages and disadvantages of placing the axial wall finishing margins supragingival as shown in Fig. 6.5A?

ii. Do you know what the black lines are adjacent to the finishing margins of the six prepared teeth as shown in Fig. 6.5B?

- *Preparation margin–shape:* The cross-sectional shape of the margin between the indirect restoration and the tooth should be a *chamfer* or a *rounded shoulder* configuration. This is dependent on:
    1. The type of material used to fabricate the restoration. Gold and other metal alloy margins can be manufactured to finer tolerances, thus reducing the amount of tooth preparation required at the interface between the restoration and the tooth. Ceramics require a greater bulk of material for strength and aesthetics, resulting in heavier marginal tooth preparation (Figs. 6.5C and 6.6).
    2. The amount of tooth structure/core restoration present. The most tooth-preserving, minimally

invasive margin preparation is a minimal chamfered finish, which may be desirable where remaining tooth structure is at a premium and not easily accessible.

3. The position of the margin. When lingual, distal or palatal, margins can be finished in metal without aesthetic compromise, thus needing only a minimally invasive chamfer finish. Indeed, circumferential indirect restoration margins may have different configurations dependent upon their anatomical position (labial vs. proximal vs. lingual/palatal).

The different margin configurations are prepared using end-cutting burs with a rounded tip (half depth) to achieve a chamfer (Fig. 6.6), and a squared-off tip profile to achieve a shoulder.

- *Adhesive resin cement:* Modern adhesive cements have chemical moieties that can bond to ions in the tooth as well as oxides and other chemical groups within the restorative material, thus providing some chemical adhesion (Fig. 6.6). This permits greater leeway in the mechanical accuracy of the tooth preparation (including the degree of taper of the axial walls, their surface finish and their surface area).

6.6 ANSWERS TO SELF-TEST QUESTIONS

Q6.2: What practical difficulties might be encountered when trying to restore the tooth shown in Fig. 6.2?
A: (1) Difficult physical instrument access to the distal of the UR7; (2) difficult moisture control (hard to place rubber dam); (3) difficult to modify cavity form at the base of the shear fracture; and (4) difficult to place restorative material at the base of the fracture (adhesive or otherwise). A possible solution to improving the restorability of the tooth would be to carry out a crown-lengthening procedure to relocate the gingival margin apically, thus improving access to the base of the cavity.

Q6.3: Look at Fig. 6.3
i. What other restorative materials could be used to fill the endodontic access cavity shown in Fig. 6.3A?
A: GIC, resin composite.
ii. Look at Fig. 6.3B. Why should the post diameter not exceed one-third of the root diameter?
A: If the post is wider than this ratio, there is an increased risk of root fracture, especially with metal-based posts which do not dissipate stresses evenly through the root length.
iii. Why should the post extend to 1 to 2 mm below the incisal edge/occlusal surface of the definitive restoration in Fig. 6.3C?
A: So that there is enough space afforded to the core restoration to cover the post. When the core restoration is prepared for a crown, up to 2 mm of clearance may be needed occlusally/incisally. There is a risk that the post may be exposed during crown preparation and this can potentially weaken the core structure or even the fibre post.
iv. Look at Fig. 6.3D. Can you suggest any alternative materials used to cement a root canal post?
A: GIC-based cements.
v. What is the C-factor of the provisional restoration shown in Fig. 6.3E?
A: The C-factor is calculated as the ratio of the bonded surface area to the dentine vs. the nonbonded surface of the resin composite restoration. As you can see from the series of images, the bonded surface is small compared to the

rest of the restoration, so this is a favourable configuration. Thus stress concentrations at the interface will be minimal.
vi. Look at Fig. 6.3G. Why should the post length within the root canal exceed the length of the final restoration it supports?
A: Mechanically, this provides the best distribution of occlusal loading forces on the postrestoration tooth complex. If the post length is shorter than its supported restoration, unfavourable fulcrums of force can be generated leading to crown or root fracture in clinical use.

Q6.4: What clinical clues in the patient shown in Fig. 6.4 might help you gain an insight into the patient's caries risk, prior to when the image was taken?
A: The presence, site and number of tooth-coloured adhesive restorations and the apparently untreated buccal carious lesion on the LR5.

Q6.5: Look at Fig. 6.5
i. What are the advantages and disadvantages of placing the axial wall finishing margins supragingival as shown in Fig. 6.5A?
A: Advantages: No trauma to the gingiva during preparation; easier recording of margins in the final impression; easier to construct accurate temporary crowns; easier for the laboratory to accurately fabricate fitting crowns; less chance of the periodontium being adversely affected, thus leading to later recession or periodontal disease; easier for the patient to clean the restoration margins. Disadvantages: Anteriorly, aesthetics may be compromised as the margins may be visible in a patient with a high lip line.
ii. Do you know what the black lines are adjacent to the finishing margins of the six prepared teeth as shown in Fig. 6.5B?
A: A gingival retraction cord, placed carefully into the periodontal pocket, that helps keep the gingival tissue away from the tooth during impression taking. This helps dry the field and stops any bleeding, especially if the margins are subgingival (due to the astringent the cord is soaked in).

MIOC Domain 3: Restorative Materials Used in Minimally Invasive Operative Dentistry

7.1 INTRODUCTION

Modern restorative dental biomaterials can be classified in terms of their:

- Retention mechanism (e.g., chemical [covalent, ionic, metallic bonds], physical [Van der Waals forces, hydrogen bonds] or mechanical [macro-, micro- or nano-mechanical]); that is, whether retention is direct or a separate adhesive is required
- Constituent chemistry (e.g., resin-based, calcium silicate, setting reaction, filler particle type and configurations, bioactivity/bio-interactivity)
- Clinical properties (e.g., aesthetics, strength, wear, handling characteristics)

As part of the 'golden triangle' for achieving an optimal bio-interactive clinical tooth-restoration complex, it is essential that (1) the chemistry of the materials is considered in conjunction with (2) the histological tissue substrate to which the materials will adhere and interact with and (3) their intricacies in clinical handling and placement techniques, to fully appreciate the complexities of each system and thus optimise their potential clinical uses, advantages and disadvantages.

This chapter will outline and discuss aspects of dental biomaterials science to enable the reader to understand and appreciate its link with relevant histology and relate this to the clinical aspects of minimally invasive operative dentistry. Also discussed is dental amalgam. While dental amalgam is still a popular restorative material among many dentists worldwide, clinical indications for its use are becoming more limited as minimally invasive treatment rationales change and adhesive materials improve. This section of the chapter will require additional input from suitable dental histology and detailed, focused dental material science texts.

7.2 DENTAL RESIN COMPOSITES

Dental resin composites are aesthetic, plastic adhesive restorative materials that consist of copolymerised methacrylate-based resin chains embedding inert filler particles to confer strength and wear resistance and requiring a separate adhesive or bonding agent to micro-mechanically or nano-mechanically bond them to either enamel or dentine, respectively. However, as not all modern dental composites are based purely on methacrylate resin chemistry (see Section 7.2.6), the term *composite resin* is a less technically accurate descriptor.

7.2.1 History

Resin composites have undergone development over the past 50+ years, after the introduction of the acid-etch technique (Buonocore, 1955) and methacrylate monomers (Bowen's resin [Bis-GMA (1971)], discussed shortly).

7.2.2 Chemistry
7.2.2.1 Resin Matrix

The uncured resin composite consists of a mixture of several different types of resin dimethacrylate monomers, most of which are *hydrophobic* or water repelling in nature (Fig. 7.1).

The resin monomer chain length affects certain properties of a resin composite:

- *Viscosity or flowability*: This is important to minimise voids trapped within the uncured resin composite during its clinical placement and packing within the depths of a cavity; the stiffer the consistency, the

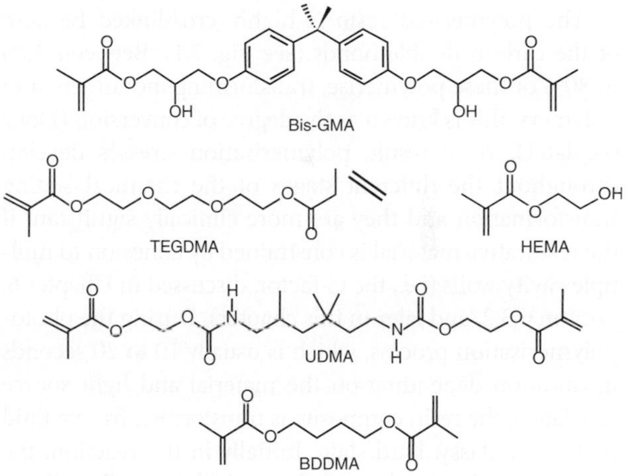

Fig. 7.1 Examples of dimethacrylate resins used more commonly in dental resin composites, with polymerisable C=C terminal double bonds. Note how TEGDMA has a shorter chain length than the others. More dental resins nowadays do not contain Bisphenol A (BPA) due to its possible associated deleterious health effects (including the brain and prostate gland of foetuses, infants and children. It might also affect children's behaviour. Additional research suggests a possible link between BPA and increased blood pressure, type 2 diabetes and cardiovascular disease). *BDDMA*, 1,4-butanediol dimethacrylate; *HEMA*, hydroxyethyl methacrylate. (From Sampaolese B, Lupi A, Di Stasio E, et al. Inhibition of telomerase activity in HL-60 cell line by methacrylic monomers. In: Calhoun FC, ed. *Dental Composites*. Nova Science Publishers, 2011.)

Q7.1: What physical properties of the resin composite material does the monomer chain length affect?

greater the risk of trapping air voids. Likewise, the shorter the uncured monomer chain lengths (and the lower the molecular weight), the less overall viscosity of the material. Often, methacrylate monomers that are shorter and lower in molecular weight form the primary constituent of the resin chemistry in the clinical category of *flowable* resin composites. Indeed, other diluent molecules may be added (see Table 7.1).

• *Volumetric polymerisation shrinkage and stress*: The setting process of a resin composite is a light-activated, free-radical addition, polymerisation chain reaction. As the linear dimethacrylate monomer chains shrink in length, more of them need to join per unit volume with a greater amount of inter-molecular space closure, resulting in the relatively increased shrinkage exhibited towards the centre of the restoration (ranging from <1%–5% vol depending upon the precise formulation and curing conditions; Fig. 7.2).

The polymerised resin is highly crosslinked because of the carbon double bonds (see Fig. 7.1). Between 35% to 80% of these polymerise, transforming monomers into polymers; this is known as the degree of conversion (DoC; see later). As a result, polymerisation stresses develop throughout the different stages of the chemical setting transformation and they are more clinically significant if the restorative material is constrained by adhesion to multiple cavity walls (i.e., the C-factor, discussed in Chapter 6, Section 6.3.2, and later in this chapter). During the photo-polymerisation process, which is usually 10 to 20 seconds in duration depending on the material and light source (see later), the resin composite is transformed from a fluid paste to a glassy, hard state. Initially in the reaction, the resins have the freedom to flow, which partially relieves

stress buildup. As light exposure continues, the monomers become reactive to form a polymer chain and the distance between the monomers reduces to form a cross-linked network. This leads to an increase in viscosity and loss in polymer fluidity; also known as the *gel point*. However, the elasticity may remain low enough at this stage to help dissipate any internal stresses produced. Finally, the resin composite will change into a rigid, glassy state—the *vitrification point*—with concurrent increases in the modulus of elasticity and shrinkage and a reduction in stress relaxation. Thus it is this stage of the setting process that results in the buildup of internal stresses.

Reducing the polymerisation shrinkage can be afforded by:

• Modifying the material's formulation, such as the resin matrix chemical composition or the filler particle content (see later)
• Clinically applying incremental layering techniques to directly place the conventional resin composites
• Using a layered or sandwich restoration technique to provide a base layer in a deeper cavity that might better relieve the internal stresses of the overall restoration
• Using bulk-fill resin composites with larger increments
• Modifying light-activation protocols

7.2.2.2 Filler Particles

Inert, dispersed filler particles are made from silica, quartz, barium or strontium glass derivatives, introducing the quality of radio-opacity useful for identification on dental radiographs. These are embedded in and bound to the resin matrix using an organo-silane coupling agent (e.g., γ-methacryloxypropyltrimethoxysilane [γ-MPTS]). Over the past 40 years, manufacturers have attempted to pack in various sizes, shapes and formulations of particles in increasing numbers per unit volume in an effort to affect the clinical properties of resin composites (see Fig. 7.3A–B). The more space that is taken up by irregular and spherical-shaped filler particles, the less space there is for native resin monomers, leading to a reduction in overall shrinkage on light-curing. Conversely, the more filler particles that are loaded into the resin composite, the more viscous it becomes, so there is a fine line between balancing the filler load and its resin content, depending on the specific properties required of the material. The filler particles confer several properties on the cured resin composite material:

• *Wear resistance:* Increasing the density of larger, harder and more irregularly shaped filler particles will tend to

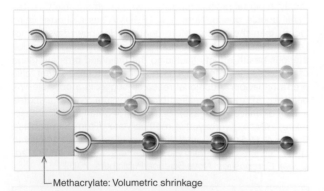

Methacrylate: Volumetric shrinkage

Fig. 7.2 A diagrammatic representation of linear monomers undergoing addition polymerisation leading to volumetric shrinkage. (Courtesy 3M.)

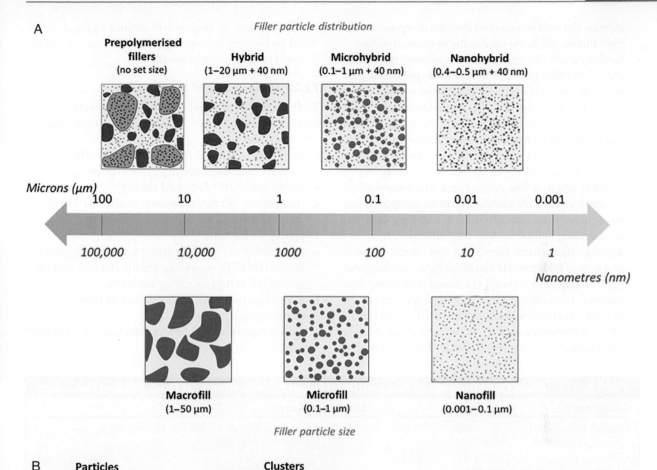

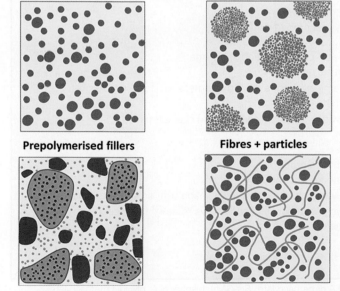

Fig. 7.3 (A) The size range of filler particles and their distribution within the resin matrix of modern dental resin composites. (B) Diagrams showing four different types of filler particle morphology found in modern resin composites. These may be used in different combinations within the resin matrix. The colour-coded particles relate to the filler particle size scale in (A).

increase the wear resistance of the resin composite as less resin matrix will be exposed at the restoration surface.

- *Surface polish*: The smaller, softer and more spherically shaped the filler particles are, the more polishable (but less wear resistant) the resin composite will be.
- *Aesthetics*: The finer the filler particles are, the more aesthetic the resin composite will be as the optical properties can be made to more accurately match that of enamel. Modern resin composites can have numerous shades (using pigments and various degrees of opacity) or just a few, relying on a 'chameleon' effect whereby a relatively translucent resin composite can encompass several tooth shades, blending into the surrounding natural colours very effectively by transmitting colour from them. The size, shape, amount and type of filler particle can affect light scattering and light propagation through the cured resin composite material, thus affecting its aesthetic properties as well as light transmission during photo-curing (see later).
- *Physical properties, such as compressive, shear strength and elasticity*: The correct balance of filler particle to resin content is required to ensure optimal physical properties, attempting to match those of natural tooth structure where possible.

7.2.2.3 Other Chemical Constituents

Table 7.1 lists additional chemical ingredients found in dental resin composites. These small fractions include:

- *Inhibitors* (butyl-4-hydroxytoluenes [BHT]) to increase material longevity prior to photocuring
- Photo-initiators (discussed shortly)
- *Accelerators* (dimethylaminobenzoates [DMAB]) to increase the reactivity of the photoinitiator, thus accelerating curing time
- *Photostabilisers* (2-hydroxy-4-methoxybenzophenone [HMBP]), providing colour stability by eliminating UV action on amine initiators
- *Radio-opacifiers* such as aluminium, titanium or zirconium oxides
- *Colour pigments* including various ferric and titanium oxides

TABLE 7.1 Main Constituents of Conventional Resin Composites and Their Clinical Relevance

Component	Examples	Clinical Relevance
Organic resin matrix; primary monomer	Bis-GMA Bis-EMA UDMA	Main resin monomer that forms resin polymer matrix
Organic resin matrix; diluent monomer	TEGDMA UDMA	Reduces viscosity of primary monomer; improves handling properties
Inorganic filler	Quartz Silica-based glasses Amorphous silica Ytterbium fluoride	Physical properties Viscosity of material Affects polymerisation shrinkage Optical properties
Coupling agent	γ-MPTS UDMS	Chemically bonds resin monomers to filler; aids physical properties
Initiator system	Camphorquinone TPO Ivocerin	Provides setting properties and characteristics
Inhibitor system	BHT MEHQ	Handling properties Material working time
UV-stabiliser	Oxybenzone	Prevents change in material shade over time due to oxidation
Radiopacifiers	Barium salts Strontium salts Lithium salts	Changes radiopacity and allows material to be seen on radiographs
Pigments	Iron Titanium dioxide	Aesthetic and optical properties

BHT, Butyl-4-hydroxytoluenes; *Bis-EMA*, ethoxylated bisphenol A dimethacrylate; *Bis-GMA*, bisphenol A, glycidyl methacrylate; *MEHQ*, monomethyl ether hydroquinone; *TEGDMA*, triethylene glycol dimethacrylate; *TPO*, trimethylbenzoyl-diphenylphosphine oxide; *UDMA*, urethane dimethacrylate; *UDMS*, urethane dimethacrylate silane; *γ-MPTS*, gamma- methacryloxypropyltrimethoxysilane.

7.2.2.4 Polymerisation Reaction

The setting (i.e., curing) process in resin composites is either light-activated (470 nm wavelength visible blue light) or dual-cured, light and chemical activation (initiated by 0.5% benzoyl peroxide, an aromatic tertiary amine and activated using dimethyl-p-toluidine). Light-cured resin composite contains a photoinitiator, α-diketone (camphorquinone) and an amine, which under the activation of visible blue light generates the free radicals by homolytic cleavage of their low-energy bonds. This is required to initiate the cross-linking polymerisation chain reaction.

Some factors related to the setting reaction of resins include:

- *Degree of monomer conversion (35%–80%)*: Not all free monomer polymerises on curing, leaving some to potentially leach out of the cured resin composite. This contributes to the long-term degradation of the material in terms of moisture ingress and possible sensitisation issues with some patients, especially in deep cavities closer to the pulp where the uncured monomers might cause direct irritation to pulp cells with a concomitant inflammatory cellular reaction.
- *Shrinkage on curing (<1%–5%)*: Fig. 7.2 illustrates how shrinkage occurs during polymerisation towards the centre of the restoration bulk and light source, thus causing the resin composite to pull away from cavity margins and increasing the risk of marginal leakage at the tooth restoration interface.
- *Shrinkage stress at the resin composite–tooth interface (3–8 MPa)*: The stresses generated by the polymerisation process can be high at cavity margins depending on the cavity C-factor (the ratio of bonded vs. unbonded restoration surfaces; see Chapter 6, Section 6.3.2), the bulk of the material and the structural compliance of the cavity walls. This can lead to debonding and/or tooth cracking or fracture of the weakened marginal tissues.
- *Water absorption*: Water is absorbed hygroscopically during and after the curing process, leading to initial expansion, long-term resin composite degradation and potential for long-term colour instability and staining.
- *Air-inhibited surface layer of uncured resin*: The free-radical addition polymerisation reaction is inhibited by air. After an increment of resin composite is cured, a glossy film of uncured resin is retained on its surface and the monomers in this layer are used to provide adherence for the next increment placed upon it. In this way, resin composites can be

added to incrementally within a cavity to build up the final restoration as an additive process.

- *Depth of cure*: Conventional resin composites can be cured to a depth of 2 mm, depending on the translucency of the material. A thicker section will not cure sufficiently at its base, because the 470 nm light does not penetrate sufficiently at those depths to permit activation of the polymerisation reaction. The resulting restoration may then be described as having an uncured or 'soggy' bottom. Note that conventional resin composites cure most efficiently closest to the 470 nm light source. The light source ideally should be placed as close as possible to the uncured resin composite which should be built up within deeper cavities, in smaller (<2 mm thick), angled increments.
- *Light-/photo-curing*: Effective photopolymerisation is a significant contributing factor for the quality and long-term clinical success of light-activated resin-based composite restorations. The changes in light transmission throughout polymerisation of a light-curable resin composite are complex and are significantly affected by the constituents and chemistry of the material and the light-curing unit (LCU) itself. The measured light irradiance (i.e., the radiant flux, or power) received by a material surface per unit area (often measured in mW/cm^2) is a critical parameter that determines the extent of cure. This is often inappropriately or inaccurately measured at the light-curing unit tip, using a radiometer device. Most modern LCUs use light-emitting diodes (LEDs) in various fibre-optic tip configurations and distributions to allow more controlled light emission wavelengths to be achieved whilst optimising their energy efficiency and longevity. Modern trends in LED-LCU manufacture include broad spectrum units which incorporate multiple LEDs to deliver light in the visible-violet (~385–410 nm), blue (~450–515 nm) as well as intermediate ranges of violet-blue wavelengths (~410–450 nm), enabling activation of a wider range of incorporated chemical photoinitiators within the resin matrix. There is also a trend towards ever higher claimed irradiance values under the premise that shorter exposure times at higher irradiance levels deliver sufficient energy for optimal polymerisation. The clinical state of the LCU tip surface (whether it is sound or chipped/scratched), its cleanliness (whether there are deposits of adhesive, restorative material or clinical debris on the tip surface), its diameter (7–13 mm), its surface area (30–>100 mm^2) and its actual distance from the resin composite surface (e.g., light curing the depths

of a proximal box) will all have a potentially detrimental effect on the *actual* irradiance level incident at the resin composite surface. Within the material itself, the filler particle size, shape, material and density, along with the colour pigments and other additives, including the photoinitiators, will all affect light transmission within the material, potentially increasing its scattering, absorption or reflectance properties, thus reducing the effective photon energy left to polymerise the resin monomers. This in turn can reduce monomer conversion rates as well as the overall depth of cure of the material.

- *'Bulk-fill' resin composites:* These materials are available, described by manufacturers as a 'dentine replacement' for the restoration of deep cavities. They can exhibit a relatively low viscosity, 'flowable' consistency so that they achieve good adaptation to the deep cavity floor and walls, almost 'self-levelling' within the cavity. Mechanical properties, such as toughness, may be compromised to a degree to achieve this effect, but this may

be an acceptable compromise when used in bulk and within the depths of a large cavity, especially if overlaid with a more wear-resistant material. Their depth of cure is achieved by the use of alternative monomer combinations and the creation of a relatively translucent material, often achieved with large filler particle clusters, thus allowing better light transmission through the material and hence improved monomer conversion at deeper levels within the material. There are also more viscous, heavily filled versions of these materials, which can be placed in bulk, with better handling and adaptation characteristics at contact points and the development of occlusal anatomy, but there may also be compromises such as achieving adequate adaptation on the cavity floor (leading to an increased risk of voids).

7.2.3 The Tooth–Resin Composite Interface

Table 7.2 highlights some of the more clinically important histological features of sound enamel and dentine relevant to the restoration of tooth surfaces with

TABLE 7.2 Clinically Relevant Dental Histology Interacting With Chemistry of Modern Adhesive Restorative Materials

	Mineral (*Inorganic*)	Matrix (*Organic*)	Structural Arrangement
Enamel	Calcium hydroxyapatite crystallites ($Ca_{10}(PO_4)_7(OH)_2$ – $40 \times 70 \times 170$ nm) 97% weight, 89% vol.	No collagen. Enamelins (MW 55 kDa), Amelogenins (MW 25 kDa) – 1% weight, 2% vol. Water – 3% weight, 9% vol.	10,000 crystallites arranged into *prisms* (US - rods); EDJ to surface; ameloblasts – Tomes' processes; 4 –7 μm diameter; undulation, decussation; keyhole pattern in cross-section; prism cores / boundaries exist due to change in orientation of crystallites. Aprismatic layer at tooth surface on eruption (Fig. 7.4A). Gradually eroded away over time.
Dentine	Calcium hydroxyapatite crystallites (with Mg and CO_3 substitutions – $5 \times 30 \times 80$ nm) β-octocalcium phosphate crystals.	90% collagen: Type I ($[\alpha1(I)]_2\alpha2(I)$) with trace amounts of type I trimer ($[\alpha1(I)]_3$), 300 nm rod-shaped triple helical collagen molecules linearly aligned and cylindrically grouped as fibrils. Parallel fibrils gathered into fibres. 10% non-collagenous proteins (phosphorylated phosphoproteins (MW 140 kDa), Gla-proteins, macromolecular proteoglycans, plasma proteins, acidic glycoproteins), water.	*Tubules* (EDJ to pulp chamber); approximately 19 – 45,000 per mm²; coronal sigmoid curvature; 1 – 5 μm diameter; anastomosing branches evident (0.5 μm – 25 nm diameter); odontoblasts and processes.

EDJ, Enamel–dentine junction; *kDa,* kilo-Daltons; *MW,* molecular weight.

TABLE 7.3 **Clinical Properties Dental Hard Tissue Confers on a Tooth And Properties Ideal Restorative Material Should Mimic**

	Enamel	Enamel–Dentine Junction	Dentine
Clinical properties	Rigidity/brittleness High compressive strength Wear resistance Translucency Dry	Scalloped Optical tint Limits crack propagation/catastrophic failure Approx. 50 MPa natural bond strength	Bulk Slight elasticity/flexibility Shade Dynamic hydration–wetter, closer to the pulp (affect bonding ability)
Closest restorative 'replacement' or 'equivalent' material	Dental resin composite ceramics	Dentine bonding agent Dynamic chemical bond	Glass-ionomer cement Resin-modified glass-ionomer cement Biodentine

adhesive materials. An understanding of the interactions between the chemistry of the materials and this relevant histology is vital to optimise the qualities of the adhesive restorative systems available, including resin composites. Table 7.3 outlines the clinical properties that each layer of dental hard tissue confers to the crown of a tooth and those properties that a restorative material should exhibit to act as an ideal replacement material for each.

7.2.3.1 The Resin Composite–Enamel Interface

Hydrophobic resin composites adhere to inherently dry enamel micro-mechanically and the prismatic, crystalline ultrastructure of enamel permits this to happen successfully, reliably and strongly (20–50 MPa tensile bond strengths in laboratory studies). Three stages are required to develop the bond between resin composite and enamel after the enamel has been prepared mechanically during cavity preparation:

1. The first stage is acid etching (be aware of the alternative US term, *conditioning*). This is the process of placing 37% orthophosphoric acid etch gel onto the prepared enamel surface for 20 seconds. This:
   - Dissolves surface contaminants (saliva, proteinaceous substances) and the smear layer (a tenacious surface layer of organic and inorganic cutting debris <20 μm thick) and increases surface area for bonding.
   - Produces micro-irregularities and micro-porosities in the prismatic enamel surface. This microscopic surface roughness will provide micro-mechanical retention for the flowable resin to penetrate and lock into (Fig. 7.4B).
2. After washing the acid etch gel off and drying the enamel thoroughly, a layer of fluid, unfilled hydrophobic

bonding resin (i.e., essentially the resin without filler particles) was traditionally placed onto the etched enamel surface. This step has now been superceded by modern dental adhesives (discussed shortly). This bond can flow easily into the micro-undercuts and porosities created by the etching process, and it is then photo-polymerised. Note that the chemistry of the unfilled fluid bonding resin is not precisely the same as that for a dentine bonding agent (see later).

3. The final resin composite can then be placed directly on the layer of photo-cured bonding resin, coupled to the air-inhibited layer, in small angled increments (to lessen the effects of polymerisation shrinkage) and photo-cured, to form the final contoured restoration (Fig. 7.5).

When bonding to enamel, consideration must be given to the quality of the prismatic structure as this is critical to adhesion. Unprepared young enamel of newly erupted teeth may still retain a surface layer of *aprismatic* enamel—the final layers of enamel to be laid down before completion of tooth crown development (Fig. 7.4A). This layer is void of enamel prisms as the elongated Tomes processes of the enamel-producing cells, the ameloblasts, had already retracted as enamel deposition was nearing completion. Up to 20 microns in thickness, this layer is removed in normal function due to the normal causes of tooth surface loss (erosion, abrasion and attrition; see Chapter 1, Section 1.2). Prisms that have been sectioned, cracked or pulled apart during tooth preparation with rotary instrumentation and do not reach the enamel–dentine junction (EDJ) intact are described as being *unsupported*. These prisms are inherently weak and if bonded to will pull apart physically under the stresses exerted on them by the curing resin composite shrinkage. This will lead to relatively

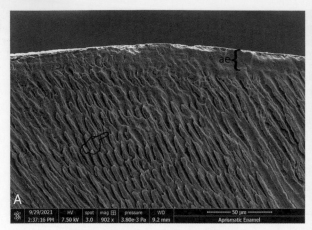
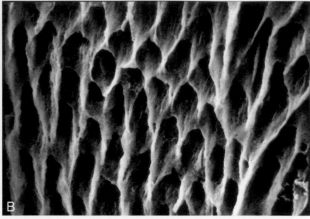

Fig. 7.4 (A) A scanning electron microscope image of transversely sectioned buccal enamel showing an approximately 20 μm thick layer of aprismatic enamel (ae) overlying the deeper prismatic layer. (Courtesy Prof S Sauro, Universidad CEU-Cardenal Herrera, Valencia, Spain.) (B) The tooth's view of an acid etch-retained resin bond. The enamel was etched, washed, bonded and then dissolved away using a strong acid. The acid-resistant resin layer was retained. It can be seen to have flowed into the prism boundary regions (field width 80 μm). (Courtesy Prof A Boyde.)

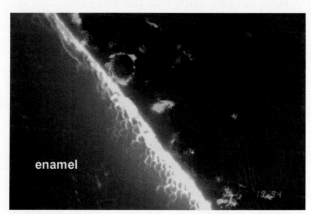

Fig. 7.5 The interface between etched and bonded enamel prisms and a restoration. The bonding agent has been labelled with a yellow fluorescent dye (fluorescein) and its penetration around the horseshoe-shaped enamel prisms can be seen. Enamel prisms are separated easily from one another in the lateral walls of a cavity such as this, especially if the restoration shrinks (field width 500 μm).

short-term marginal failure within the enamel: that is, *cohesive enamel failure*. In theory, if supported prisms are cut at or close to 90 degrees to their long axis (i.e., clinically, the enamel margin is lightly bevelled) then the deleterious effects of shrinkage stress at the margins may be reduced as prisms possess greater tensile and compressive strengths along their c-axes (long axes), as opposed to perpendicular to the c-axes. Enamel that has lost much of the underlying dentine beneath it (*undermined* enamel) will need to have this replaced with a

suitable material prior to the resin composite–enamel bond being created.

7.2.3.2 Resin Composite – Dentine Interface: Dentine Bonding Agents/Dental Adhesives

The fundamental clinical problem to overcome is to achieve intimate compatibility of two immiscible substrates: dentine is hydrophilic (likes water and is innately wet) whereas methacrylate resins are hydrophobic (water-repelling). Therefore a *dentine bonding agent (DBA) or dental adhesive* is required as a coupling agent between the two. DBAs have three generic components:

- *Acid etch*: The first stage of the process, which has the following effects on dentine:
  - Dissolves the dentine smear layer created by the cavity preparation process (Fig. 7.6)
  - Helps to unblock and widen the dentine tubule orifices
  - Demineralises the dentine surface, thus exposing the network of collagen in the dentine matrix (Table 7.2)
- *Primer*: A bifunctional coupling molecule (e.g., hydrophilic HEMA [hydroxyethylmethacrylate]) which has one functional group that is hydrophilic and thus is compatible with the moist collagen in dentine and another that is hydrophobic and thus is compatible with the bond/resin composite. The primer is carried into the moist collagen fibrillar network using a solvent such as water, acetone or

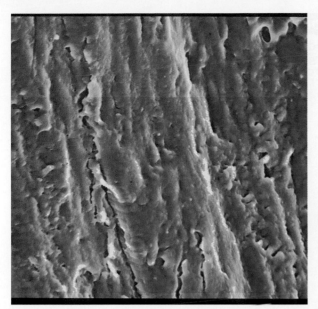

Fig. 7.6 Dentine smear layer (a tenacious layer of organic and inorganic cutting debris usually <20 μm thick) imaged using scanning electron microscopy: this can be a barrier to good bonding and is normally removed or modified using acids (field width 500 μm).

> **Q7.6:** How is the smear layer created?

alcohol, displacing the water molecules from the collagen and permitting the primer to enter into the micro- and nano-spaces created around the collagen fibrils after the etching process. Other monomers that have been shown to promote successful bonding to hydroxyapatite and calcium ions include the MDP monomer (10-methacryloyloxydecyl dihydrogen phosphate). This has a terminal double bond group for polymerisation, a hydrophobic alkylene group to maintain the balance between hydrophobic and hydrophilic properties and a hydrophilic phosphate group for acid demineralisation and chemical bonding to tooth structure.

- *Bond*: This can be considered simplistically as the resin component of the composite without the filler particles. A mixture of low-viscosity monomers capable of penetrating the spaces not occupied by the primer monomers, the bond can be photo-cured in the conventional way and then the resin composite placed incrementally (chemically cross-linking to the monomers in the air-inhibited layer of the bond) and the restoration completed.

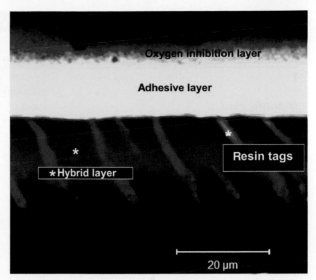

Fig. 7.7 A fluorescent micrograph of a dentine bonding agent on sound dentine, showing penetration of the red-labelled (rhodamine) primer into the collagen network and tubules in dentine, forming the hybrid zone up to 15 μm thick (nano-retention) as well as resin tags (microretention). The yellow-labelled (fluorescein) adhesive uses its oxygen-inhibition layer to help adherence to the composite. (Courtesy Prof S Sauro, Universidad CEU-Cardenal Herrera, Valencia, Spain.)

Each of these stages needs to be accomplished in optimal clinical conditions to enable a successful bond to be created between resin composite and dentine. The status of the collagen network on the cut dentine surface is of prime importance: it is the penetration of the primer and bond into these micro-/nano-spaces that provides the integrity of the seal and bond between the resin composite and dentine. This zone of collagen penetration is known as the *hybrid zone* and can be between 0.5 μm and 15 μm thick. Note that the thickness of the hybrid zone is less important than its continuity and integrity along the entire bonding surface. Any significant gaps in the hybrid zone will reduce the quality of the seal and ultimately the bond. Penetration of the bonding agent into the dentine tubules (so-called *resin tag formation*) plays only a small part in reinforcing the bond strength (Fig. 7.7). DBAs are used on enamel instead of the unfilled bonding resin described in the previous section to simplify the overall bonding process, but note that the chemistries of unfilled bonding resin (for enamel only) and DBAs (for both dentine and enamel) are different. There are numerous clinical presentations of DBAs from different manufacturers. A simple classification system

TABLE 7.4   **Classification System for Modern Dentine Bonding Agents (Dental Adhesives)**

Type of Dentine Bonding Agent	Generation	Effect on Smear Layer	Etching Technique	Clinical Steps	Components	Substrate Adhesion	Examples
1 (3-bottle, etch and rinse)	4th	Total removal	Total-etch (etch and rinse)	3	3-Etch, Prime and Bond	Enamel and dentine	Adper Scotchbond Multi-Purpose, Optibond FL, ProBond
2 (2-bottle, etch and rinse)	5th	Total removal	Total-etch (etch and rinse)	2	2-Etch, Prime and Bond	Enamel and dentine	Prime & Bond NT, I bond Total Etch, Adper Scotchbond 1XT
3 (2-bottle, self etch)	6th	Dissolved and incorporated	Self-etch Selective-etch	2	2-Etch, Prime and Bond	Enamel and dentine	Clearfil SE Bond 2, Adper Scotchbond Self-Etch
4 (1-bottle, self etch)	7th	Dissolved and incorporated	Total-etch (etch and rinse) Self-etch Selective-etch	1	1-Etch, Prime and Bond	Enamel and dentine	Xeno V, Adper Easy One, G-Bond, G-aenial Bond
5 (Universal/ multimode)	8th	Dissolved and incorporated	Total-etch (etch and rinse) Self-etch Selective-etch	1	1-Etch, Prime and Bond	Enamel and dentine Resin composites Ceramics Metal alloys	Scotchbond Universal, Scotchbond Universal +, Prime & Bond Universal, Futurabond U, GC G-Premio Bond, G2-Bond, Clearfil Universal Bond

Note: Data indicate the effect on the smear layer, presentation options of the three stages, etch, primer and bond, with some UK market examples current at the time of publication.

dependent on the three stages described earlier is presented in Table 7.4. In Chapter 8, a more detailed table is presented outlining the differences in the clinical techniques employed for each type of system (Table 8.12).

7.2.4 Classification of Dental Adhesives

7.2.4.1 Type 1: Three-Bottle or Three-Step Bonding Systems

In this group the three clinical steps described previously are completed separately. Ideally, dentine should be etched for 10 to 15 seconds and enamel for 20 seconds using 37% orthophosphoric acid, which is then washed away thoroughly (10 seconds) and dried until the enamel appears frosty white. As the primer contains water, any overdried exposed collagen on the dentine surface will rehydrate up to a point, thus permitting the primer and then the bond to penetrate the collagen network. However, overetching coupled with incomplete rehydration of the collagen might leave unfilled micro-/nano-porosities within the depth of the hybrid zone, and subsequent fluid movement in the dentine might lead to post-operative sensitivity and bond degradation over time. Even though sensitivity with the clinical technique is greater for these type 1 systems due to the three separate clinical steps, it is still accepted that type 1, three-bottle systems provide a good-quality, reliable bond and have been used for many years as the gold standard for dentine bond strength measurements in laboratory (*in-vitro*) studies.

7.2.4.2 Type 2: Two-Bottle or Two-Step, 'Total Etch' or 'Etch and Rinse' Adhesives

The clinical stages have been simplified into two steps in this group: an initial etch which is rinsed away, thus removing the smear layer. In type 2 systems it is imperative not to overdry the exposed collagen network as this cannot be rehydrated by the contents of the second bottle containing both the primer plus solvent and the bond (Fig. 7.8A–C). A technique of *moist bonding* must be employed after washing the etchant gel off, wicking the 'puddles' of excess surface water away using cotton wool pledgets, paper points or very gentle air drying (see Chapter 8, Table 8.12, for practical considerations). This will ensure the collagen network remains erect and supported, and thus more conducive for bond nano-penetration (Fig. 7.9A–C). The primer and bond are combined and it is essential to evaporate the solvent carrier (acetone or alcohol-based) as any remnants will contaminate and weaken the final bond. This evaporation procedure also thins the adhesive on the cavity walls and the operator must ensure enough adhesive is present before the photo-curing stage (the cavity walls must appear shiny). Therefore multiple applications of the adhesive (primer and bond together) may be required prior to placing the resin composite restoration.

7.2.4.3 Type 3: Weaker Self-Etching Primers

In this third group, the acidic phosphate monomers in the primer act as the etchant, so no separate acid etch/rinsing/drying phase or moist bonding technique is required. The dentine is etched sufficiently to partially dissolve the smear layer and expose the collagen network. Uncut enamel margins may be etched less efficiently, however, leading to a possibility of stained enamel margins of restorations in the long term (see Fig. 7.10A–B).

Q7.8: What are the dark irregular shapes outlined within the rhodamine-labelled (red) portion of Fig. 7.8C?

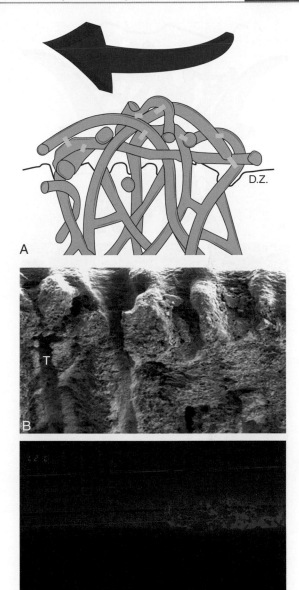

Fig. 7.8 (A) Diagram showing collagen fibres in dentine that have been overdried after etching. They have collapsed, so neither the primer nor the bond can penetrate into the nano-spaces within the collagen network *(red arrow)*. (Courtesy D Ziskind.) (B) A scanning electron micrograph (field width 75 µm) showing an overdried cut dentine surface with a collapsed collagen network (*T*, dentine tubule cut longitudinally). (Courtesy of Jorge Perdigão.) (C) Fluorescent confocal microscopic image (field width 250 µm) showing the bonding agent labelled with rhodamine *(red)*. The resin composite can be seen in the top half of the image and the barely visible outlines of dentine tubules in the bottom half. Note that as the dentine has been overdried (A), there has been no penetration of the collagen network or tubules and the resulting bond and seal will be poor.

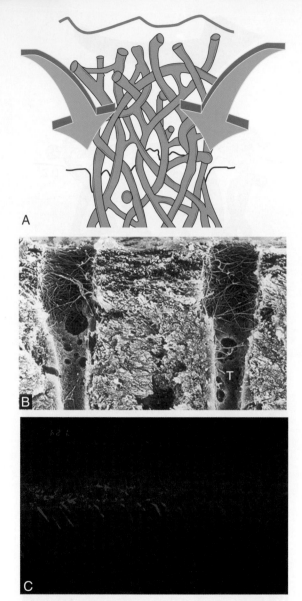

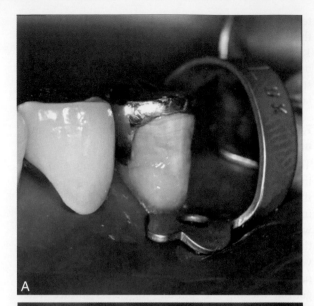

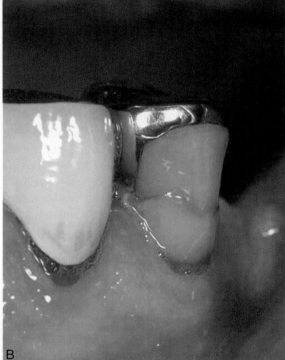

Fig. 7.9 (A) Diagram showing collagen fibres in dentine that have been kept moist so that the network is upright with micro-/nano-spaces available to accept the primer and bond *(green arrows)*. (Courtesy D Ziskind.) (B) An environmental scanning electron micrograph (field width 75 μm) showing moist collagen on the cut dentine surface. Individual collagen fibrils can be easily detected and the orifices of two tubules have been clearly widened by the etching process (*T*, dentine tubule cut longitudinally). (Courtesy of Jorge Perdigão.) (C) Fluorescent confocal microscopic image (field width 250 μm) showing the bonding agent labelled with a red dye penetrating the moist collagen network on the dentine surface (nano-mechanical retention) and into the tubules (micro-mechanical retention). Note the thin red diffuse band at the interface between the dentine and composite. This is the *hybrid zone* (10 μm thick).

Fig. 7.10 (A) Resin composite class V buccal cervical restoration of the LL5 placed using a type 3 self-etching primer dentine bonding agent. (B) The same restoration 10 years later.

Q7.10: Can you spot the difference between the two images of the same restoration and explain the reason for the difference?

This issue may be prevented by pre-etching the enamel margins with 37% orthophosphoric acid for 20 seconds, converting the whole clinical process to one similar to a type 1, three-stage system (Chapter 8, Section 8.3). The solvent again must be evaporated thoroughly after the acidic primer is agitated onto the dentine surface as in the type 2 systems.

7.2.4.4 Types 4 and 5: Self-Etching All-in-One/Universal Systems

Clinically, these are the simplest to use as there is a single application step where the three bonding stages (etch, prime and bond) are incorporated into one. Laboratory studies on sound enamel and dentine show not only favourable bond strengths, but also the presence of water blisters in the adhesive layer as it acts as a semi-permeable membrane, drawing water from the wet dentine tubules. As hydrolysis of polymeric dentine bonds occurs, there is evidence that marginal discolouration is potentially more of an issue with these adhesives. However, vigorous evaporation of the water-based solvent in the adhesive may reduce this problem. Longer-term clinical data have shown the clinical acceptability of these materials. The type 4 category of such adhesives is distinguished by the fact that these contain only acidic monomer chemistry with relatively strong self-etching capability depending on the product (pH 0.7–2.4), thus allowing adhesion to tooth structure and resin composites only. The type 5 adhesives contain additional, manufacturer-specific, bifunctional phosphate monomers (e.g., PENTA (dipentaerythritol penta-acrylate phosphate, amongst others)), which enables them to adhere not only to tooth structure and resin composites but also ceramics and metal alloys. They also have a milder self-etching pH range compared to the type 4 all-in-one adhesive systems (pH 2–2.7).

7.2.5 Clinical Issues With Dentine Bonding Agents/Dental Adhesives

- *Technique sensitivity*: The steps involved in dentine bonding require high levels of moisture control intra-orally and appropriate handling of the dental materials themselves. For example, if volatile solvents are allowed to naturally evaporate from bottles of adhesive when lids are not replaced after dispensing chairside, the chemistry is irreversibly adversely affected and therefore bonding will be impaired. The use of single-use doses might help alleviate this problem. Primers and bonds need to be agitated well into the tooth surface,

and all of these procedures must be followed to obtain a successful bond. Avoid the temptation to take clinical shortcuts and to omit stages of the bonding procedure—or indeed, of any restorative procedure!

- *Packaging instructions*: Familiarisation with the steps in the bonding process is essential and teamwork with your nurse is vital to place the various materials in the correct order and with speed and precision. Single-dose capsules, foils and bubble packs can be of assistance, reducing material wastage and improving infection control procedures. However, biodegradable packaging should be considered with regards to environmental sustainability during the manufacture and waste disposal processes.

- *Shelf life*: If kept refrigerated, the shelf life of most DBAs is approximately 1 to 2 years. Volatile solvents need to be kept tightly stoppered, and as many material components are light-sensitive, blacked-out bottles and packaging are advised.

- *Suitable substrate*: Most in-vitro research studies on DBAs use sound enamel and dentine as the tooth surface to which to bond, often on extracted teeth. The histological properties of teeth *in vivo* may be quite different and also the quality of the hard tissues will vary depending on the amount of carious tooth structure that has been retained. Therefore a comprehensive understanding is required of the state of the collagen network and mineral levels prior to using the DBA. More recent publications have used caries-affected dentine substrates *in vitro* and show clinically acceptable bond strengths of many different systems (15–28 MPa). It must be stressed again that the clinician's operative skills and understanding of the chemistry of the materials they are using, along with their handling characteristics and appreciation of tissue histology ('the golden triangle'), is paramount in conjunction with the patient's standard care primary prevention regimens for the optimal outcome of the final restoration.

- *Hydrolysis*: This is the major factor in the long-term degradation of the bond interface. The residual uncured monomers will be affected by the water transition through vital dentine, thus ultimately compromising the seal and bond. Therefore a good-quality peripheral enamel seal is essential for the long-term success of adhesive bonding. Matrix metalloproteinases (MMPs) and cathepsins released from the exposed collagen (see Chapter 1, Section 1.1.6) and activated in the caries acidic environment may account for the failure of the adhesive bond in both caries-affected and sound dentine by accelerating collagen fibril cleavage. This in turn will cause a breakdown of the hybrid zone, thus jeopardising the long-term adhesive seal and bond of the restoration.

- *Sensitisation*: These chemicals are designed to penetrate living tissue, and latex or nitrile gloves do not offer protection from resin-based materials. Therefore the dentist and nurse need to follow a 'no-touch' regimen when handling these materials.

7.2.6 Developments

The world of dental biomaterials is constantly evolving and by the time this book is published new materials will be available to be used clinically. Some of the ongoing challenges and developments are discussed in this section.

7.2.6.1 Reducing Shrinkage Stress and Strain

Manufacturers can alleviate the problem of significant volumetric shrinkage (often leading to increased marginal stress and/or material strain) by producing low-shrink materials, or materials that impart little strain on the tooth during their setting and maturation process. Historically, one such system used siloxane-oxirane (silorane) chemistry as opposed to conventional methacrylates. In this system, the monomers, instead of being linear, were ring-opening; therefore, during the cationic polymerisation process, less shrinkage occurred (0.9%). This chemistry required a separate bonding agent which was very hydrophobic, thus minimising water transition through the adhesive. Another system is a dimer-acid nanohybrid composite (based on dimer dicarbamate dimethacrylates), which exhibits polymerisation-induced phase separation (expansion) on curing, thus reducing some of the effects of polymerisation shrinkage. Whilst these low-shrink materials have been shown to be effective, commercially it seems, dentists are still using conventional resin composites, perhaps indicating that the clinical manifestations of shrinkage stress can be mitigated by careful operative handling. Conversely, the 'bulk-fill' material developments (Section 7.2.2.4) indicate that low-stress/low-viscosity composites that simplify restoration placement can become popular. Clinical studies are now showing favourable results with these materials and they are gaining in popularity.

7.2.6.2 Dentine Bonding Agents

With the advent of low-shrink composites, the importance of direct bond strengths may lessen and more emphasis placed on the ionic interaction between the materials and tooth structure. Medicinal ions could be transferred from the adhesive to help remineralise the enamel or dentine or act as antibacterial agents. Enzyme-inhibitor molecules have been introduced in an attempt to reduce enzymatic MMP-induced breakdown of collagen in the hybrid zone. Time will tell regarding their clinical efficacy and uptake by the profession.

7.2.6.3 'Self-Adhesive Composite'

The ultimate development, a simple-to-use, self-adhesive composite hybrid restorative material, both self- and light-cured, has been developed and marketed at the time of publication (Surefil One, Dentsply Sirona). This classification of material uses a modified polyacid system that promotes bonding to tooth structure while also acting as a copolymerising crosslinker between the covalent and ionic structural network in the set material. Even though laboratory testing data indicate at least an equivalent performance of this material compared to other clinical restorative materials (in terms of in-vitro mechanical strength, dimensional stability, wear resistance, marginal integrity and adhesive performance to sound enamel and dentine), further long-term clinical evaluation is required in the form of randomised controlled clinical trials to ascertain whether these in-vitro data can be extrapolated to the clinical environment. In this area of materials research, the boundary between resin composite and glass-ionomer chemistry is becoming more blurred.

7.3 GLASS-IONOMER CEMENT

Glass-ionomer cement (GIC – polyalkenoates) is a water-based, plastic direct dental restorative cement formed from an acid–base reaction between a polyalkenoic acid and ion-leachable fluoro-calcium (strontium) aluminosilicate glass particles.

7.3.1 History

GIC was developed as a biocompatible, chemically adhesive plastic restorative material by Wilson and Kent in the UK in 1972.

7.3.2 Chemistry

- *Powder*: Calcium fluoro-aluminosilicate glass particles with strontium (to increase radio-opacity). The silica (SiO_2 – affecting transparency), alumina (Al_2O_3 – affecting opacity, setting time and can increase the compressive strength of the set cement) and calcium fluoride (CaF_2 – the fluoride ions reduce the fusion temperature, increase strength of the set cement, enhance translucency and have a therapeutic effect) are the key components. These are structured ionically as a tetrahedral complex with a centrally located aluminium ion and closely localised alkaline earth cations (sodium, potassium, calcium and strontium) to maintain electro-neutrality.

- *Liquid-polyacid*: Itaconic acid copolymer solution in water plus tartaric acid (5%–15%, maintains working time and assists setting reaction). Anhydrous forms have vacuum-dried polyacrylic acid incorporated into the powder and are mixed with water ± dilute solution of tartaric acid.
- *Setting reaction*: Acid–base reaction with three stages (Fig. 7.11):
  1. *Dissolution*: Sol forms from the outer layers of the glass particles as they are attacked by the polyacid and calcium, strontium, aluminium and fluoride ions are released.
  2. *Gelation and hardening*: Primarily calcium ions bind to carboxylate groups (4–5 minutes) producing a clinically hard surface (initial set) and a siliceous hydrogel is formed, maturing over 24 hours, with further cross-linking with aluminium ions, up to 7 days. This process causes volumetric shrinkage of up to 3%. Surface protection at this stage is advisable to ensure regulation of water molecules in and out of the hydrogel, thus permitting maturation to occur.
  3. *Hydration*: Associated with stage 2, this maturation continues over several weeks, gradually improving the physical properties of the material. The gradual uptake of water leads to expansion, thus reducing any ill effects of the initial shrinkage that occurred.

7.3.3 The Tooth–GIC Interface

GICs have the ability to adhere chemically to mineralised dental tissues. They do this by the dynamic processes of diffusion and adsorption.

7.3.3.1 Enamel

GIC polyacid displaces phosphate and divalent Ca^{2+} ions from enamel hydroxyapatite and these ions become incorporated into the GIC matrix which sets. Subsequently the pH rises, and reprecipitation of minerals at the GIC–tooth interface occurs, forming an ion-enriched layer so firmly bound that when GIC restorations fail, this can be cohesive within the GIC material itself (Fig. 7.12A–B). If the enamel prisms have been damaged, fractured or pulled apart in preparing the cavity, the mineralised component of the interface can also fail cohesively due to the initial shrinkage stresses generated by the setting GIC (Fig. 7.13).

7.3.3.2 Dentine–Collagen

Adhesion to collagen may occur through hydrogen bond formation or metallic ion bridging between carboxyl groups of the polyacid and collagen.

7.3.3.3 Dentine–Tubules

There is limited evidence to argue for any significant micro-mechanical retention by the GIC penetration into dentine tubules. The penetration depth is limited (<5 μm) and the tensile strength of GIC in this dimension is poor, so it is unlikely to contribute significantly towards its retention within the cavity.

7.3.3.4 Surface Conditioning

Conditioning is the process by which both enamel and dentine are 'freshened' or pre-activated prior to the placement of freshly mixed GIC. The acid used is 10% polyacrylic acid for 10 seconds, which is then washed off and the surface dried gently, in order to:

- Remove/modify the smear layer and expose calcium and phosphate ions on the mineralised tooth surface
- Increase the surface energy of the tooth surface to allow improved wettability of the GIC as it is placed on the tooth surface

Dentine conditioner is mildly acidic, so it neither demineralises the dentine excessively nor opens up dentine tubules significantly. Note that this conditioning step is not the same as the 'conditioners' used in resin composite adhesion; that material, even though sharing the same nomenclature (especially in the United States), is a much stronger acid etchant (37% orthophosphoric acid).

7.3.4 GIC Surface Protection

These can be of three types:

1. Emollients such as petroleum jelly (Vaseline, Unilever, UK) and cocoa butter (GC Cocoa Butter, GC Corp, Japan)
2. Solvent-based waterproof varnishes such as GC Fuji Varnish (GC Corp, Japan) and Ketac Glaze (3M)

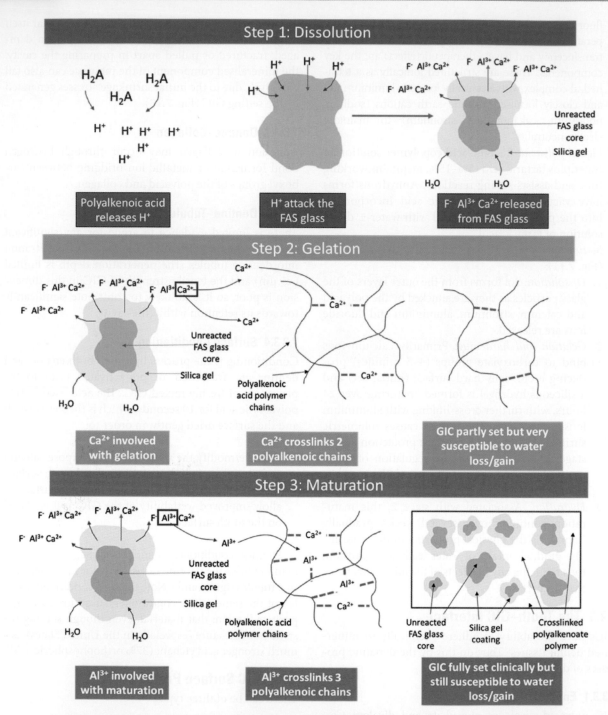

Fig. 7.11 Simplified schematic of the GIC setting process. Dissolution occurs within the first few seconds after mixing, gelation occurs within the first couple of minutes, while maturation occurs from 24 hours to up to several weeks after placement. (From Mylonas P, Zhang J, Banerjee A. Conventional glass-ionomer cements; a guide for practitioners. *Dent Update.* 2021;48:643-650. doi:10.12968/denu.2021.48.8.643.)

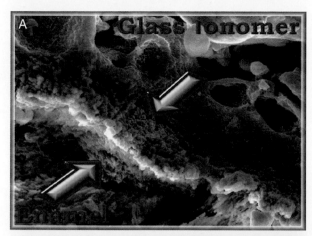

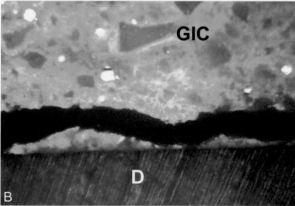

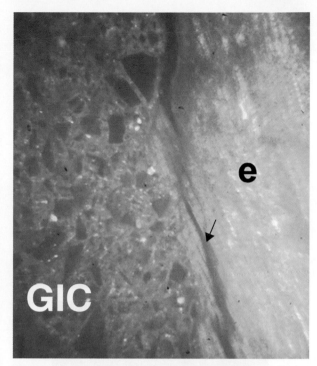

Fig. 7.13 Photomicrograph of glass-ionomer cement having pulled apart enamel prisms and caused cohesive failure in the enamel *(e; black arrow)* (field width 100 μm).

Fig. 7.12 (A) Scanning electron microscopy image showing interface between glass ionomer and enamel. The section surface has been etched lightly and a raised area (between the arrows) shows the ion-enriched layer at the tooth-restoration interface (field width 10 μm). (Courtesy Prof Hien Ngo.) (B) Fractured GIC–tooth interface *(D)* showing the cohesive failure common to these materials. The ion-enriched layer is still attached to the tooth (field width 300 μm).

> **Q7.13:** What are the irregular-shaped particles within the GIC?

> **Q7.12:** What is responsible for the cohesive fracture in Fig. 7.12B?

3. Light-cured, resin-based coatings such as EQUIA Coat (GC Corp, Japan) and Riva Coat (SDI, Australia)

Emollients can be petroleum- or lipid-based products, similar to those used for therapeutic management of dry skin conditions. Solvent-based varnishes are products that are simple solutions of different polymers in solvent, which when evaporated with air leaves behind a layer of polymer on the GIC surface.

Light-cured resin-based coatings are products designed for use with their corresponding GIC brand, generally consisting of a mixture of methacrylate monomers and photo-initiators, with or without filler particles.

Studies from the early 1990s indicated that coating the freshly set GIC restoration with a resin-based material (originally the bond from a dentine bonding agent) improved the surface contour and smoothness of the restoration as well as regulating the water transport across the exposed surface, allowing the GIC to mature appropriately. The surface sheen was also improved, thus improving the overall aesthetics of the final restoration. Of course, the surface coat will eventually be eroded and abraded away in clinical function, but this coating can easily be refreshed periodically at clinical review consultations (active surveillance; domain 4 of the MIOC pathway) to improve the overall longevity of the tooth-restoration complex (see Chapter 9, Section 9.4, and Fig. 7.14A–B).

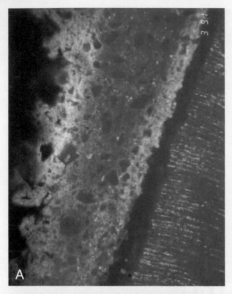

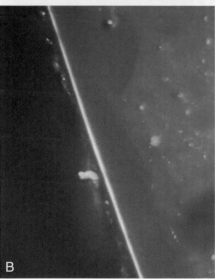

Fig. 7.14 (A) Photomicrographs of unprotected glass-ionomer cement (GIC) placed on dentine. The dentine substrate on the right side of the image shows its tubular pattern. The GIC layer has debonded from the dentine surface during sample preparation. The glass particles within the GIC are visible as dark irregular shadows, as is the exposed surface roughness on the left aspect of the image. (B) A layer of resin-based dental adhesive/dentine bonding agent that has been applied to the GIC surface. Note the close adaptation of the light-cured resin surface coat to the underlying GIC, with the resulting improvement of surface contour. (Copyright © 2023 European Journal of Prosthodontics and Restorative Dentistry. Reproduced with Permission.)

7.3.5 Clinical Uses of GIC Relating to Its Properties

GICs are used conventionally as:

- *Luting cements for indirect restorations*: In this scenario, the powder:liquid ratio is closer to 1.5:1 (less viscosity to improve fluid adaptation between the restoration and tooth).
- *Direct restorative material*: In this scenario, the powder:liquid ratio is >3:1 (stiffer, high-viscosity material), making this especially useful in high caries susceptible individuals. A useful material for carious lesion stabilisation when patients present with multiple carious lesions, direct restorative material is also used in atraumatic restorative treatment (ART) and in paediatric dentistry where the clinical environment and moisture control in particular may be compromised when trying to restore cavities in children. It is also indicated for carious lesion management in the older adult, especially those with compromised salivary quality and flow due to physiological age-related changes, polypharmacy affecting saliva output or head and neck radiation therapy. It is a useful restorative material in special care dentistry for patients with more challenging operative conditions. Many clinicians will also use GICs in deep carious lesions where the clinical environment is difficult to control, or as part of a laminate/layered/sandwich technique where indicated. Modern hybrid GICs can also be used as a core material for large posterior restorations that will be protected by a cast, indirect restoration.
- *Indirect pulp protection material*: With a powder:liquid ratio of 1.5:1, this solution is used to cover a direct pulp capping agent (e.g., setting calcium hydroxide or MTA) or in the depths of a cavity with very close proximity to the pulp, beneath an amalgam restoration (see, Chapter 5, Section 5.10). This is perhaps less indicated nowadays within the minimally invasive philosophy, where emphasis should be placed on simplifying and optimising restorative procedures.

As a direct, plastic restorative material, the best physical properties (tensile, compressive strengths and fracture toughness) of GIC are exhibited when the high-viscosity material is used in thick sections or in bulk. GICs have classically not been recommended for *long-term* stress-bearing restorations (e.g., posterior occlusal restorations). However, with the introduction of glass-hybrid GICs and other GIC-reinforced technologies, clinical trials are starting to produce medium-term longevity data for their successful use in occlusal posterior load-bearing restorations. Studies are ongoing for Class II restorations, so watch this space! Internal cavity line angles should be smooth and rounded prior to placement.

- *Fracture resistance/toughness*: Original GICs were brittle and prone to fracture under heavy occlusal loading. Modern high-viscosity derivatives have improved fracture toughness and clinical evidence is building as justification for them being used routinely as *long-term* restorations in the posterior load-bearing dentition, especially Class I cavities.
- *Abrasion/wear resistance*: Again, generally poorer than resin composites or dental amalgam but the use of resin-based surface-coating systems (e.g., G-Coat Plus, GC Japan) help regulate the long-term water uptake and provide a protective and aesthetic coating, thus improving this quality. The use of such resin-based surface coatings should be considered a mandatory part of clinical operative protocol.
- *Physical properties*: Compressive, shear, flexural strengths, thermal expansion and diffusivity have all improved with developments in GIC science. Modern materials appear to have some properties more closely approaching those of natural dentine.
- *Fluoride release*: Fluoride ions are released initially at high levels which fall away within 4 weeks after placement. The fluoride ions are captured within the siliceous hydrogel matrix and can pass in and out of this to the tooth surface, thus prompting the description of its 'fluoride reservoir' characteristic, recharging from high doses of professional fluoride application. There is contrary evidence, however, arguing that the fluoride release effect is of subclinical value after initial placement and setting and is more of a laboratory finding.
- *Aesthetics*: Significant improvements have been made with better shade and translucency of modern GICs. Water uptake and high solubility affect the long-term stability of colour and translucency in restorations, but resin-coating the surface just after placement or veneering the surface with resin composite at a later date are potential pragmatic clinical solutions (Fig. 7.15).

7.3.6 Developments

As with dental resin composites, GIC material science is continuously evolving. Developments include:

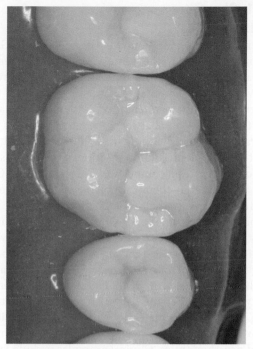

Fig. 7.15 Mesio-occlusal (Class II MO) restoration of the UR6. This material is a glass hybrid GIC (GC Equia Forte plus G Coat showing the high-quality aesthetics that can now be achieved with this material). (Courtesy B Dawett.)

- The speed, control and conversion rate of the initial set, with fast-setting materials on the market taking <90 seconds to reach a carvable stage
- Improving the physical properties to enable more reliable use in posterior, load-bearing cavities with the potential use of ceramic nanofiller technology, glass hybrid technology or developing the use of N-vinyl pyrrolidone-containing polyacids (NVPs) in the matrix polymer
- Improving the wear resistance, polishability and aesthetics of the final restoration with advances in resin-based coating systems, applied after finishing the restoration
- Greater use of the ionic exchange potential to introduce other ions to help remineralise and repair tooth structure and confer antibacterial effects.

7.4 RESIN-MODIFIED GLASS-IONOMER CEMENT AND POLYACID-MODIFIED RESIN COMPOSITE (COMPOMER)

The description of these materials as 'light-cured GICs' should be avoided.

7.4.1 Chemistry
7.4.1.1 RM-GICs

Resin-modified glass-ionomer cements (RM-GICs) essentially contain the same chemistry as conventional GICs with the addition of the hydrophilic resin, HEMA (hydroxyethylmethacrylate), Bis-GMA and other photoinitiators. They set with a combination reaction: acid–base between the glass particles and polyalkenoic acid (as previously described) and also light-cured polymerisation reaction of the resin (similar to that of a resin composite). The resin in RM-GICs can also undergo chemical polymerisation due to an intrinsic redox (reduction-oxidation) reaction, thus autocuring over time (approximately 1 month) into a fully set material. Because the HEMA resin is hydrophilic, there is a risk that after the initial snap-setting process, water is absorbed which might lead to medium- to long-term degradation and colour instability when used as the definitive restorative material (Fig. 7.16). These materials at a low powder:liquid ratio form the basis of widely used luting systems in fixed prosthodontics. Clinical examples include Fuji II LC (GC Corp), Vitremer (3M) and Ketac Nano (3M).

7.4.1.2 Polyacid-Modified Composites

These are materials that are primarily resin-based, with some GIC chemistry incorporated but not enough to promote a significant acid–base setting reaction. These materials essentially require light activation to promote the polymerisation chain reaction. They cannot adhere chemically to tooth structure as do conventional GICs, as the acid–base reaction only occurs over a prolonged time, after the initial set of the resin component. Therefore dentine bonding agents are a prerequisite for retention of these materials within a cavity. The original example of this class of material is Dyract (Dentsply).

7.4.2 Clinical Indications

Both of these materials can be used as provisional or definitive, shade-matched, tooth-coloured adhesive restoratives. However, there is some evidence that the colour stability of RM-GICs might be suspect over longer periods due to the extent of water absorption that occurs (Fig. 7.16).

RM-GICs may also be used as a base in an adhesive *layered/laminate/'sandwich'* restoration with an overlying resin composite completely covering the RM-GIC base (a closed restoration). However, there is clinical

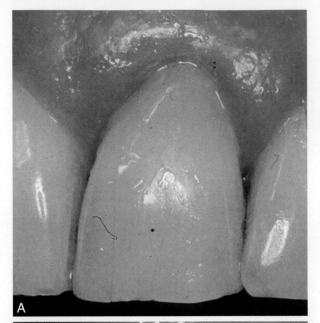

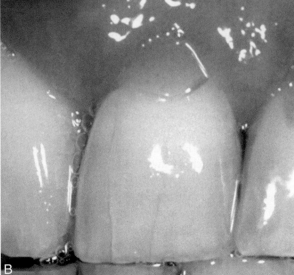

Fig. 7.16 (A) Resin-modified glass-ionomer cement buccal cervical Class V restoration of the UL1 with good aesthetic properties initially. (B) The same restoration 7 years later showing clear intrinsic discolouration due to water absorption.

evidence that these types of restoration are more prone to long-term failure, especially at the interfaces between the differing materials. Evidence shows that the layered/laminate/sandwich restoration should be limited to the placement of a resin composite veneer over the exposed, occlusal surface of large GICs/RM-GICs at least 6 months after the GIC restoration has been placed to allow for its full maturation, thus maximising its physical and chemical properties. Indeed, modern RM-GICs can be used to fully restore a cavity for several years' duration, before the exposed surface(s) requires refurbishing, possibly with a resin composite (see Chapter 9, Section 9.4).

When indirect chairside or laboratory-made restorations are constructed, some form of cementation (or luting) is required and the use of self-etching low-viscosity derivatives of the RM-GIC technology has become popular for such an application. Whilst the adhesive bond strengths of these materials may be inferior to those of a multistage light- and self-cured resin adhesive system, when measured in laboratory studies and used in conjunction with low-viscosity dual-cured composite luting cement, their handling simplicity will help potentially achieve a more reliable everyday clinical outcome when used by skilled operators. An example of this type of material is RelyX Unicem (3M).

With a push towards bio-interactivity and bio-activity of modern materials, and with the global phasedown and eventual phaseout of the use of dental amalgam (see Section 7.5), industry partners are pursuing further research and development into this area, trying to simplify and bridge the gap between the different classes of adherent tooth-coloured plastic restorative biomaterials to find a suitable and improved dental amalgam alternative. As one example amongst many, Pulpdent has marketed a range of bio-active restorative materials under the brand name Activa. This classification of material combines resins (aliphatic urethane dimethacrylate and other multimethacrylate monomers without Bis-GMA or bisphenol A [BPA] derivatives) and polyalkenoate chemistries with novel moieties including methacrylate-functionalised calcium phosphate (MCP) bio-active fillers, in an attempt to maximise the collective advantages of the restorative materials discussed earlier, including remineralisation potential and improved wear resistance, whilst minimising their clinical and physical disadvantages. As with all newly developed materials, medium- to long-term clinical data from randomised controlled clinical trials are needed and expected by the profession to ascertain whether these materials can reproduce the promising findings from controlled *in vitro* studies, in the variable clinical environment, before they can be clinically recommended. One way to collate such data in primary care is for practitioners to carefully select suitable cases and then place such materials judiciously and record their long-term outcome. This form of experience-based evidence is just as important as data from trials.

7.5 DENTAL AMALGAM

Dental amalgam, one of the oldest direct plastic restorative materials still in use, is an alloy of one or more metals including silver (Ag), tin (Sn), zinc (Zn), copper (Cu) and tiny amounts of some minor elements (palladium, platinum, indium) with mercury (Hg). Its use is now on the decline worldwide as:

- Patients demand more aesthetic restorations and can appreciate the benefits of simple tooth preserving restore/repair cycles of minimally invasive operative dentistry (MID: clinical domain 3 of MIOC).
- Health and safety and environmental issues have been raised against the mining extraction, use and disposal of mercury-containing products. The latter can be mitigated against by the use of appropriate traps in surgery waste water systems (compulsory in the UK). The United Nations Environmental Programme (UNEP) 2013 Minamata Convention on Mercury has declared that the use of dental amalgam will be phased down, and eventually phased out, as caries prevention strategies should be reinforced (administered through the MIOC delivery framework) and research into alternative restorative materials develop. At the time of publication, all four constituent nations of the UK have published an intent to phase down the use of dental amalgam in line with the European Union (EU) Regulation 2017/852 on Mercury (Article 10 [3]) and ambitions of the Minamata Convention. Indeed, a phase out may be enforced as early as 2027 or thereafter.
- Adhesive biomaterials are continuously being developed with significantly improved bonding capabilities to sound and caries-affected tooth structure.
- Principles of minimally invasive operative dentistry (MID) are being embraced, producing smaller, less mechanically retentive cavities to restore, thus advocating the use of adhesive, bio-interactive, tooth-coloured materials.
- Caries control and management strategies have evolved with a better understanding of the histopathology of the disease, as well as evolving preventive behaviour management strategies.

7.5.1 Chemistry

- Silver (70%–75%), tin (27%–29%), copper (<7% low Cu, >12% high Cu) and trace metallic elements (<1%) are presented as phases—γ gamma (Ag_3Sn), ε epsilon (Cu$_3$Sn) and d dispersant (Ag-Cu eutectic alloy)—and mixed with mercury (triturated in an amalgamator unit) to form an alloy (amalgamation reaction), thus producing the intrinsic strength and mechanical properties of the set material.

- Metal phases are presented as ingots which are then made into lathe-cut particles. Alternatively, molten alloy is sprayed into an inert atmosphere and atomised into spherical particles. The final powder may be an admix of the two particle types. The particle size and shape have an effect on the ease of packing the triturated amalgam into a cavity; spherical particle alloys require less force to condense into a cavity, resulting in fewer voids.
- Modern alloys are high-copper alloys with >12% Cu (single composition or dispersion-modified Cu-enriched alloys). The inclusion of copper improves corrosion and creep resistance and strengthens the set material by reducing unwanted Sn-Hg γ_2 (gamma 2) phase in the set amalgam.
- Compositions of >0.01% zinc were introduced to scavenge oxygen when casting the metal ingots. The use of an inert atmosphere in the manufacture of spherical particles makes the inclusion of zinc redundant. Inclusion of zinc led to increased hygroscopic expansion due to water contamination during placement but may increase marginal strength.

7.5.2 Physical Properties

- *Strength*: High compressive and tensile strengths are exhibited several days after placement. Care is required when checking the occlusion immediately after condensation and carving as the amalgam may be brittle at this stage. High Cu alloys have a greater strength and are used in large load-bearing posterior restorations. Amalgam is weak in thin section and requires at least 2 mm thickness to support itself. Therefore cavity design is important for this reason as well as for mechanical retention via undercuts as well as support.
- *Corrosion*: An electrochemical breakdown occurs due to the interaction between any metal and its surroundings. Low Cu amalgams corroded more quickly and extensively, thus sealing any micro-gaps between the cavity wall and restoration. Commonly used high Cu alloys are more resistant to corrosion and corrosion fatigue at the margins. Amalgam surfaces can oxidise over time, leading to surface corrosion

or even breakdown and then to pitting and surface deficiencies.

- *Rigidity*: The modulus of elasticity of amalgam is high but not as rigid as enamel.
- *Dimensional changes*: After minor setting contraction, water uptake during setting (especially in low Cu, Zn-containing alloys) can lead to hydrogen production and expansion, leading to pain. Thermal expansion can also occur to a degree further than normal tooth structure, so fine surface polishing, where friction will generate heat, should be undertaken with due care and coolant water irrigation.

7.5.3 Bonded and Sealed Amalgams

Amalgam restorations obtain retention within a cavity macro-mechanically, achieved by making undercut preparations (where the base of the cavity is wider than its opening) or using slots and grooves cut into the cavity walls or floor using burs, root canal posts or the pulp chamber and root canal orifices themselves (Nayyar core, Fig. 7.17; see Chapter 5, Table 5.10). All of these require

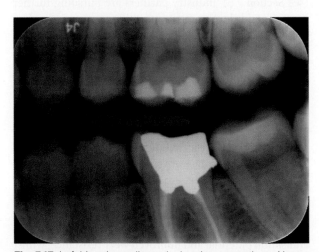

Fig. 7.17 Left bitewing radiograph showing an amalgam Nayyar core of the LL6. Note how the 'amalgam pins' extend into the coronal aspects of the endodontically treated root canals to aid retention, after the gutta percha was removed. The bulk of amalgam will also confer strength to the restoration. For the clinical steps to place a Nayyar core, see Chapter 8, Section 8.10.

Q7.17: What problem can you see with this restoration and how may it be treated? What do you think should be considered as part of the long-term management of this tooth?

excessive amounts of tooth structure to be removed or damaged to some extent, thus ultimately weakening the remaining tissue—not particularly minimally invasive! Dentine pins have historically been used to retain dental amalgam in larger cavities where cusps are missing. There is clear evidence that even correct placement of dentine pins tends to significantly increase the stresses in an already weakened tooth, leading to ultimate catastrophic failure of the restoration and tooth. Clinical evidence clearly indicates that dentine pins should not be used in modern minimally invasive operative dentistry as alternative methods and materials now exist, including self-curing adhesive luting cements to couple the cavity walls to the amalgam restoration.

7.5.3.1 Bonded Amalgams

An adhesive, chemically cured resin-based luting cement is used to seal the exposed dentine tubules after cavity preparation, bonding to the dentine mineral and collagen (as with resin composites) and micro-mechanically interlocking simultaneously with the freshly condensed dental amalgam as they both set (see Chapter 8, Section 8.9). Chemical bonds with metal oxides forming in the set dental amalgam may form, but these have little clinical significance for retention in the long term. The clinical evidence for their routine use continues to be inconclusive, but the procedure might be beneficial when repairing old, large, fractured amalgams with new amalgam (see Chapter 9, Section 9.4.1).

7.5.3.2 Sealed Amalgams

As modern high-copper alloys corrode less and so do not adequately seal the spaces at the tooth–amalgam interface over time, a flowable resin/dentine bonding agent can be used to coat the surface of the tooth–amalgam interface after condensation, shaping and finishing. This can penetrate into and seal any micro-gaps at the marginal interface which form during the setting process, thus reducing the chance of marginal leakage and the risk of subsequent CARS (caries associated with restorations and sealants, or secondary caries). A dentine bonding agent or dental adhesive may also be used to seal the dentine cavity walls prior to placement of the amalgam restoration.

7.5.4 Contemporary Indications for the Use of Dental Amalgam

In the current climate of the ever-increasing availability of more clinically and physically acceptable tooth-coloured, but not perfect, biomaterial alternatives alongside the

practise of minimally invasive dentistry skill sets as well as the ever stronger pushback due to the environmental concerns over the extraction, safety and disposal of mercury, the clinical indications for using dental amalgam are becoming more limited. Scandinavian countries banned the use of dental amalgam over 2 decades ago. In 2018, Article 10(2) of EU Reg. 2017/852, a European Union–wide dental amalgam phaseout for vulnerable populations came into force. The intent of this directive remains in place despite the UK having left the European Union. The directive applies to pregnant or breastfeeding women and children under 15 years of age. However, there is a clear exemption that dental amalgam can be placed when deemed '*strictly necessary by the dental practitioner based on the specific medical needs of the patient*'. Aligned with the 2018 European Union (EU) Regulation and ambitions of the Minamata Convention, all four constituent nations of the UK have published an intent to phase down the use of dental amalgam, possibly as soon as 2025 after further EU directives recently published. This is in addition to the restrictions on the use of dental amalgam in the specified patient groups mentioned above.

The use of dental amalgam may reasonably be restricted to large posterior load-bearing restorations or as a core material for crowns (Fig. 7.18; see Chapter 8, Section 8.9), even though adhesive biomaterial alternatives do now exist for this purpose. Repairs to existing restorations, especially in scenarios where moisture control is difficult to achieve clinically (e.g., subgingival cavities) or in patients where achieving a dry clinical field required for adhesive restorations is fraught with patients' physical disability and/or behavioural challenges, may also be indications for the limited ongoing use of dental amalgam.

7.6 TEMPORARY AND PROVISIONAL (*INTERMEDIATE*) RESTORATIVE MATERIALS

7.6.1 Characteristics

Temporary restorative materials ideally should:

- Be simple for both the operator and nurse to handle clinically
- Be easy to remove to allow final placement of the definitive restoration
- Not interfere with the setting or bonding chemistry of any definitive restorative material or luting cement

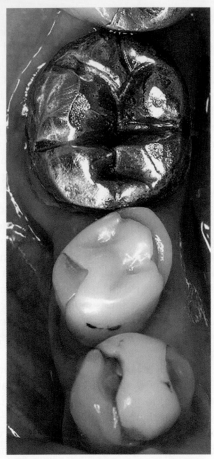

Fig. 7.18 Broken down LR6 mandibular molar restored with a large load-bearing amalgam restoration. (From MacKenzie L, Banerjee A. Minimally invasive direct restorations: a practical guide. *Brit Dent J.* 2017 Aug 11;223(3):163-171. doi:10.1038/sj.bdj.2017.661.)

Q7.18i: At what stage of restoration placement has this photograph been taken and what stage is left to complete?

Q7.18ii: What is the clinical status of the tooth-coloured restorations in the LR4 and LR5?

- Be durable enough to last in the oral cavity for several weeks
- Be inexpensive and biocompatible

In addition to exhibiting the preceding qualities, provisional restorative materials ideally should:

- Be durable enough to last in the oral cavity for several months
- Be as aesthetically pleasing as possible

The differences between a provisional and definitive restorative material can be blurred nowadays as many adhesive restorative materials combine all of these qualities.

7.6.2 Chemistry

- Radio-opaque, polymer-reinforced zinc oxide-eugenol cements (e.g., Kalzinol, Sedanol, pre-mixed Intermediate Restorative Material or IRM). Quick setting and easy to spatulate and load into cavities, but must not be used where resin composites will follow as the eugenol can affect the polymerisation chain reaction adversely.
- Glass-ionomer/RM-GICs (see previous sections).
- Zinc polycarboxylate cements (Poly F Plus): Water-soluble, low-molecular-weight polymers of acrylic or methacrylic acid that form solid, insoluble products when mixed with specially prepared zinc oxide powder. The resulting cement adheres to dental enamel and can also be used as a luting agent.

7.7 CALCIUM SILICATE CEMENTS

7.7.1 History

Calcium silicate cements were introduced to operative dentistry in 1993 when Mahmoud Torabinejad developed a formula based on ordinary Portland cement which was intended primarily for use as an endodontic material (e.g., in root end/perforation repairs). As a mineral trioxide aggregate (MTA) that is composed principally of tricalcium silicate, dicalcium silicate, tricalcium aluminate and tetracalcium aluminoferrite, its operative dental applications were limited somewhat due to the protracted working and setting time of several hours.

In 2010, Biodentine (Septodont, France), a quicker-setting calcium silicate restorative cement, was introduced. This cement was developed as a dentine replacement material, a novel clinical application of this family of materials, intending it to function as a direct coronal restoration. The comparatively shorter working and setting time (approximately 12 minutes) enables the use of this cement for clinical restorative procedures, which is impossible with modern MTAs that achieve only an initial set in 3 to 4 hours.

7.7.2 Chemistry and Interactions With the Tooth

The faster-setting (12 minutes) calcium silicate cement (Biodentine/injectable Biodentine XP) is principally composed of a highly purified tricalcium silicate powder that is synthetically prepared in the laboratory *de novo*, rather than derived from a clinker product of cement manufacture. Additionally, Biodentine contains dicalcium silicate, calcium carbonate and zirconium dioxide as a radio-opacifier. The powder is dispensed in a two-part capsule to which is added an aliquot of hydration liquid, composed of water, calcium chloride (to accelerate the setting reaction) and a reducing agent.

Similar to ordinary Portland cement, calcium silicate-based dental cements set via a hydration reaction. Although the chemical reactions taking place during the hydration are more complex, the conversion of the anhydrous phases into corresponding hydrates can be simplified as follows:

$$2Ca_3SiO_5 + 6H_2O \rightarrow 3CaO.2SiO_2.3H_2O + 3Ca(OH)_2$$
$$+ \text{energy}$$

C_3S + water $\rightarrow$ CSH + CH

$$2Ca_2SiO_4 + 5H_2O \rightarrow 3CaO.2SiO_2.4H_2O + Ca(OH)_2$$
$$+ \text{energy}$$

C_2S + water $\rightarrow$ CSH + CH

This setting reaction is a dissolution-precipitation process that involves a gradual dissolution of the unhydrated calcium silicate phases (C_3S and C_2S) and formation of hydration products, mainly calcium silicate hydrate (CSH) and calcium hydroxide (CH). The CSH precipitates as a colloidal material and grows on the surface of unhydrated calcium silicate granules, forming a matrix that binds the other components together, gradually replacing the original granules. Meanwhile, calcium hydroxide is distributed throughout water-filled spaces present between the hydrating cement species.

The setting cement attains a high pH and this has a novel effect on the dentine. Any organic substrate that is directly in contact with the fresh, setting cement (e.g., demineralised collagen in caries-affected dentine at the base of a cavity) will be 'caustically etched' by the alkaline cement and subsequently subjected to calcium ion release and crystal precipitation from the cement. This alkaline environment is conducive for mineralisation to occur within the cement–dentine interface, so this material might be termed 'bio-interactive' (see Fig. 7.19). Equally important is the direct cellular therapeutic effect on the pulp elicited by the release of calcium hydroxide, leading to reparative (tertiary) dentine formation, in cases of direct pulp protection—a 'bio-active' quality.

7.7.3 Clinical Applications

The presence of large amounts of calcium hydroxide within the set material makes this material potentially

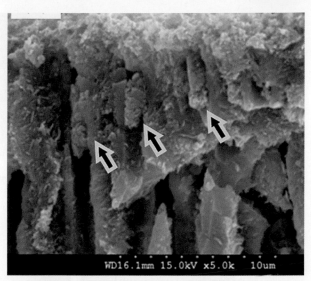

Fig. 7.19 A scanning electron micrograph showing the Biodentine–dentine interface. The patent, vertically oriented dentine tubules are evident in the lower portion of the image. The Biodentine residue is located at the top surface. Arrows indicate an example of the tubular infill of crystallites generated by precipitation of mineralising ions, such as calcium, from the Biodentine material. (Courtesy A Atmeh.)

useful for its therapeutic pulp effects, being more robust and resistant to dissolution when compared with the traditional calcium hydroxide pulp protection materials. The faster-setting calcium silicate cement described has sufficient compressive strength to act as a bulk replacement of dentine (approximately 200 MPa), but it is not appropriate for long-term exposure to wear or occlusal loading in the mouth. As such, it has an appropriate use as a provisional restorative material especially when restoring deep carious lesions, offering indirect pulp protection (Fig. 7.20), prior

---

Q7.20: What other management regimens would you put in place to manage this patient?

Q7.20A: What signs are evident on the radiograph that the LR7 has been resisting the caries process as it has gradually progressed through the tooth?

Q7.20C: What are the classic symptoms of an acute reversible pulpitis?

Q7.20D: What is Carisolv gel? How does it work? What quality of enamel and dentine has been retained at the base of this cavity and why?

Q7.20I and J: How would you describe the resin composite veneer overlaying the Biodentine: open or closed 'sandwich'? What do you think might be the cause of the radiolucent line in the radiograph beneath the Biodentine restoration?

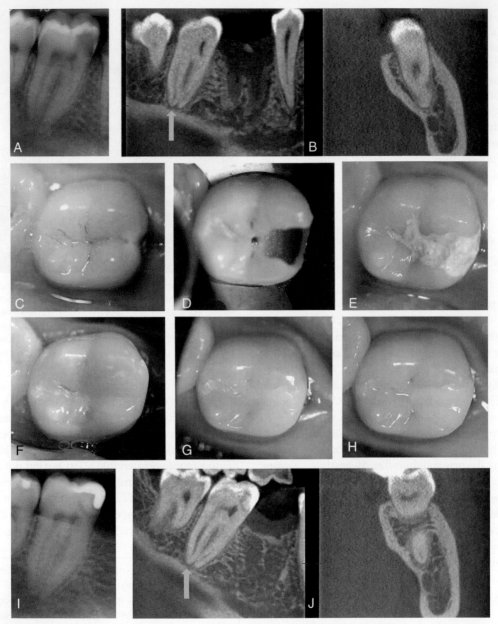

Fig. 7.20 (A) Long cone periapical radiograph at presentation revealing a large carious lesion on the mesial aspect of the lower right 7 with apparently healthy periapical tissues. (B) Cone Beam Computer Tomography (CBCT) at presentation revealing radiolucency around the apex of the distal root *(yellow arrow)*. (C) Clinical photograph of the tooth at presentation, before operative intervention. The tooth offered positive pulp sensibility to an electric pulp test and exhibited the classic symptoms of an acute reversible pulpitis. A clinical decision was made to restore it minimally invasively as it was cavitated mesially. (D) The lesion accessed from the mesio-occlusal aspect. Dental burs and then Carisolv gel were used to excavate the deepest carious dentine. No pulp exposures were created. (E) Biodentine application. (F) After 1 month (T1) following cutback of Biodentine and placement of resin composite (N'Durance, Septodont) restoration. (G) After 6 months (T6). (H) After 12 months (T12). (I) Long cone periapical radiograph at T12 revealing the Biodentine restoration and the veneering resin composite restoration, with healthy periapical tissues. Note the thin radiolucent line beneath the Biodentine restoration in the radiograph. (J) CBCT at T12 revealing resolved radiolucency around the apex of the distal root *(yellow arrow)*. (Courtesy D Hashem.)

to reducing the cement height and veneering the occlusal and proximal surfaces with a material such as resin composite. The relatively slow set and maturation of this material precludes the placement of the resin composite veneer immediately onto the newly placed, initially set cement. GICs should also be avoided in this regard, especially as their setting chemistry and that of Biodentine are incompatible and each will compromise the other. It is optimal to leave it for at least 1 week to mature enough to improve the bond of the resin composite to the Biodentine.

- Biodentine should be mixed carefully, adhering fully to the manufacturer's instructions (as with all materials). Any change in the number of drops of liquid will adversely affect the mix and setting chemistry of the material. Biodentine XP removes this handling issue as it is presented as a pre-packaged cartridge system that requires its own specific high-speed oscillating mixer to ensure an optimal clinical mix is achieved every time.
- Once mixed, Biodentine should be gently placed into the cavity using a suitable carrier instrument. As the setting reaction starts immediately, care should be taken not to forcibly pack the material into the cavity as this action will impair the internal crystallisation process. Biodentine XP can be syringed directly into the cavity, from the cavity base to the tooth surface, precluding the use of a carrier or any force being applied.
- Once the cavity is fully filled with Biodentine, the occlusal shaping should be carried out simply and quickly using the gentle use of flat plastic instruments and ball burnishers. The material should then be left alone to set for the remaining time. The rubber dam can be removed as some moisture from the oral cavity will aid the setting reaction. Pooled saliva of course must be removed using adequate suction.
- Ideally at the second visit, usually a few weeks after initial placement when the pulp status has been checked, the cut surface of a mature Biodentine surface should be given a 15-second acid etch, either with 37% orthophosphoric acid (followed by thorough water rinsing) or using a strong self-etching adhesive, treating the cement surface much as one would dentine.
- The interface between the overlying resin composite and cement will be micro-mechanical in nature in a similar manner to the interface between GICs and resin composites.
- The potential for the long-term acid dissolution of exposed cement under a biofilm on a proximal restoration surface would indicate that the 'closed

sandwich' type of restoration would be favoured, where clinically achievable (Fig. 7.20).

Biodentine can also be used directly on a vital exposed pulp, that may sometimes occur during tissue removal in the depths of a deep carious cavity (as a direct pulp capping agent).

7.8 MATERIALS AND TECHNIQUES FOR RESTORING THE ENDODONTICALLY TREATED TOOTH

7.8.1 Root Canal Posts

Root canal posts can be made using metals such as stainless steel, titanium and gold and can be directly fabricated chairside by the dentist or indirectly cast in the laboratory, techniques and materials that have been used for many years. Fibre-reinforced posts are also popular (see Chapter 6, Section 6.3). These posts consist of very fine glass fibres extruded through the long axis of the post and shaped within a matrix of resin, normally an epoxy or methacrylate which is then fully polymerised, but retaining a roughened surface to aid retention of the cement luting material. The shape of the post is designed to mimic the tapered anatomy of the enlarged root canal space, thus reducing the need for unnecessary root dentine removal during placement. Clinical studies have reported that direct fibre-reinforced composite posts outperform cast and metal posts in general.

Compared to metal posts, fibre posts (due to their flexibility and closer match to the elastic modulus of dentine) would seem to protect the root against fracture especially when there is extensive coronal tissue breakdown or loss. The most common type of failure with fibre-reinforced composite posts is debonding, which normally permits re-restoration of the tooth. The current available evidence does not rule out the use of cast posts made in the dental laboratory. However, since the use of cast posts may result in a significantly greater loss of tooth structure during preparation and on failure compared to fibre posts, their application should be limited to those cases in which no additional dentine has to be removed to allow for their cementation.

7.8.2 Root Canal Post Cementation

Fibre and metal posts can be cemented into the root canal using all types of adhesive systems. The use of conventional two- and three-step bonding systems can be challenging due to the difficulty in light-curing the adhesive within the depths of the root canal space. There are also polymerisation shrinkage stresses likely to develop in the root canal, which is a very confined space with an unfavourably high C-factor (see Chapter 6, Section 6.3.2). For this reason, self-etching adhesive cements based on resin-modified GIC technology have become very popular as they are easy to use, create a uniform layer of cement along the root canal walls and still allow the use of conventional two- and three-step adhesive systems to more effectively bond the resin composite core to the residual coronal tooth structure.

7.9   ANSWERS TO SELF-TEST QUESTIONS

Q7.1: What physical properties of the dental composite does the monomer chain length affect?
A: The viscosity of the uncured material and the degree of polymerisation shrinkage (see text).

Q7.6: How is the smear layer created?
A: By the friction generated from any cutting instrument on the tooth surface (hand instrument or rotary); air-abrasion produces a layer similar to a smear layer created from organic/inorganic chip debris and abrasive particles.

Q7.8: What are the dark irregular shapes outlined within the rhodamine-labelled (red) portion of Fig. 7.8C?
A: These are the irregular silica-based filler particles within the resin composite.

Q7.10: Can you spot the difference between the two images of the same restouration and explain the reason for the difference?
A: Note the dark discolouration on the superior margin of the restoration–enamel interface. This is due to the enamel not being as efficiently etched by the weaker self-etching primer. This has led to a less well sealed adhesive bond which has gradually picked up stain over the last decade of use. Pre-etching the enamel with 37% orthophosphoric acid etch can alleviate this problem.

Q7.12: What is responsible for the cohesive fracture in Fig. 7.12B?
A: Phase 2 of the setting reaction with the formation of calcium and aluminium cross-links coupled with potential dehydration of the GIC.

Q7.13: What are the irregular-shaped particles within the GIC?
A: Unreacted fluoro-calcium aluminosilicate glass particles.

Q7.17: What problem can you see with this restoration and how can it be treated? What do you think should be considered as part of the long-term management of this tooth?
A: Note the distal amalgam overhang, caused by inadequate adaptation of the matrix band when originally packing the cavity. This may be removed using fine burs (if clinical access is available) and interproximal amalgam finishing strips. If not, the long-term management of the tooth may involve the placement of an indirect full-coverage cast restoration (e.g., a metal ceramic or full gold crown) and during the tooth preparation for this, the overhang will be automatically removed.

Q7.18i: At what stage of restoration placement has this photograph been taken and what stage is left to complete?
A: Just after the amalgam has been packed, circumferential matrix band removed and the restoration finished. This means that margins, contour, surface finish, contact points and occlusion have all been checked. The next stage might be to polish the restoration to smooth the surface, thus reducing potential plaque accumulation. However, polishing techniques must use water-cooling to avoid an increase in frictional heat causing damage to the pulp.

Q7.18ii: What is the clinical status of the tooth-coloured restorations in the LR4 and LR5?
A: These older resin composite restorations have ditched margins. There is no caries associated with these margins, there are no pain symptoms from the patient and the biofilm control is adequate as the marginal gaps are accessible to oral hygiene aids. There is no structural or functional compromise of these tooth-restoration complexes, therefore the only potential issue is their aesthetics which might indicate restoration repair using the "5Rs" approach (see Chapter 9, Section 9.4).

Q7.20: What other management regimens would you put in place to manage this patient?
A: A preventive regimen consisting of oral hygiene instruction (OHI), dietary advice and use of fluoride. Also, ensuring that the caries risk/susceptibility of this patient is brought under control, with regular review consultations to assess the patient's adherence to the behavioural change advice given by the oral healthcare team as well as to check the progress (or not) of further disease (active surveillance).

7.9   ANSWERS TO SELF-TEST QUESTIONS—cont'd

Q7.20A: What signs are evident on the radiograph that the LR7 has been resisting the caries process as it has gradually progressed through the tooth?

A: Note the reduced size of the pulp chamber directly adjacent to the lesion. This is tertiary dentine that has been laid down in response to the gradual caries process.

Q7.20C: What are the classic symptoms of an acute reversible pulpitis?

A: Short, sharp, poorly localised pain of a few seconds' duration, stimulated by hot/cold/sweet stimuli.

Q7.20D: What is Carisolv gel? How does it work? What quality of enamel and dentine has been retained at the base of this cavity and why?

A: Read Chapter 5, Section 5.8.5 for revision about chemomechanical excavation gels. There is caries-affected dentine retained on the cavity base. The enamel margin is sound. If the cavity was to be excavated to sound dentine

(yellow and hard) there would be a significant risk of unnecessary pulp exposure and the restoration margin would end up being very subgingival, thus questioning the actual restorability of the tooth/viability of placing a restoration.

Q7.20I and J: How would you describe the resin composite veneer overlaying the Biodentine: open or closed 'sandwich'? What do you think might be the cause of the radiolucent line in the radiograph beneath the Biodentine restoration?

A: This is an open sandwich restoration as some Biodentine has been left exposed to the oral cavity on the mesial aspect of the restoration. Please read Chapter 2, Section 2.5.3 for the answer to the second part. As Biodentine caustically etches the dentine due to its high pH, it is possible that this radiolucency has been created by this process and only time will tell (with review radiographs) if this gains mineral and therefore becomes more radio-dense like the surrounding sound dentine.

MIOC Domain 3: Minimally Invasive Operative Dentistry (MID), a Step-by-Step Clinical Guide

CHAPTER OUTLINE

8.1 INTRODUCTION

This chapter illustrates several tertiary preventive, minimally invasive operative dentistry procedures (one of the clinical domains of the minimum intervention oral care (MIOC) delivery framework) used for the successful placement of direct plastic restorations in the posterior and anterior dentition. The procedure list cannot be and is not exhaustive, but has been selected to give the reader the broadest application of the minimally invasive techniques described. The techniques shown are not exclusive; there are many varied operative techniques to remove caries and place suitable bio-interactive restorations (see Chapters 5 and 7), but the methods described are simple and achievable for most clinical abilities and in most clinical situations. The experienced skilled clinician is able to adapt the myriad skills outlined in these examples to best fit the

developing clinical situation presented to them. It is important to emphasise that this is not a 'one size fits all' operative approach to placing restorations in a purely standardised manner.

8.1.1 Cavity/Restoration Classification

There are several classifications of cavities in the dental literature attempting to correlate site, size of lesion and disease activity. The oldest, simplest and probably most universally accepted is Black's classification (Table 8.1). This classification was originally used to denote the most common sites for carious lesions to develop, thus helping to assess the individual's caries risk/susceptibility and for clinical notation. Nowadays, it is used to describe the site of the cavity or restoration and is useful for descriptive purposes, communicating between clinicians or annotations in dental

TABLE 8.1	Black's Classification of Carious Lesions
Black's Class	**Site**
I	Posterior lesion contained within the occlusal surface
II	Posterior lesion including a proximal surface
III	Anterior lesion including a proximal surface
IV	Anterior lesion involving the incisal edge
V	Buccal cervical lesion

Note: Black's classification of carious lesions is often misappropriated by clinicians as a purely descriptive analysis of the restoration site. With the increased use of adhesive restoratives, many restorations may involve several of the listed surfaces and therefore need more specific, accurate descriptions.

records. It must be understood that cavities in teeth should not be cut with pre-determined geometric shapes according to this classification but the classification used according to the final restoration placed, which will be governed by the biological extent of the caries, the type of material used and other factors (e.g., amount/strength of tooth structure retained, occlusal factors, etc.).

8.1.2 Restoration Procedures

The remainder of this chapter is dedicated to describing and illustrating the practical stages in placing certain types of restoration, outlining in detail the clinical procedures involved (Tables 8.2–8.11). Discussion of the separate steps will be found throughout the preceding chapters and these links are highlighted throughout. It is assumed that the clinical need for such interventions have been appropriately ascertained, documented and communicated to the patient and any necessary local analgesia has been administered prior to commencement of the restorative procedures outlined. As you will see, the procedures are classified with regard to tissue structures being prepared, as opposed to the restorative material used, *per se*.

8.2 PREVENTIVE FISSURE SEALANT

TABLE 8.2 Outline of Fissure Sealant Procedure

Operative Procedure	Indication (Chapters 2 and 3)	Pre-op Procedures/ Isolation (Chapter 5)	Caries Removal/ Cavity Preparation (Chapter 5)	Cavity Modification (Chapter 5)	Bonding Steps (Chapter 7)	Restorative Steps	Finishing Steps
Preventive fissure sealant (FS) **Resin composite (RC)**	High caries risk/ susceptibility, deep fissure patterns, stagnating plaque, poor OH. Newly erupting molars.	Pre-op occlusal check with articulating paper. Rubber dam. (Cotton wool rolls + aspiration if rubber dam placement not possible).	Fissure debridement with prophy paste and rotating brush. Sodium bicarbonate air-polishing. Bio-active glass air-abrasion.	Wash and dry using 3-1 syringe (10 sec).	*Resin composite*: 37% orthophosphoric acid-etch enamel fissures (20 sec), wash and dry (10 sec).	*Resin composite*: FS flowed into fissure pattern, 470 nm light cure for 20 sec.	Remove isolation. Check margins with probe. Check occlusion with articulating paper/remove high spots.
GIC/RM-GIC					*GIC/RM-GIC*: 10% polyacrylic acid conditioning of enamel fissures (15 sec), wash and dry (10 sec).	*GIC/RM-GIC*: applied into fissure pattern, autocured/light-cured (470 nm, 20 sec).	

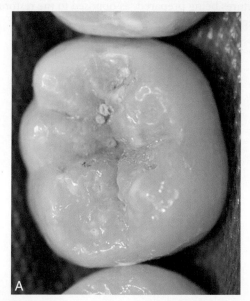

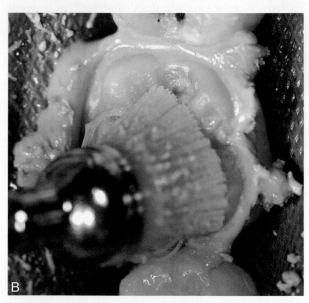

Fig. 8.2A Pre-operative image of the occlusal surface of the LR6 with deep fissures in a high caries risk individual. Remember to check pre-op occlusion with articulating paper.

Fig. 8.2B LR6 occlusal surface debrided using rotating bristle brush in a slow-speed handpiece and prophy paste.

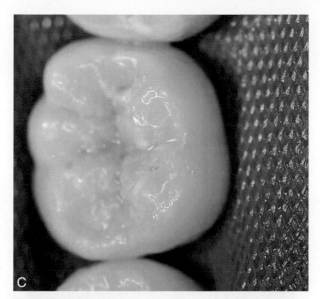

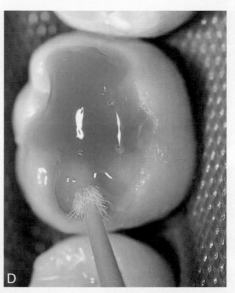

Fig. 8.2C LR6 post-cleaning, washing and drying using a 3-1 air/water syringe.

Fig. 8.2D A 37% orthophosphoric acid etch gel rubbed onto the enamel occlusal surface of the LR6 for 20 seconds using a microbrush.

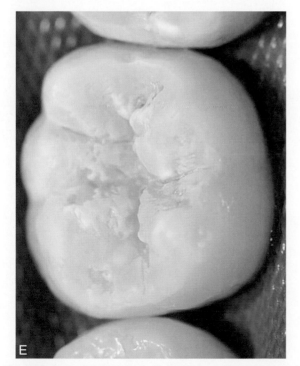

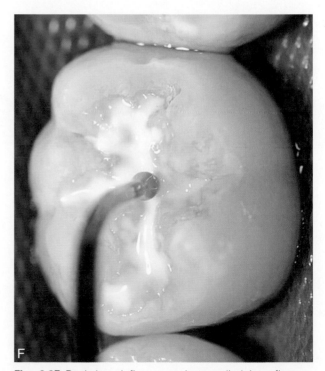

Fig. 8.2E Etchant gel washed off for 10 seconds and air-dried using the 3-1 air/water syringe. Note the frosty appearance of etched occlusal enamel, indicating creation of micro-porosities, which aid the micro-mechanical retention of the resin-based fissure sealant.

Fig. 8.2F Resin-based fissure sealant applied into fissures using a ball-ended dental probe. The sealant flows easily into the fissure pattern.

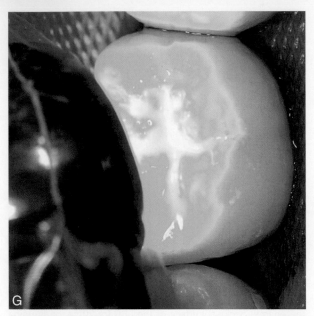

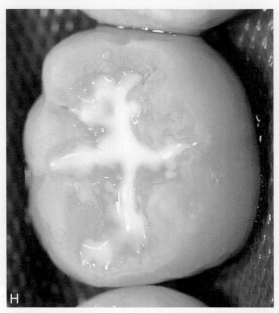

Fig. 8.2G Resin-based fissure sealant is light-cured (470 nm wavelength light for 20 seconds) to initiate the addition polymerisation reaction of the resin monomers.

Fig. 8.2H Completed occlusal fissure sealant on the LR6. Check margins for any rough catches with sharp explorer and post-op occlusion with articulating paper.

8.3 THERAPEUTIC SEALANT RESTORATION/PREVENTIVE RESIN RESTORATION: TYPE 3 ADHESIVE (ENAMEL PRE-ETCH; See Chapter 7)

TABLE 8.3 **Outline of Therapeutic Sealant Restoration/Preventive Resin Restoration**

Operative Procedure	Indication (Chapters 2 and 3)	Pre-op Procedures/ Isolation (Chapter 5)	Caries Removal/ Cavity Preparation (Chapter 5)	Cavity Modification (Chapter 5)	Bonding Steps (Chapter 7)	Restorative Steps	Finishing Steps
Therapeutic fissure sealant... **Sealant restoration** **(preventive resin restoration (PRR))**	Same as for FS but evidence of early enamel demineralisation (mICDAS 1, 2)	Pre-op occlusal check with articulating paper. Rubber dam. (Cotton wool rolls + aspiration).	Enamel fissure lesion excavated to enamel–dentine junction with 330 TC bur, minimal prep burs, air-turbine handpiece. (Air-abrasion– bio-active glass, alumina). Debride remaining sound fissures with prophy paste/ rotating brush.	Wash and dry using 3-1 syringe (10 sec).	Resin composite (RC): 37% orthophosphoric acid-etch enamel fissures (20 sec), wash and dry (10 sec).	Resin composite: resin flowed into cavity/widened fissure, 470 nm light cure for 20 sec. Remaining fissure pattern sealed with flowable resin-based fissure sealant.	Remove isolation. Check margins with probe. Check occlusion with articulating paper and remove high spots.
					GIC: 10% polyacrylic acid conditioning of enamel fissures (15 sec), wash and dry (10 sec).	GIC: applied into widened fissure, autocured/light-cured (470 nm, 20 sec).	

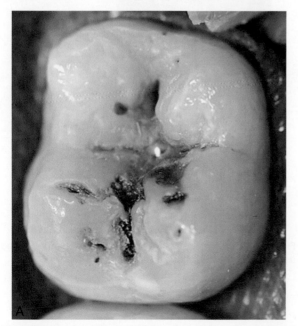

Fig. 8.3A Isolated LR7 with deep stained fissures, cavitated and carious in places in a high caries risk/susceptible individual (mICDAS 3/ICCMS moderate). Pre-op occlusion must be checked with articulating paper.

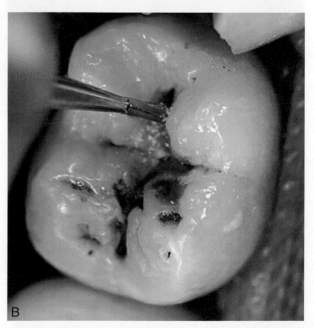

Fig. 8.3B Cavitated occlusal fissures are explored gently using an irrigated 330 TC bur in an air-turbine handpiece.

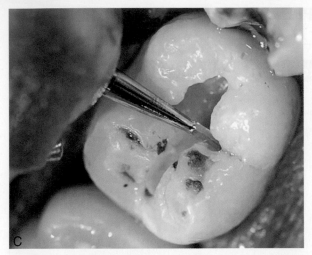

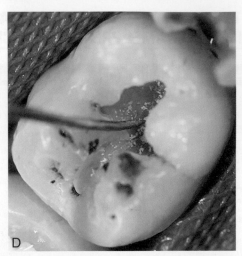

Fig. 8.3C Fissures are minimally widened and caries-infected dentine is removed distally (soft, sticky). The mesial extent of the fissures widened minimally within enamel only (this step may not always be required and the remaining fissure pattern may be suitably debrided only (as per 8.2 – PFS)).

Fig. 8.3D Fissure pattern is fully opened distally with caries-affected dentine retained at the cavity floor (scratchy but flaky–leathery, to a sharp dental explorer scratched across the dentine surface).

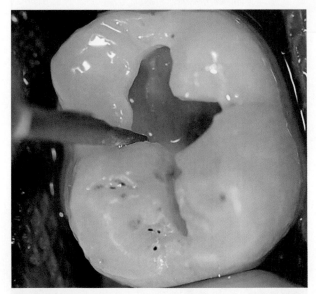

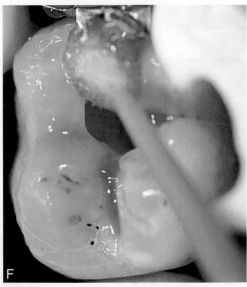

Fig. 8.3E A fine diamond bur is used to remove any grossly unsupported peripheral enamel and lightly bevel the margins.

Fig. 8.3F The LR7 occlusal enamel margins only pre-etched using 37% orthophosphoric acid etch gel for 15 seconds.

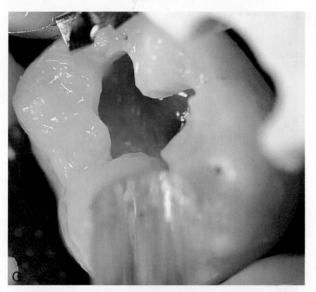

Fig. 8.3G Gel is washed off for 10 seconds and the tooth is gently air-dried (2–3 seconds).

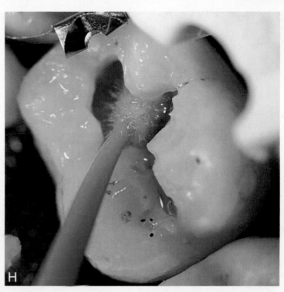

Fig. 8.3H Type 3 adhesive/dentine bonding agent (DBA) is applied (2-step, self-etching primer). Self-etching primer is agitated into all cavity surfaces for 10 seconds with a microbrush.

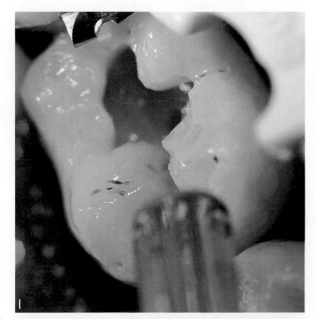

Fig. 8.3I Tooth is air-dried for 5 to 10 seconds to evaporate the solvent (and thin the layer) until there is no visible 'rippling' of primer on the tooth surface (rippling will be visible through dental loupe magnification with an LED headlight with an orange filter).

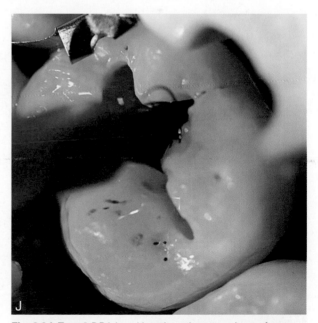

Fig. 8.3J Type 3 DBA bond is agitated onto cavity surfaces.

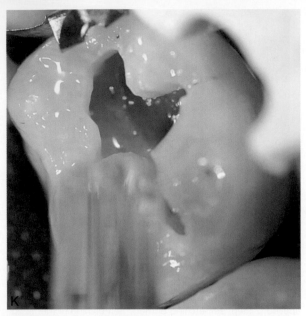

Fig. 8.3K Type 3 DBA bond is air-thinned as in Fig. 8.3I. Note the shiny cavity floor surface which should be seen before light-curing (470 nm, 20 seconds).

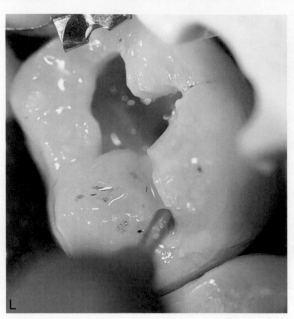

Fig. 8.3L Flowable resin composite (or resin-based fissure sealant) is introduced directly into the mesial fissure and light-cured.

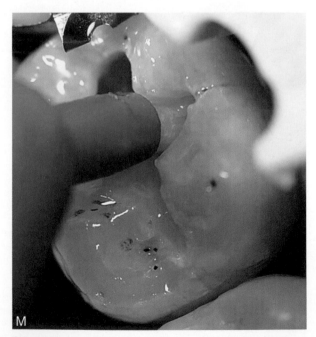

Fig. 8.3M Dentine shade resin composite is introduced into the distal cavity from the compule.

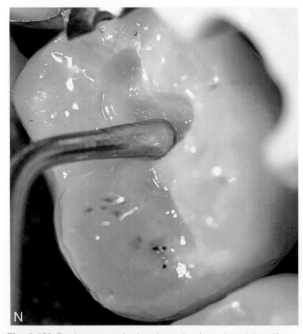

Fig. 8.3N Resin composite is adapted using a burnisher (2 mm increment), leaving space for the next enamel shade increment. This is light-cured, leaving an uncured air-inhibited layer on the resin composite surface ready to accept the next increment.

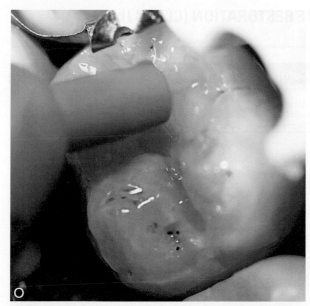

Fig. 8.3O Enamel shade resin composite is directly introduced into the cavity.

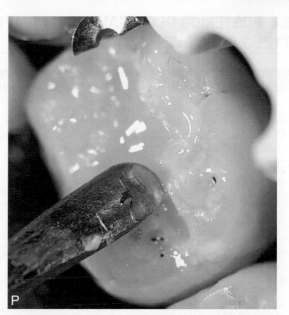

Fig. 8.3P Resin composite is shaped and contoured using a Ward's carver/pear-shaped burnisher and subsequently light-cured.

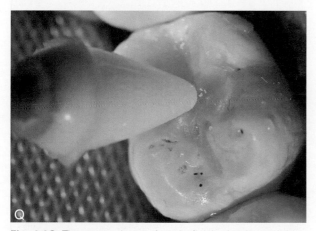

Fig. 8.3Q The restoration surface is finished using polishing points and cups.

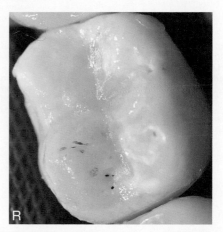

Fig. 8.3R The final finished therapeutic sealant/PRR restoration on the LR7. Once the rubber dam is removed, the post-op occlusion is checked with articulating paper.

8.4 POSTERIOR OCCLUSAL RESIN COMPOSITE RESTORATION (CLASS I): TYPE 3 ADHESIVE

TABLE 8.4   Outline of Posterior Occlusal Resin Composite Restoration

Operative Procedure	Indication (Chapters 2 and 3)	Pre-op Procedures/ Isolation (Chapter 5)	Caries Removal/ Cavity Preparation (Chapter 5)	Cavity Modification (Chapter 5)	Bonding Steps (Chapter 7)	Restorative Steps	Finishing Steps
Posterior occlusal adhesive restoration: **(Class I)** **All GIC** **All resin composite (RC)**	High caries risk/ susceptibility pt (mICDAS 2); cavitated lesion (mICDAS 3,4). Consider pulp response to sensibility tests. Radiographic assessment of lesion depth/pulp proximity.	Check occlusion with articulating paper, pre-op. Select tooth– material shade (Vita guides). Place rubber dam.	Remove unsupported demineralised enamel with tungsten carbide (TC)/diamond bur, air-turbine. Leave sound enamel margin. Peripheral dentine caries excavation (carbon-steel (CS), slow-speed rose-head bur, hand excavator) to sound dentine (lesion depth-dependent). Excavate infected dentine overlying pulp with hand excavator/avoid pulp exposure.	Lightly bevel sound enamel margins using fine diamond bur, air-turbine. Gently round off internal cavity line angles using slow-speed CS rose-head burs. Wash and dry cavity (10 sec).	*GIC*: 10% polyacrylic acid conditioner rubbed onto cavity walls with microbrush (15 sec), wash and dry (10 sec)—removes smear layer and exposes Ca^{2+} ions for bonding.	Mix/dispense *GIC* into cavity, filling from base upwards (to prevent voids/improve adaptation to cavity walls). Slightly overfill cavity initially. After 60 secs pack GIC into the cavity with burnisher/flat plastics, ensuring adequate condensation. Occlusal morphology adapted with flat plastics and excess material removed whilst GIC still malleable.	*GIC:* wait 3 min for initial set. Check margins/ occlusion with articulating paper. Final occlusal adjustments made with diamond burs/stones/ sharp scalpel blade. Finish with diamond polishing paste and coat with lightly filled resin for GIC surface protection (dry surface, paint on resin and light cure (470 nm for 20 sec)).
Existing posterior occlusal GIC veneered with RC	Assess occlusal integrity/wear/ marginal failure of >6-month-old posterior GIC restoration.		Remove 2 mm thickness of old, occlusal GIC with diamond/TC bur, air-turbine. Leave sound enamel margins.		*RC:* dependent on which DBA (Types 1–4) used (Table 8.12).	Place *RC* in 2 mm increments in stacked angles from base outwards, light-curing each increment (20 sec). Ensure uncured monomer of the oxygen-inhibited layer on surface of each increment is undisturbed to allow adhesion of next increment. Shape final occlusal morphology.	*RC:* Remove rubber dam. Finish surface morphology/ margins with fine diamond burs/discs, check margins/ occlusion with articulating paper, polish using diamond grit-impregnated cups/discs.

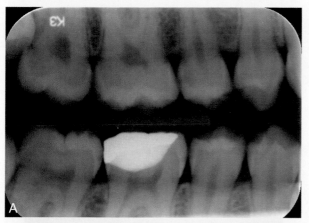

Fig. 8.4A Right bitewing radiograph showing multiple early enamel lesions in a high caries risk patient. Can you spot any radiographic changes in the LR7?

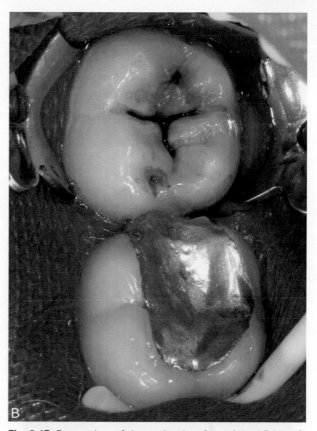

Fig. 8.4B Pre-op view of the occlusal surface of the LR7 (mIC-DAS 2). Note the heavily stained fissure pattern, biofilm accumulation and remnant of an old fissure sealant. Rubber dam isolation is in place, held anteriorly with a medium widget *(yellow)*. The occlusion was checked and the resin composite shade was taken prior to placement of the rubber dam, whilst the tooth was still fully hydrated.

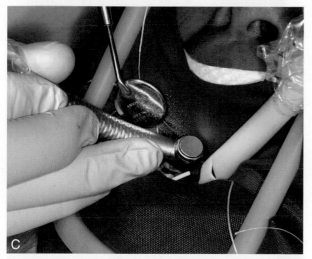

Fig. 8.4C Operating view showing the rubber dam cut away from the nose with a paper towel beneath to protect from skin irritation *(white)*. Note that the operator's finger rests on the patient's lower incisors.

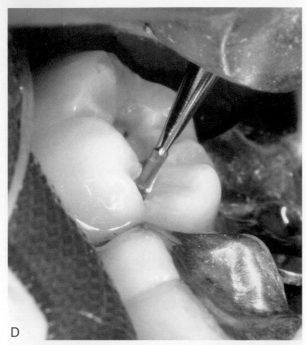

D

Fig. 8.4D A 330 TC bur in an air-turbine handpiece with water irrigation is used to gain access to the enamel. A rosehead bur in a slow-speed handpiece and hand excavators are used to remove softened, caries-infected dentine.

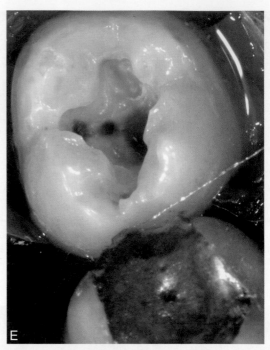

E

Fig. 8.4E Cavity preparation of the occlusal LR7, with caries-affected dentine retained over pulp. Note the clear enamel–dentine junction.

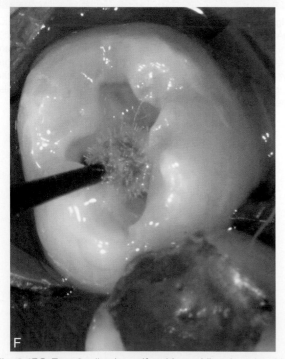

F

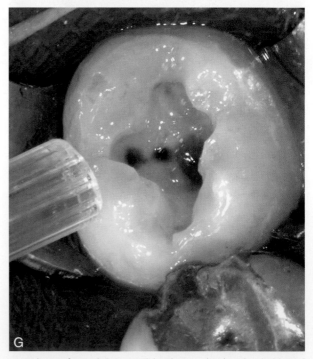

G

Fig. 8.4F,G Type 3 adhesive self-etching acidic primer is rubbed onto cavity surfaces (10 seconds) using a microbrush, air-thinned for 5 seconds to evaporate solvents.

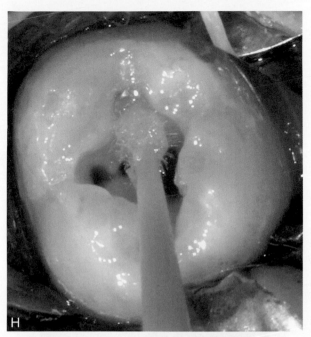

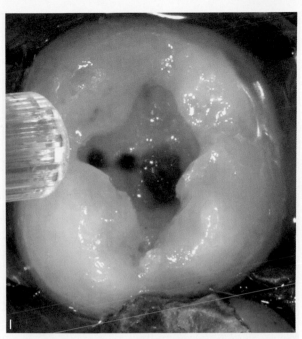

Fig. 8.4H,I Type 3 adhesive is agitated onto cavity surfaces for 10 seconds, air-thinned for 5 seconds and finally light-cured (20 seconds; 470 nm).

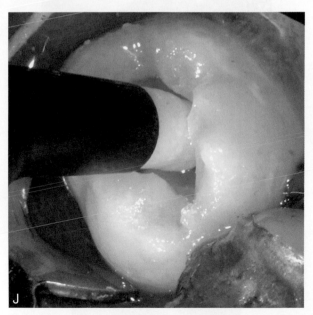

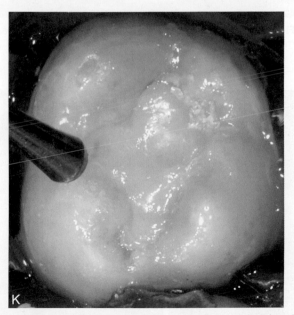

Fig. 8.4J,K Resin composite (RC) is placed directly into the cavity and adapted using pear-shaped burnishers. This can be placed incrementally for conventional RCs, with each increment being photo-cured, or in one increment with bulk-fill RCs.

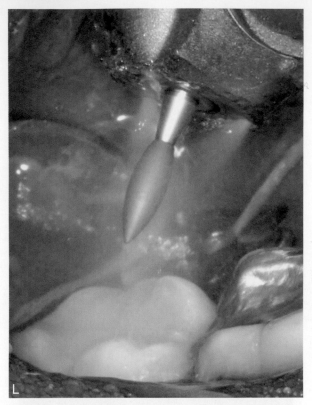

Fig. 8.4L Occlusal resin composite is adjusted using a fine diamond rugby ball–shaped bur with water irrigation.

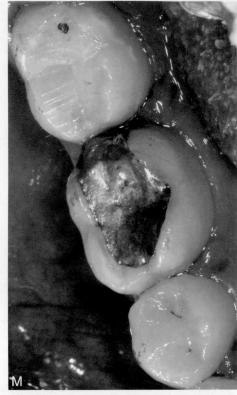

Fig. 8.4M The rubber dam is removed and the occlusion is checked with articulating paper. Note the high spot marked in red on the distal aspect LR7.

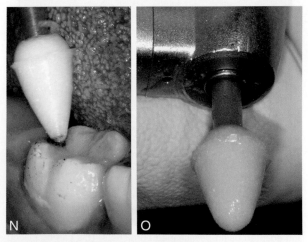

Fig. 8.4N,O The high spot is removed and the restoration is finished using silica-impregnated points/cups. Note how the finishing point has blunted in use. More pressure increases the abrasiveness of the point but simultaneously increases its wear.

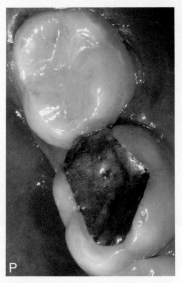

Fig. 8.4P Final resin composite restoration of the LR7.

8.5 POSTERIOR PROXIMAL RESTORATION (CLASS II)

8.5.1 Type 2 Adhesive, 'Moist Bonding'

TABLE 8.5   Outline of Posterior Proximal Adhesive Restoration

Operative Procedure	Indication (Chapters 2 and 3)	Pre-op Procedures/ Isolation (Chapter 5)	Caries removal/ Cavity Preparation (Chapter 5)	Cavity Modification (Chapter 5)	Bonding Steps (Chapter 7)	Restorative Steps	Finishing Steps
Posterior proximal adhesive restoration (Class II) Contact point present	Proximal cavitated lesion/ mICDAS 3,4. PA radiograph to ascertain depth; pulp response to sensibility tests.	Check occlusion with articulating paper, pre-op. Select tooth–material shade (Vita guides). Place rubber dam. Pre-wedge adjacent teeth to aid rubber dam placement. Ensure dam can be placed and held firmly cervical to the base of the carious lesion (clamps, wedgets, floss).	Remove unsupported enamel with TC/ diamond bur (air turbine) accessing proximal lesion through occlusal surface, just medial to the relevant marginal ridge. Having gained access to proximal infected dentine, remove undermined marginal ridge with excavator or bur. Fender wedge to protect adjacent proximal tooth surface. Peripheral caries excavation (CS bur, hand excavator) to sound dentine (lesion depth, moisture control-dependent)– 'box' preparation. Excavate infected dentine overlying pulp with hand excavator/ avoid exposure. Leave sound enamel periphery, bevel if possible/avoid gingival papilla trauma.	Wash away debris with water from 3-1 syringe and dry (10 sec total). Place sectional ideally, or circumferential metal matrix band interproximally ensuring tight adaptation cervically with wedges and contact point formation. Circumferential band/retainers may interfere with rubber dam clamps.	*RC:* dependent upon the DBA used (Types 1–4; see Table 8.12). *GIC (if difficulty gaining moisture control):* 10% polyacrylic acid conditioner rubbed onto cavity walls with microbrush (15 sec), wash and dry (10 sec)	Place *RC* in 2 mm increments in stacked angles from base of box outwards, adapting against walls and matrix band, light curing each increment (470 nm, 20 sec). Ensure uncured monomer of the oxygen-inhibited layer on the surface of each cured increment is uncontaminated, allowing adhesion of next increment. Shape occlusal morphology with carving instruments. Mix/dispense *GIC* into box base upwards (prevent voids/ improve adaptation to cavity walls). After 60 sec pack GIC into cavity with burnishers/flat plastics ensuring adequate condensation. Occlusal morphology adapted with flat plastics.	*RC:* Remove rubber dam. Finish resin composite surface with fine diamond burs/discs/ proximal finishing strips, check margins/occlusion with articulating paper, polish using diamond grit-impregnated cups/discs. *GIC:* wait 3 min for initial set. Check margins/ occlusion with articulating paper. Adjustments made with diamond burs/ stones/sharp scalpel blade. Finish with diamond polishing paste and coat with lightly filled resin for GIC surface protection.
If proximal lesion directly accessible by instruments (e.g., no adjacent tooth, rotated tooth), then treat as buccal cervical restoration (see Section 8.8)							

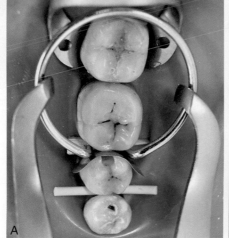 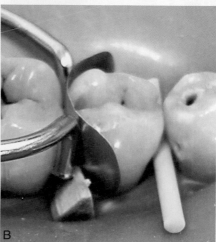

Fig. 8.5A,B LR5 distal-occlusal cavity (Class II), isolated with a rubber dam (wingless clamp LL7 and medium rubber wedget, mesial LL5). A sectional matrix band is wedged gingivally and retained with an oval ring.

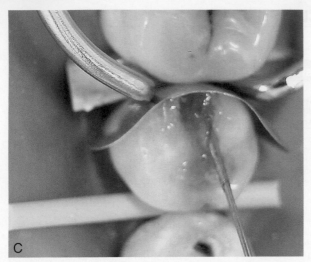

C

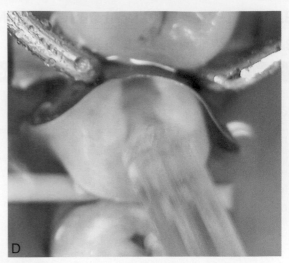

D

Fig. 8.5C Cavity is acid-etched with 37% orthophosphoric acid for 20 seconds.

Fig. 8.5D Cavity is washed thoroughly for 10 seconds.

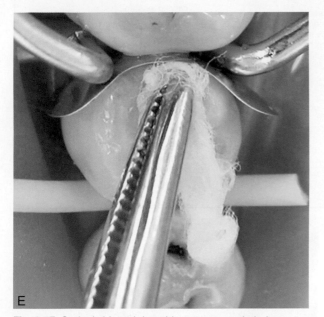

E

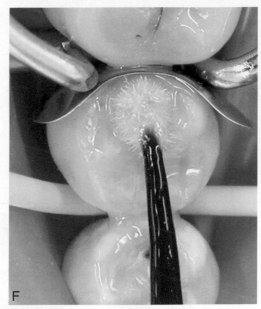

F

Fig. 8.5E Cavity is blotted dry with a cotton wool pledget.

Fig. 8.5F Type 2 adhesive (primer and bond plus solvent) is rubbed onto the cavity walls for 5 seconds.

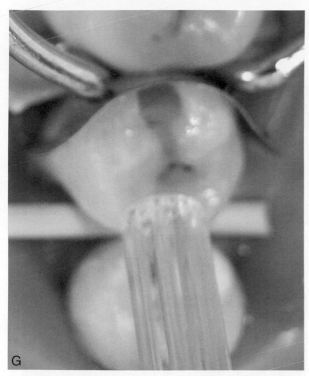

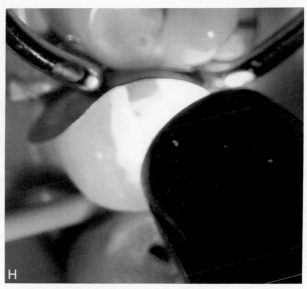

Fig. 8.5H Type 2 adhesive is light-cured (470 nm; 20 seconds).

Fig. 8.5G Type 2 adhesive is air-thinned and solvent is evaporated for 5 seconds. Look for a shiny film on the cavity walls and a loss of rippling on 2 adhesive surface (aided with the use of dental magnification and LED lighting).

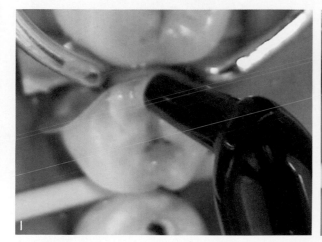

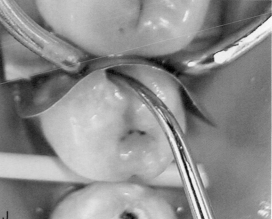

Fig. 8.5I,J Resin composite is placed and adapted into the distal box using a pear-shaped burnisher. Increments are light-cured.

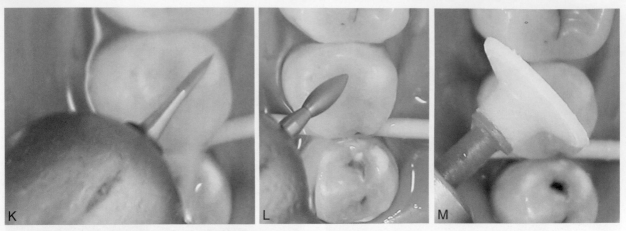

Fig. 8.5K,L,M Resin composite is trimmed and finished using fine diamond finishing burs and abrasive polishing discs.

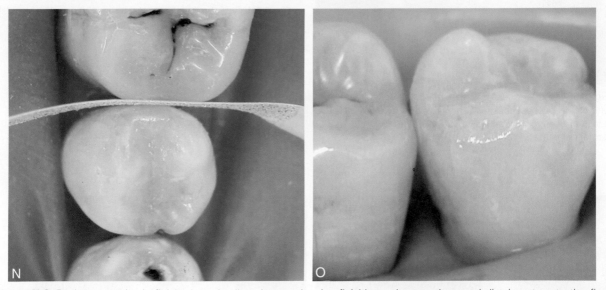

Fig. 8.5N,O Resin composite is finished proximally using an abrasive finishing strip, ensuring good distal contour to the final restoration.

8.5.2 Type 3 Adhesive (Enamel Pre-etch; See Chapter 7)

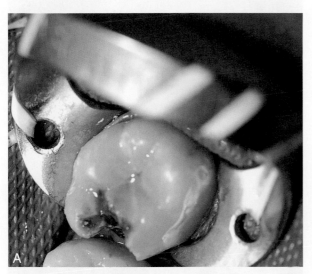

Fig. 8.5A Cavitated LR8 with mesio-occlusal caries (mICDAS 4/ICCMS extensive) and a lesion present in the distal-occlusal pit (mICDAS 2), both requiring operative intervention. The tooth is isolated with a rubber dam using a steel wingless molar clamp (threaded with dental floss to enable retrieval in case the clamp dislodges from the tooth or fractures). A pre-op occlusal check with articulating paper was carried out prior to rubber dam placement as was the shade match for the resin composite whilst the tooth was hydrated.

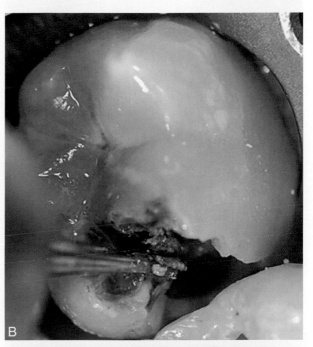

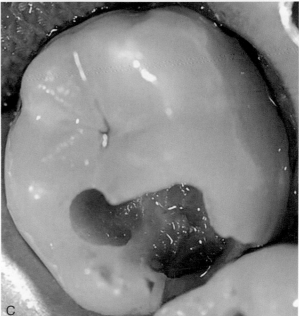

Fig. 8.5B,C Using a 330 TC bur in an air-turbine handpiece with water irrigation, access to dentine caries is improved by removing grossly unsupported and undermined enamel at the cavity margins.

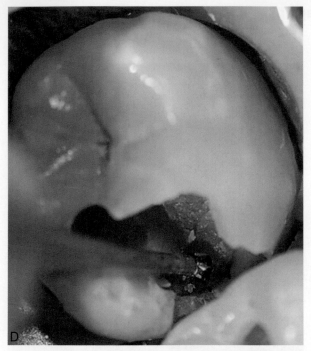

Fig. 8.5D A size 3 rosehead carbon steel bur in a slow-speed handpiece removing peripheral caries at the enamel–dentine junction.

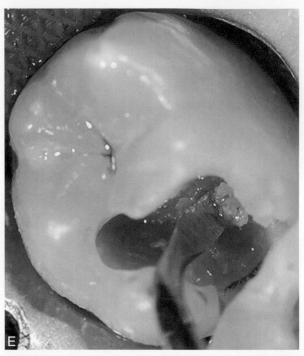

Fig. 8.5E Pulpal caries-infected dentine (soft and wet) is carefully removed using a spoon excavator.

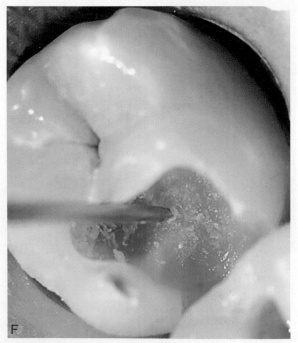

Fig. 8.5F The cavity floor is scratchy and flaky, indicative of leathery caries-affected dentine over the pulp.

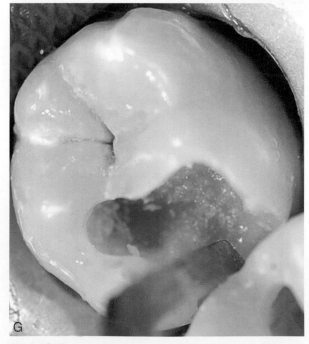

Fig. 8.5G The enamel margin at the base of the mesial box can then be finished using a gingival margin trimmer.

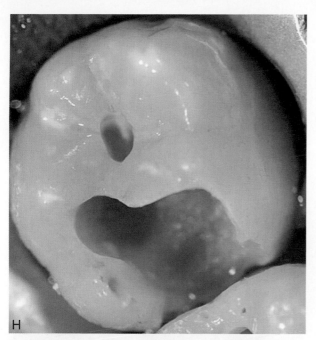

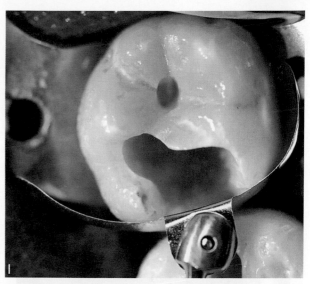

Fig. 8.5I Placing the sectional metal matrix band to reconstitute the mesial wall of the restoration (see Chapter 5). The precurved, contoured band is worked interproximally.

Fig. 8.5H The enamel margins are lightly bevelled using a multifluted tungsten carbide bur. Note how the distal occlusal pit lesion has been accessed in a similar fashion to the preventive resin/sealant restoration shown previously (Fig. 8.3).

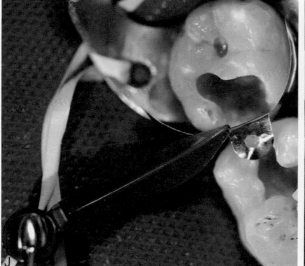

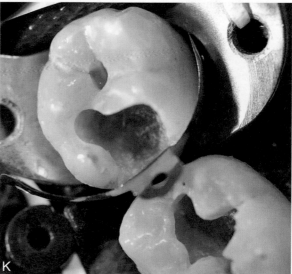

Fig. 8.5J,K A gingivally contoured plastic wedge is selected and inserted buccally to maintain tight adaptation of the band to the mesial surface of the LR8.

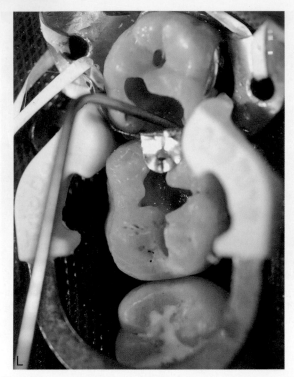

Fig. 8.5L An oval retainer with curved tines is placed to secure and adapt the band to the LR8. This is checked using a sharp dental explorer at the base of the mesial box, ensuring there is no space through which restorative material can extrude. A liquid dam/caulk can be used to help adapt the sectional band.

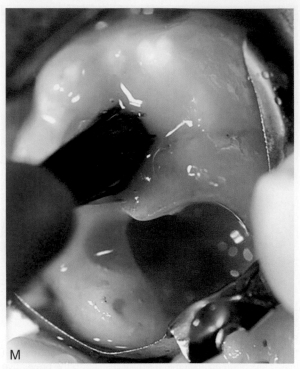

Fig. 8.5M Enamel margins are pre-etched with 37% ortho-phosphoric acid etch gel for 20 seconds, washed off for 10 seconds and gently air-dried for 2 to 3 seconds.

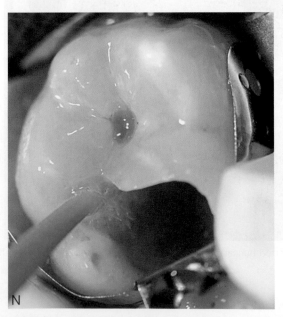

Fig. 8.5N Self-etching primer (Type 3 dentine bonding agent) is rubbed onto the cavity walls for 10 seconds.

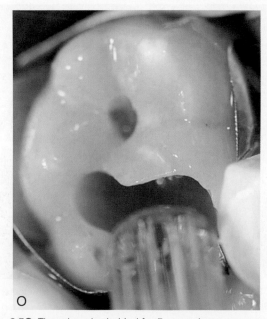

Fig. 8.5O The primer is air-dried for 5 seconds to evaporate the solvent carrier until there is no 'rippling' of the primer film on the tooth surface (visible using dental magnification loupes plus an LED headlight with orange filter).

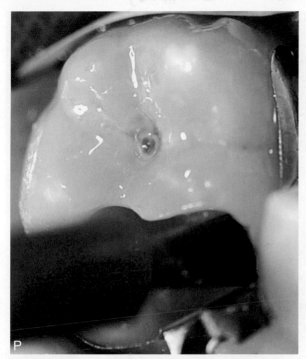

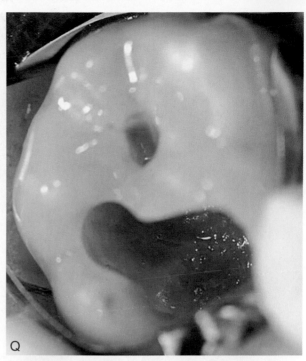

Fig. 8.5P Type 3 bond is applied to the cavity walls for 10 seconds, air-thinned using a 3-1 air/water syringe and light-cured for 20 seconds (470 nm).

Fig. 8.5Q This results in shiny cavity surfaces which must be present prior to placing the first increment of resin composite.

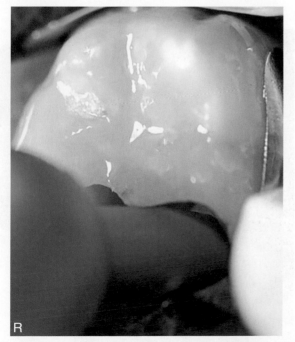

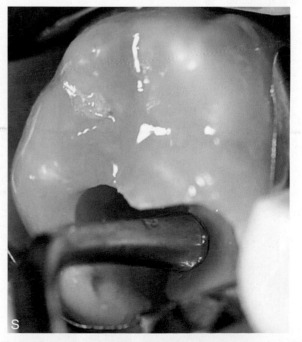

Fig. 8.5R Occlusal cavity is restored with flowable composite. Dentine shade resin composite is directly introduced into the mesio-lingual aspect of the LR8 cavity.

Fig. 8.5S The first increment is adapted using a pear-shaped burnisher and then light-cured for 20 seconds (470 nm).

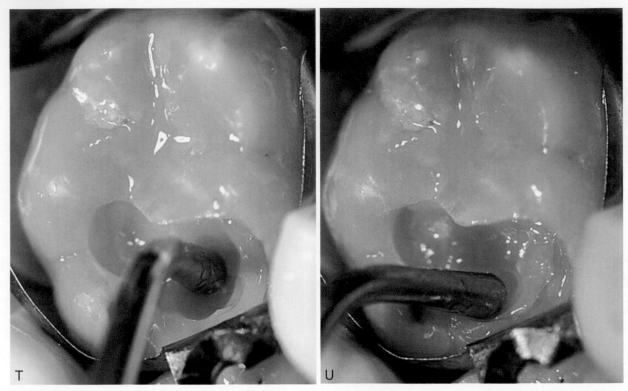

T

U

Fig. 8.5T,U Further 2 mm increments are placed and adapted to form the mesial wall of the restoration against a firm matrix band and light-cured.

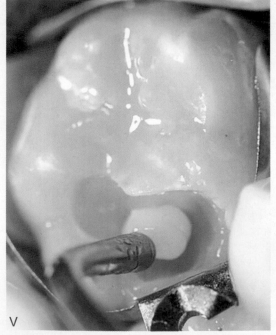

V

Fig. 8.5V Final increments are placed, adapted and light-cured, leaving space for the enamel shade resin composite to be placed.

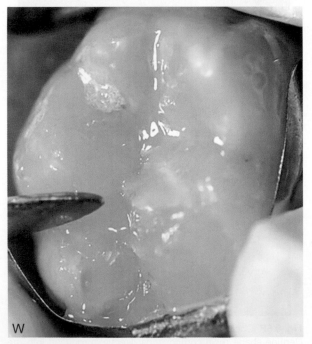

W

Fig. 8.5W Using Ward's/Half-Hollenback carvers, occlusal morphology is introduced in the enamel composite, including the mesial marginal ridge, fossae and fissure pattern.

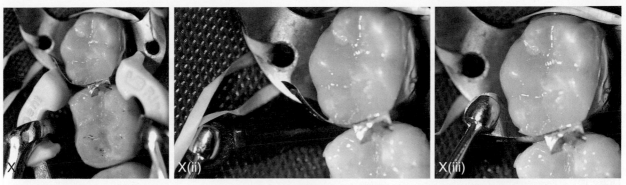

Fig. 8.5X The retainer is removed with a clamp, the wedge is removed buccally and the sectional matrix is teased from the inter-proximal area using special tweezers.

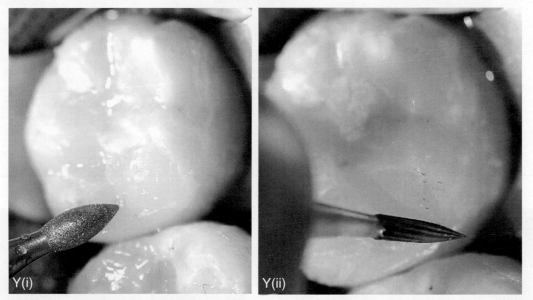

Fig. 8.5Y Fine diamond grit/multifluted tungsten carbide burs are used to adjust the occlusal/axial surfaces of the restoration after checking the occlusion with articulating paper. Proximal surfaces are finished with strips and checked with floss.

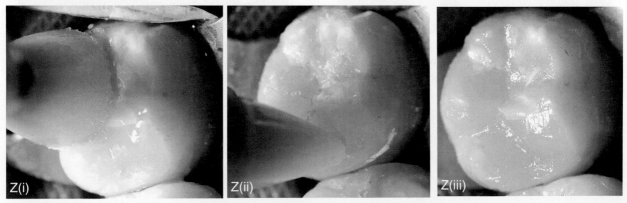

Fig. 8.5Z The resin composite surface is then finished using silica-impregnated cups and points of reducing coarseness. Diamond polishing pastes can help achieve a high lustre. The final completed restoration.

8.6 CLASS III ANTERIOR RESTORATION: TYPE 2 ADHESIVE (also see Chapter 5, Fig. 5.51 A–C)

TABLE 8.6   Outline of Class III Anterior Restoration

Operative Procedure	Indication (Chapters 2 and 3)	Pre-op Procedures/ Isolation (Chapter 5)	Caries Removal/ Cavity Preparation (Chapter 5)	Cavity Modification (Chapter 5)	Bonding Steps (Chapter 7)	Restorative Steps	Finishing Steps
Anterior proximal adhesive restoration **(Class III)**	Cavitated carious lesion/mICDAS 3,4/pulp response/ plaque stagnation. Replacement of discoloured/failed tooth-restoration complex.	Check palatal guiding (protrusive) occlusion with articulating paper, pre-op. Select tooth–material shade (Vita guides– dentine/enamel shades). Place rubber dam. Prewedge adjacent teeth to aid rubber dam placement. Ensure dam can be placed and held firmly cervical to the base of the carious lesion (clamps, wedgets, floss).	Caries: remove unsupported/ undermined demineralised enamel with TC/diamond bur from palatal aspect (air turbine). Preserve labial enamel wall if possible to aid aesthetics. Leave sound enamel margin (may be difficult cervically). Peripheral dentine caries excavation (CS bur, hand excavator) to affected/sound dentine (lesion depth dependent). Avoid gingival trauma. Excavate infected dentine overlying pulp with hand excavator/ avoid exposure.	Lightly bevel sound enamel margins using fine diamond bur, air turbine. Wash away debris with water from 3-1 syringe and dry (10 sec total). Place 15 mm long, clear matrix strip interproximally and wedge cervically (contact point, cervical adaptation of restorative material).	*RC:* dependent upon the DBA used (Types 1–4; see Table 8.12).	Place *RC* in 2 mm increments in stacked angles from base of cavity outwards, light-curing each increment (470 nm, 20 sec). Consider aesthetic layering techniques with dentine and enamel shades. Ensure uncured monomer of the oxygen-inhibited layer on the surface of each cured increment is uncontaminated prior to placement of the next to allow adhesion of next increment. Shape palatal morphology with flat plastic instruments, removing excess prior to curing.	Remove wedge, clear matrix band and rubber dam. Finish resin composite surface morphology/ margins with fine diamond burs/ discs/interproximal finishing strips. Check margins with probe/ protrusive guiding occlusion with articulating paper. Polish using diamond grit-impregnated cups/ discs.

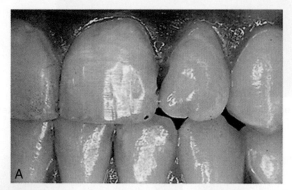

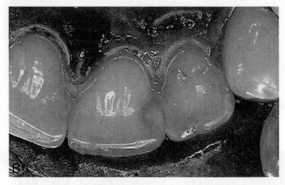

Fig. 8.6A Anterior view of a proximal carious lesion (mICDAS 2; ICCMS mild/moderate) on the distal surface of the UL1. Check pre-op occlusion with articulating paper, anterior protrusive movements included.

Fig. 8.6B The same lesion on the UL1; note palatal shadowing.

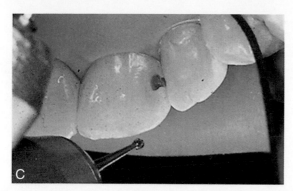

Fig. 8.6C After taking the shade, rubber dam isolation is placed and disto-palatal access is cut through enamel using a small round bur in an air-turbine handpiece.

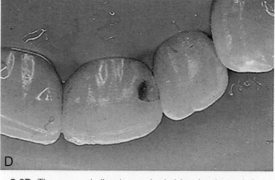

Fig. 8.6D The enamel distal marginal ridge is cleared through the contact area with the adjacent UL2. Note the brown, caries-infected dentine still present.

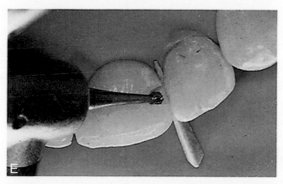

Fig. 8.6E All stained dentine is excavated (to prevent aesthetic shine-through), leaving yellow hard sound dentine at the cavity base for aesthetic reasons, preventing shadowing beneath the final restoration. Labial enamel is preserved. This complete caries removal is acceptable here as the lesion has not encroached upon the pulp.

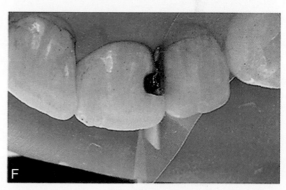

Fig. 8.6F A clear plastic matrix strip is placed interproximally and wedged against the tooth surface. The cavity is etched for 20 seconds using 37% orthophosphoric acid etch.

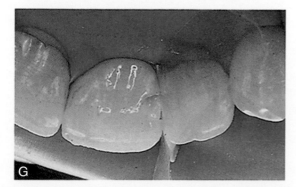

Fig. 8.6G Etch is rinsed away (10 seconds) and blotted dry gently with cotton pledgets ('moist bonding technique') before applying the dentine bonding agent and light-curing for 20 seconds.

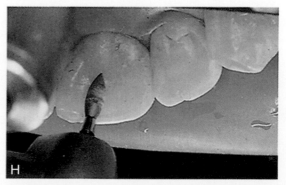

Fig. 8.6H A dentine/enamel shade resin composite is placed incrementally and light-cured. The palatal surface contour is smoothed with a rugby ball–shaped fine diamond resin composite finishing bur.

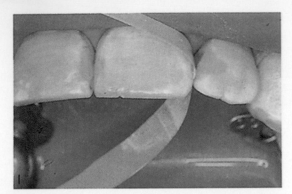

Fig. 8.6I The proximal surface is finished using an abrasive finishing strip (coarse then fine). Take care to preserve the contact point.

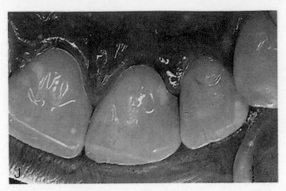

Fig. 8.6J Final Class III distal restoration of the UL1. Once the rubber dam has been removed, the palatal occlusal articulation is checked with articulating paper, intercuspal position as well as in protrusive guidance.

8.7 ANTERIOR INCISAL EDGE/LABIAL VENEER COMPOSITE (CLASS IV): TYPE 3 ADHESIVE (WITH ENAMEL PRE-ETCH)

TABLE 8.7 Outline of Anterior Incisal Edge/Direct Veneer Restoration

Operative Procedure	Indication (Chapters 2 and 3)	Pre-op Procedures/ Isolation (Chapter 5)	Caries Removal/ Cavity Preparation (Chapter 5)	Cavity Modification (Chapter 5)	Bonding Steps (Chapter 7)	Restorative Steps	Finishing Steps
Anterior incisal edge (Class IV) Direct labial veneer restoration	Replacement of discoloured/failed restoration. Traumatic fracture of coronal enamel/ dentine. Aesthetic masking of intrinsic staining, minor alteration of labial morphology. Toothwear lesions with superimposed caries; high-risk patients.	Check palatal/ protrusive guiding occlusion with articulating paper, pre-op. Select tooth–material shade (Vita guides–dentine/ enamel shades depending on the composite system). Place rubber dam. Prewedge adjacent teeth to aid rubber dam placement. Ensure dam can be placed and held firmly cervical to the base of the carious lesion (clamps, wedgets, floss).	Remove old resin composite restoration with diamond/TC bur, air turbine or bioactive glass/ alumina air abrasion. Excavate soft caries-infected and stained caries-affected dentine with excavators/CS rosehead burs. Remove extrinsic staining with sodium bicarbonate air-polishing, bioactive glass air abrasion. Achieve sound enamel margins at periphery of cavity.	Long, undulated bevel cut into sound enamel on labial surface, fine long-tapered diamond bur, air turbine. Short bevel placed on the palatal aspect. Sharp line angles rounded off. Wash away debris with water from 3-1 syringe and dry (10 sec total). Place 15 mm-long clear matrix strip interproximally and wedge cervically.	RC: dependent upon the DBA used (Types 1–4; see Table 8.12).	Place RC in 2 mm increments in stacked angles from palatal aspect of cavity labially, light curing each (470 nm, 20 sec). Can use preformed rigid acrylic/putty matrix outlining the palatal contour, incisal/ mesial/distal margins; interproximal strips cannot be used with matrices. Consider aesthetic layering techniques with dentine and enamel shades. Ensure uncured monomer of the oxygen-inhibited layer on the surface of each cured increment is uncontaminated to allow adhesion of next increment. Shape morphology with Ward's/Half-Hollenback carver removing excess.	Remove wedge, clear matrix band and rubber dam. Finish resin composite surface morphology/ margins with fine diamond burs/discs/ interproximal finishing strips. Check margins with probe/ protrusive guiding occlusion with articulating paper. Polish using diamond grit-impregnated cups/discs.

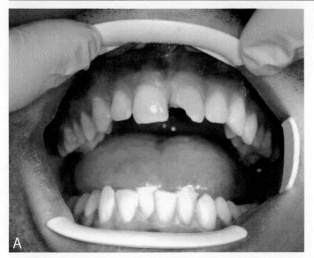

Fig. 8.7A A UL1 mesio-incisal enamel-dentine fracture (Class IV) causing sensitivity and a clear aesthetic concern.

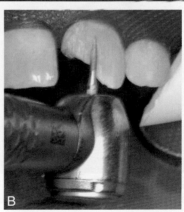

Fig. 8.7B Resin composite shade is selected under natural light with hydrated teeth, occlusion is checked, anterior teeth are isolated with a rubber dam and enamel margin is prepared with a long, undulating light bevel on the labial enamel. This is done to prevent a straight line junction between the tooth and final resin composite restoration which may be clinically noticeable due to the more abrupt change in light reflection and refraction at a straight line boundary/interface between the natural tooth and the resin composite.

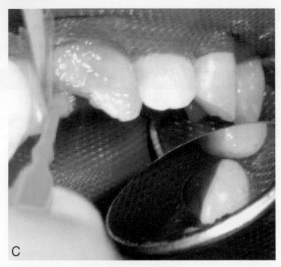

C

Fig. 8.7C 37% orthophosphoric acid etch gel is agitated over bevelled enamel margins and labial enamel for 20 seconds, washed and dried (10 seconds).

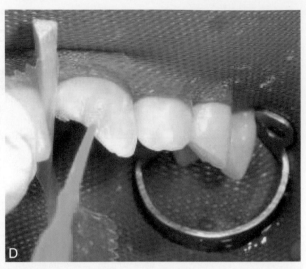

D

Fig. 8.7D Type 3 dentine bonding agent primer is rubbed over the bonding surfaces for 5 seconds.

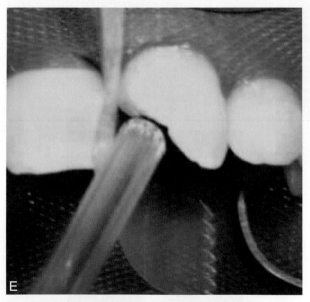

E

Fig. 8.7E Primer is air-dried until the film no longer ripples (approx. 5 seconds), removing solvent and air-thinning the film.

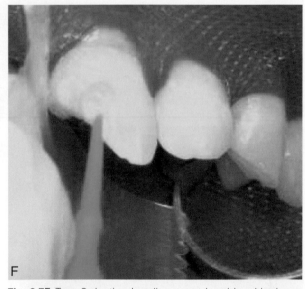

F

Fig. 8.7F Type 3 dentine bonding agent bond is rubbed over the cavity surfaces for 5 seconds, air-thinned as before and light-cured.

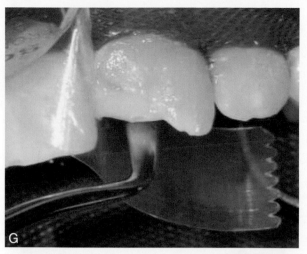
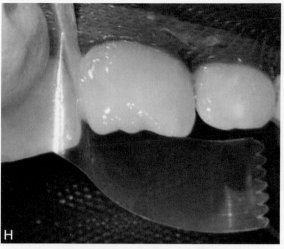

Fig. 8.7G,H Dentine shade resin composite is placed to form the palatal wall of the final restoration. Note how the clear matrix strip is wedged cervically for a better emergence profile and marginal adaptation. The underlying mamelon anatomy is mimicked with the resin composite. Brushes could be used to manipulate the resin composite in this regard. This is light-cured (20 seconds; 470 nm). See Chapter 5, Section 5.11.2 and Fig. 5.65 for an example of the use of a palatal stent/matrix to help build up the correct tooth morphology.

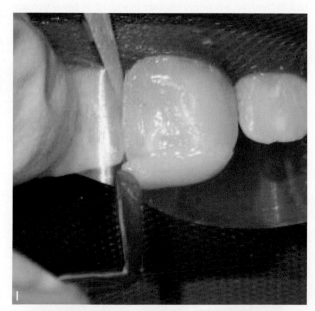
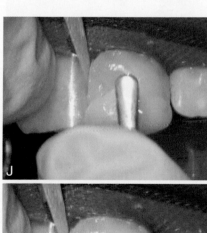
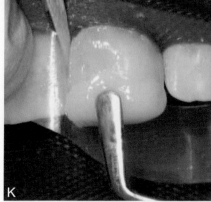

Fig. 8.7I Enamel shade resin composite is placed as a roll along the incisal edge of the UL1 using a flat plastic instrument.

Fig. 8.7J,K This roll of enamel shade resin composite is then teased cervically across the labial surface with the flat plastic instrument, thinning as it blends with the natural tooth along the previously created undulating bevel. A brush could also be used for this purpose.

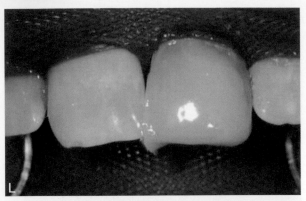

Fig. 8.7L This clinical protocol permits the placement of a smooth, thin layer of resin composite labially, without introducing voids, that is easily finished later. Excess is removed with brushes/flat plastic instruments and the resin composite is light-cured (20 seconds; 470 nm)

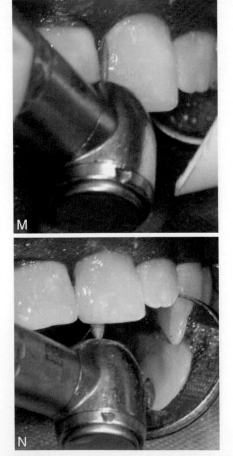

Fig. 8.7M,N Margins are trimmed using composite finishing fine diamond burs cervically, proximally and palatally (rugby ball–shaped bur).

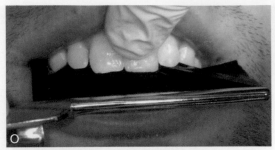

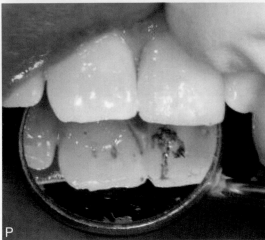

Fig. 8.7O,P Once the rubber dam is removed, incisal occlusion is assessed using articulating paper. A finger is placed on the UL1 to 'feel' for any heavy contact (*fremitus*). A heavy contact is highlighted on the mesio-palatal aspect of the UL1, with the straight line trace of protrusive guidance evident (towards the incisal edge).

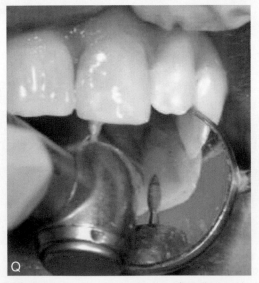

Fig. 8.7Q This is gently removed using a fine diamond bur.

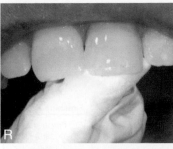
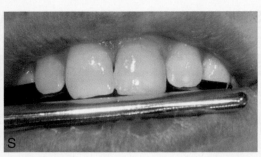
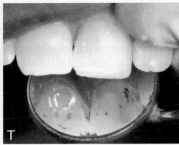

Fig. 8.7R,S,T The teeth are dried with cotton wool rolls and the occlusion is rechecked, this time showing a light contact distocervically on the UL1 (normal incisal contact).

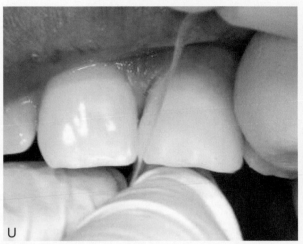
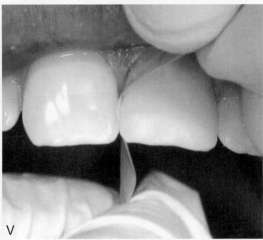

Fig. 8.7U,V Proximal coarse/fine finishing strips are worked through the mesial contact, against the restoration subgingivally to remove any excess adhesive, taking care not to open the established mesial contact point.

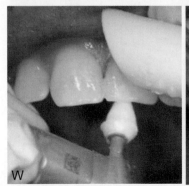
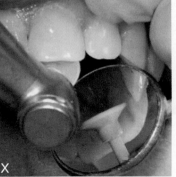
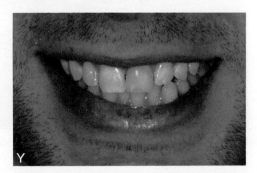

Fig. 8.7W,X Resin composite is polished with coarse to fine abrasive points and discs, achieving a final high surface lustre and surface anatomy. Polishing pastes can be used to aid this process, but care is needed using light pressure so as not to generate excessive frictional heat.

Fig. 8.7Y Final aesthetic resin composite restoration of the UL1 with the patient smiling. Note that the final shade seems slightly darker than the adjacent natural dentition. This is due to dehydration of the natural teeth, making them appear whiter. The patient should be warned about this prior to starting the procedure. This will correct itself within a few hours.

8.8 BUCCAL CERVICAL RESIN COMPOSITE RESTORATIONS (CLASS V): TYPE 2 ADHESIVE

TABLE 8.8 Outline of Buccal/Lingual Cervical Adhesive Restoration

Operative Procedure	Indication (Chapters 2 and 3)	Pre-op Procedures/ Isolation (Chapter 5)	Caries Removal/ Cavity Preparation (Chapter 5)	Cavity Modification (Chapter 5)	Bonding Steps (Chapter 7)	Restorative Steps	Finishing Steps
Buccal/ lingual cervical adhesive restoration (Class V)	Discoloured anterior/ posterior toothwear (causing plaque stagnation or risk of structural weakness). Cavitated carious lesion/ mICDAS 3,4/ pulp response?	Select tooth–material shade. Moisture control: rubber dam isolation often difficult as clamp/ dam obscures access to lesion margins. Simpler cotton wool isolation/ aspiration may be necessary.	Caries: remove unsupported and/ or undermined demineralised enamel with TC/diamond bur (air turbine). Leave sound enamel margin (may be difficult gingivo-cervically). Peripheral dentine caries excavation (CS bur, hand excavator) to affected/sound dentine (lesion depth dependent). Avoid gingival trauma. Excavate infected (contaminated) dentine overlying pulp with hand excavator/ avoid exposure. Toothwear lesion: ideally air-abrade exposed lesion surface, removing stain and surface debris.	Lightly bevel sound enamel margins using fine diamond bur, air turbine. Wash away debris with water from 3-1 syringe and dry (10 sec total).	*RC:* dependent upon the DBA used (Types 1–4; see Table 8.12). *GIC (if difficulty gaining moisture control):* 10% polyacrylic acid conditioner rubbed onto cavity walls with microbrush (15 sec), wash and dry (10 sec).	Place *RC* in 2 mm increments in stacked angles from base of cavity outwards, light-curing each increment (470 nm, 20 sec). Shape occlusal morphology with flat plastic instruments or cervical matrices, removing excess prior to curing. Mix/dispense *GIC*, filling from base up (prevent voids). Slightly overfill cavity. After 60 sec adapt GIC with burnishers/ flat plastics to ensure adequate condensation. Smooth surface may be adapted using cervical matrix.	*RC:* Remove rubber dam. Finish resin composite surface morphology/ margins with fine diamond burs/ discs, check margins and polish using diamond grit-impregnated cups/ discs. *GIC:* wait 3 min for initial set. Final contour adjusted with diamond burs/stones/ sharp scalpel blade. Finish with diamond polishing paste and coat with lightly filled resin for GIC surface protection.

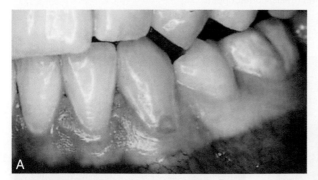

Fig. 8.8A Buccal cervical cavity in the LL3 with plaque stagnation. Gingival margin finishing on dentine.

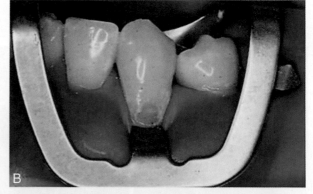

Fig. 8.8B The LL3 is isolated with a rubber dam using a Ferrier clamp to ensure good gingival adaptation of the dam. Using this clamp can cause damage to the gingival tissues, so often the use of floss ligation and/or rubber wedgets can suffice to hold the dam in place. The cavity is cleaned with prophy paste and a rotating bristle brush. Air-abrasion could also be used to freshen the cavity surface prior to bonding.

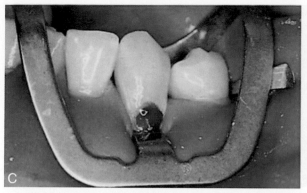

Fig. 8.8C Acid etch gel is placed on all cavity surfaces for 20 seconds, washed off (10 seconds) and air-dried for 2 to 3 seconds (moist bonding; no enamel frosting is visible). Adhesive is then rubbed onto the cavity, air-thinned for 5 seconds, checked for a shiny film and light-cured (20 seconds; 470 nm).

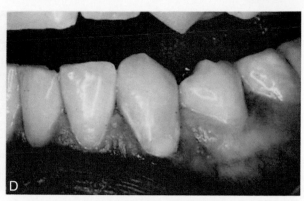

Fig. 8.8D Final buccal cervical resin composite restoration placed on the LL3. Contour is achieved using diamond finishing burs and discs. Clear cervical matrices could also aid in achieving an optimal surface contour (Chapter 5, Fig. 5.64).

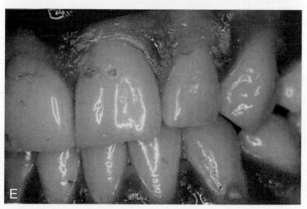

Fig. 8.8E An alternative case. Two small enamel pits on the labial surface of the UL1 causing an aesthetic concern.

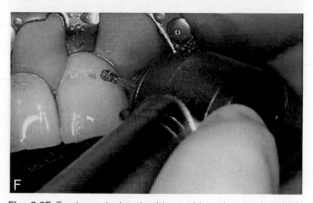

Fig. 8.8F Teeth are isolated with a rubber dam and stain is removed with a round diamond bur in the air-turbine handpiece. Again, air-abrasion could also be used here as a minimally invasive technique.

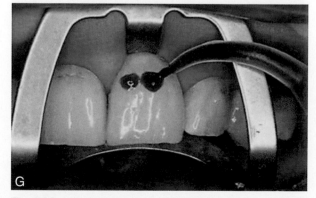

Fig. 8.8G Acid etch gel is placed on the enamel cavities for 20 seconds, washed off for 10 seconds and air-dried for 2 to 3 seconds to remove the surface water droplets (moist bonding).

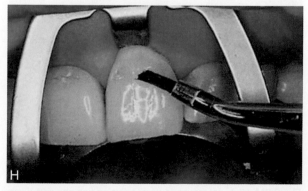

Fig. 8.8H Type 2 adhesive is agitated onto the cavity surfaces, air-thinned to evaporate solvent (5 seconds) and checked for the presence of a shiny film, then light-cured.

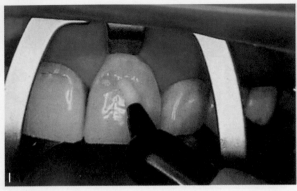

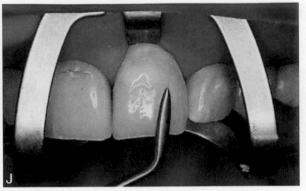

Fig. 8.8I,J Flowable resin composite (shade is assessed before rubber dam is placed) is dispensed into cavities and adapted using a titanium nitride-coated non-stick carver.

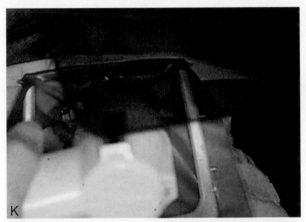

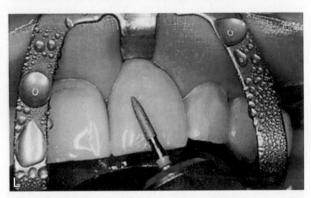

Fig. 8.8L Resin composite is adjusted using fine diamond burs with a water spray.

Fig. 8.8K Resin composite is light-cured. Note the orange filter held in front of the light to protect the nurse's and operator's eyes from the intense 470 nm light.

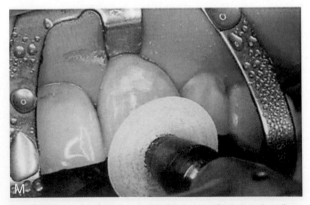

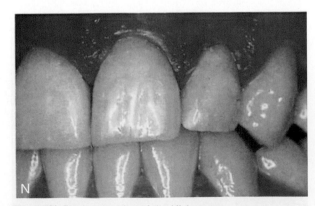

Fig. 8.8M UL1 restoration is finished using fine abrasive discs.

Fig. 8.8N Final restoration of the UL1.

8.9 POSTERIOR 'BONDED' AMALGAM RESTORATION (courtesy Dr G Palmer; also refer to Chapter 7)

TABLE 8.9 **Outline of Posterior Amalgam Restoration**

Operative Procedure	Indication (Chapters 2 and 3)	Pre-op Procedures/ Isolation (Chapter 5)	Caries Removal/ Cavity Preparation (Chapter 5)	Cavity Modification (Chapters 5 and 6)	Bonding Steps (Chapter 7)	Restorative Steps	Finishing Steps
Large posterior amalgam restoration	Heavily broken down coronal tooth structure. High load-bearing, large restoration. Core build up for posterior root-filled teeth. Difficult moisture control conditions.	Check occlusion pre-operatively with articulating paper. Cotton wool rolls/aspiration or rubber dam isolation if possible.	Cavity/defect already present– access cavity from endodontic treatment, fractured cusps. Caries– biologically excavate to sound dentine using hand excavators/CS rosehead burs. Remove undermined/ unsupported enamel (diamond/TC burs, air turbine).	Undercut dentine at diametrically opposite aspects of cavity (CS rosehead bur), if remaining tissue permits this. Round off sharp internal line angles. Smooth cavity base. IPC over blushing pulp with low viscosity GIC. Wash away debris and dry (10 sec). Place circumferential matrix band, wedging the cervical aspect interproximally.	Bonded amalgams: use auto-/dual-cure resin cement (e.g., Panavia).	Triturate high-Cu alloy, plug and condense incrementally from the base of the cavity outwards, ensuring adaptation against walls/ matrix. Slightly overfill cavity and carve back to occlusal level and morphology using carvers (Ward's, Half-Hollenback), flat plastics. Work quickly but not hastily!	Remove matrix band. Take care not to fracture/dislodge marginal ridges. Check occlusion with articulating paper/interproximal overhangs with dental floss/finishing abrasive strips. Remove high spots with excavator/ Mitchell's trimmer or amalgam finishing burs if required. Burnish occlusal surface and margins for smooth finish and good adaptation. Wipe occlusal surface with slightly damp cotton wool pledget for final surface finish.

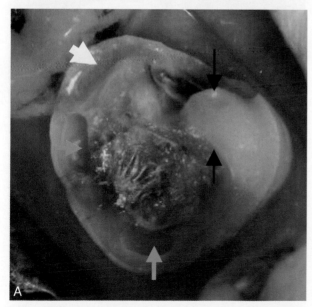

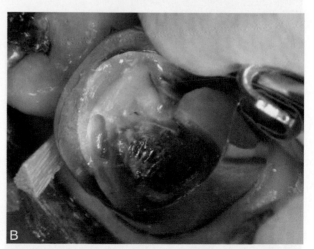

Fig. 8.9A Grossly broken down LL6 prepared for an amalgam restoration. Note the two lingual slots *(green arrows)* and relative undercuts around the mesio-buccal cusp to aid retention *(black arrows)* and the disto-buccal heavy shoulder preparation to aid distal support *(white arrow)*.

Fig. 8.9B Circumferential metal matrix band with retainer placed around tooth and wedged disto-lingually using a wooden wedge to help adaptation of the distal margin of the final restoration. The band's inner surface is lightly coated with petroleum jelly to aid its final removal after the amalgam has been placed. To aid retention, a self-etching primer has been rubbed onto the cavity surface and air-dried to thin and evaporate the solvent (note the shiny appearance of the of the cavity floor).

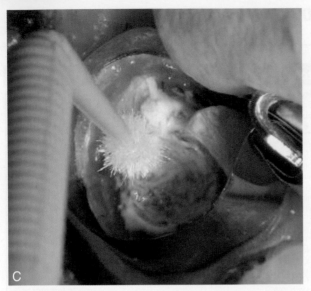

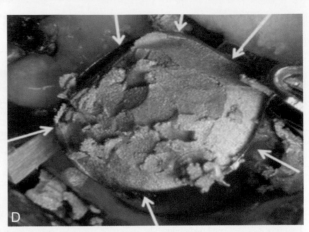

Fig. 8.9C A thin, chemically cured resin adhesive cement is applied using a microbrush onto the cavity surfaces. This technique is known as a bonded amalgam, assisting retention in such large cavities.

Fig. 8.9D The amalgam is triturated and then condensed into the cavity, filling the volume of the matrix band whilst keeping in mind the cuspal height of the adjacent teeth. The excess amalgam has been removed around the margins *(yellow arrows)*, thus exposing the edge of the band.

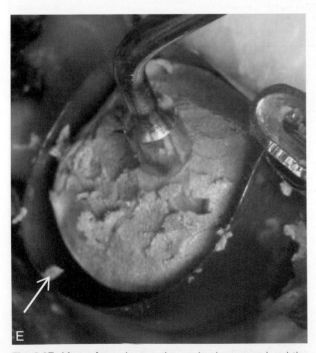

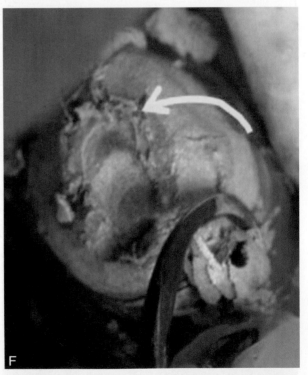

Fig. 8.9E After a few minutes, the wedge is removed and the band is loosened and pushed sideways lingually, through the contact area (note the gap, *arrowed*). The amalgam is supported with a Guy's pattern plugger as the matrix band is eased off.

Fig. 8.9F Using the curved blade of a periodontal sickle scaler, the buccal and lingual walls of the amalgam are contoured, closely following that of the adjacent teeth (curve of the yellow arrow). The height of the amalgam is reduced to the level of the final cusp tips.

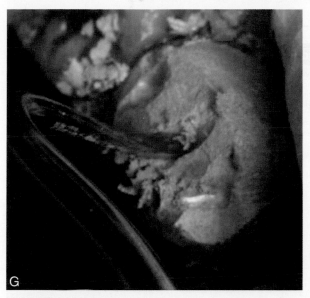

Fig. 8.9G The mesial and distal marginal ridges are carved to the height of the adjacent ridges, followed by the marginal ridge and central fossae using a spoon excavator.

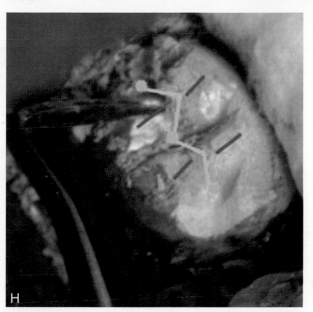

Fig. 8.9H Using a Half-Hollenback or Ward's carver, carve in the central fissure pattern *(blue line)* by joining up the three fossae *(green dots)*. To maintain cusp bulk, try to carve from the fossae up to the transverse ridge *(purple lines)* and then back down to the adjacent fossa.

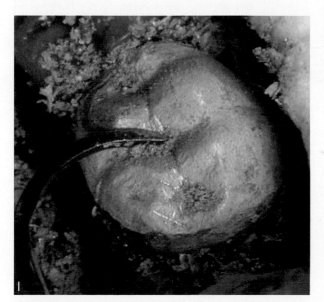

Fig. 8.9I Refine the final occlusal morphology and anatomy using carvers (Ward's or Half-Hollenback), a sickle scaler, an excavator and/or Mitchell's trimmer and check the occlusion using articulating paper.

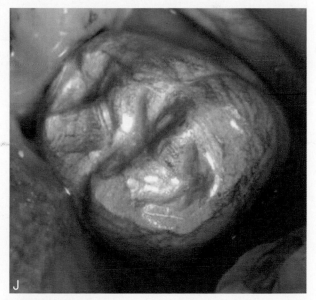

Fig. 8.9J After checking the occlusion and margins, the final restoration is burnished and a smooth surface is achieved by gently rubbing the surface with a damp cotton wool pledget.

8.10 'NAYYAR CORE' RESTORATION

TABLE 8.10 Outline of 'Nayyar Core' Restoration

Operative Procedure	Indication (Chapters 2 and 3)	Pre-op Procedures/ Isolation (Chapter 5)	Caries Removal/ Cavity Preparation (Chapter 5)	Cavity Modification (Chapters 5 and 6)	Bonding Steps (Chapter 7)	Restorative Steps	Finishing Steps
Nayyar core restoration Dental amalgam GIC Resin composite (RC)	Posterior root-filled teeth with short, curved root canals. Enough cervical coronal dentine must remain to support the final restoration. Technique provides retention and strength for the coronal restoration.	Rubber dam isolation if possible. Cotton wool rolls/aspiration.	Use already created endodontic access cavity and natural shape of the pulp chamber. Remove coronal 2–4 mm of root canal filling (e.g., gutta percha) from the obturated canals using Gates-Glidden burs.	Remove any sharp internal line angles with CS rosehead bur. Wash and dry final cavity (10 sec). Place suitable matrix as required to replace any missing coronal walls of cavity.	*Bonded amalgam:* auto-/dual-cure resin cement. *GIC:* 10% polyacrylic acid conditioner, 15 sec (wash and dry, 10 sec). *RC:* DBA, Types 1–4 (Table 8.12). Original Nayyar core described using dental amalgam, but adhesive materials may be used with their own bonding procedures.	Triturate, plug and condense amalgam into the openings created in the coronal aspect of the root canals using narrow Smith plugger/periodontal probe. Pack the remaining cavity, slightly overfill and carve back using appropriate carvers. For RC/GICs, ensure the root canal spaces are filled without voids, using a dark shade. Place fine capsule tips into canal orifice and back fill (GIC). Light cure RC increments (470 nm, 20 sec).	Remove rubber dam/matrix band. Check interproximal margins with floss and remove overhangs/finish surfaces with amalgam/composite finishing strips. Check occlusion with articulating paper and adjust high spots with carvers/amalgam burs (amalgam), fine diamond burs/discs (GIC/composite). Burnish final amalgam/finish with diamond-impregnated polishing discs (GIC/composite).

8.11 DIRECT FIBRE-POST/RESIN COMPOSITE CORE RESTORATION

TABLE 8.11	Outline of a Direct Fibre-Post/Composite Core Restoration						
Operative Procedure	Indication (Chapters 2 and 3)	Pre-op Procedures/ Isolation (Chapter 5)	Caries Removal/ Cavity Preparation (Chapter 5)	Cavity Modification (Chapters 5 and 6)	Bonding Steps (Chapter 7)	Restorative Steps	Finishing Steps
Direct fibre-post/resin composite core restoration (see Fig. 6.3, Chapter 6)	Broken down anterior (and posterior) root-filled teeth. Relatively straight root canal(s). Technique retains large adhesive coronal restoration and reinforces remaining coronal/radicular tooth structure.	PA radiograph of root-filled tooth. Choose shade of composite. Rubber dam isolation ideal. Otherwise, cotton wool and suction essential.	Remove gutta percha (GP) root filling using Gates-Glidden burs. Calculate radicular post length from original length of post minus the length of post required coronally. Take into account root canal length, ensuring a minimum of 4 mm GP is retained apically. Use LCPA. Gauge diameter of post from PA radiograph. Prepare post hole using supplied post drills (narrow–wide diameter in stages). Wash and dry post hole (paper points). Holding fibre-reinforced post with college tweezers, try post in for size and fit. Section post to required length (if necessary) using a carborundum disc, from coronal end.	Round off any sharp line angles on the coronal surface. Wash post hole with NaOCl and dry with paper points. Clean fibre-post with alcohol and air-dry for 5 sec.	Use self-etching dual-cure resin cement (e.g., RelyX Unicem (3MESPE)). Activate capsule, automix, attach fine nozzle and backfill post hole.	Insert fibre-post, hold in place, remove excess cement with flat plastic instrument and light cure (470 nm, 40 sec) or wait 5 min. Apply DBA (Types 1–4; see Table 8.12) onto coronal tooth surface and coronal portion of post. Place interproximal clear matrix strips to separate adjacent teeth/ help create contact points. Incrementally place resin composite, building up dentine/enamel shades if chosen, to provisionalise tooth. Start around post, light-cure 470 nm, 20 secs and layer next increment. Ensure post is covered with composite	Remove rubber dam/matrix strips. Check approximal margins with floss–smooth with composite finishing strips. Check occlusion with articulating paper and adjust with fine diamond bur, air-turbine/discs. Smooth/polish with diamond-impregnated cups/points/ discs.

8.12 DENTINE BONDING AGENTS/ADHESIVES: A STEP-BY-STEP PRACTICAL GUIDE FOR USE

TABLE 8.12   Dentine Bonding Agents: Types, Constituents and Tips for Clinical Use

Type	Smear layer	Etch	Primer	Bond
1 **Three-step (4th generation)** **Total etch/etch and rinse**	Remove	37% orthophosphoric acid gel painted on enamel (20 sec) and dentine (15 sec). Removes smear layer, demineralises (microporosities in enamel) and exposes dentine collagen fibres. Wash off (10 sec) and air-dry (10 sec). May notice frosted enamel.	Contains hydrophilic monomer (e.g., HEMA) acting as bifunctional molecules linking hydrophilic collagen to hydrophobic resin monomers, creating the hybrid layer. Exists with a carrier–water. Painted on cavity surface with microbrush (5 sec) and gently air-thinned (5 sec).	Contains HEMA and other, more hydrophobic monomers. Essentially acts as the unfilled (or in some cases, lightly filled) resin composite. This component is painted onto the primer for 5 sec and then light-cured (470 nm, 20 sec). A shiny cavity surface indicates the presence of the cured dentine bonding agent, ready for first increment of resin composite.
2 **Two-step (5th generation)** **Total etch/etch and rinse 'moist bonding'**	Remove	37% orthophosphoric acid gel painted on enamel (20 sec) and dentine (15 sec). Removes smear layer, demineralises (microporosities in enamel) and exposes dentine collagen fibres. Wash off (10 sec) Air-dry (2 sec). Blot away surface water droplets (cotton wool pledgets, paper points)–MOIST BONDING. If enamel appears frosted then it is likely the dentine surface is too dry and should be rehydrated.	Primer and bond mixed together in same bottle–known as the 'adhesive'. The more hydrophilic monomer (e.g. HEMA) is carried in a volatile solvent (e.g. acetone or alcohol) easing its penetration into the moist dentine collagen fibres, forming the hybrid layer. The combined adhesive is rubbed actively into the cavity surfaces using a microbrush (5 sec). The adhesive is air-dried (5 sec) to evaporate the solvent and thin the adhesive layer/prevent pooling within the cavity. Visually check the surface for a 'sheen'; a shiny cavity surface indicates presence of the adhesive. A dull surface indicates the adhesive has been blown out of the cavity or has been absorbed into the dentine. If dull, a second layer of adhesive is rubbed in (5 sec), air-dried (5 sec) and visually checked. Shiny cavity surfaces can be light-cured (470 nm, 20 sec) and are then ready for resin composite, 2 mm angled increments or bulk-fill.	
3 **Two-step (6th generation)** **Weaker self-etching primer**	Dissolve and incorporated	The etch and primer have been combined using acidic monomers, creating a self-etching primer. The acidity of these primers is considerably less than that of phosphoric acid etch. This acidic primer still contains a volatile solvent requiring evaporation, but no washing is required. The acidic primer is applied with the microbrush on the cavity walls (5 sec) and air-dried (5 sec), evaporating the solvent/thinning the pooled primer until no rippling of the applied layer is noticed. Some authorities suggest a 37% orthophosphoric acid selective etch of enamel for 20 sec, wash and dry (as above) before applying the acidic primer as described. This is to ensure an adequate bond and seal to enamel and essentially converts the clinical steps into a Type 1 system.		The bond has similar chemistry to unfilled/lightly filled resin composite with some hydrophilic monomers included. This adhesive is applied onto the self-etching primer (5sec), air-thinned for 5 sec and light-cured (470 nm, 20 sec). A shiny surface appearance indicates the dentine bonding agent is in place and ready to accept the first 2 mm increment of resin composite or bulk-fill.
4/5 **One-step (7th & 8th generations)** **Stronger self-etching primers**	Dissolve and incorporated	All-in-one systems which present the three steps (etch, prime and bond) together in one application (may need to premix constituents thoroughly, but adhesive applied as one step). With Type 4 systems, stronger acidic monomers (e.g., glycerophosphoric acid dimethacrylate) etch the tooth surface, dissolving the smear layer, demineralising and, in dentine, exposing the collagen fibres to the more hydrophilic monomers to penetrate and form the hybrid layer. Type 5 systems contain slightly weaker acidic bifunctional phosphate monomers (e.g., PENTA, 10-MDP, 4-META etc) that allow adhesion to tooth structure, indirect restorative metal alloys and ceramics. Dentine bonding agent should be premixed thoroughly to ensure all components are homogeneously distributed and rubbed into the cavity surfaces with a microbrush (5 sec). Air-thin for 5 sec, visually check for shiny surfaces/no rippling. Light-cure (470 nm, 20 sec). A shiny surface appearance indicates the dentine bonding agent is in place and ready to accept the first 2 mm increment of resin composite or bulk-fill.		

8.13 CHECKING THE FINAL RESTORATION

Once any dental restoration has been placed and finished (of varying size, shape and material), it is wise for the operator to get into the habit of running through a final clinical checklist before discharging the patient, evaluating the tooth-restoration complex for:

- *Occlusion/occlusal morphology/marginal ridge position* (assessed using articulating paper pre- and postoperatively; see Chapter 5, Section 5.13.3).
- *Marginal adaptation* (positive or negative ledges, overhangs, excess flash material, assessed using straight probe, Briault probe or dental floss proximally).
- *Tight contact areas* (for Class II/III proximal restorations, assessed by feeling for some resistance when working dental floss through the new contact area).
- *Surface finish* (smooth finish assess using a dental probe).
- *Aesthetics* (especially in the anterior aesthetic zone, colour/translucency coassessed by the patient). Do not forget to warn patients that teeth that have been isolated with rubber dam will dehydrate and therefore will appear whiter than their natural hydrated appearance. This should resolve in a few hours as the teeth rehydrate.

8.14 PATIENT INSTRUCTIONS

Depending on the type of restorative material used the patient should be given appropriate instruction on how to look after/manage the new restoration for the immediate 24- to 48-hour period. In all cases, suitable oral hygiene must be achieved as soon as is clinically possible. If local anaesthetic has been used, patients should be warned to take care regarding chewing and biting and consuming hot beverages until the anaesthetic effects have fully worn off.

- For temporary restorations and dental amalgam, care must be taken to avoid heavy occlusal loading. Ask the patient to avoid chewing too heavily on the restoration for 24 hours.
- For dental resin composites, no further instruction is required. The patient should have been forewarned of the possible shade changes as the adjacent teeth rehydrate over the few hours immediately after the rubber dam has been removed (see Fig. 8.7Y). In some cases, there might be some residual postoperative sensitivity experienced after the placement of deep resin composite restorations, close to the pulp. This again should alleviate in a few days.

Minimum Intervention Oral Care (MIOC) – Clinical Domain 4

Minimum Intervention Oral Care (MIOC) – Clinical Domain 4

MIOC Domain 4: Clinical Re-assessment, Recall and Maintenance of the Tooth-Restoration Complex

CHAPTER OUTLINE

9.1 ACTIVE SURVEILLANCE OF THE PATIENT/COURSE OF DISEASE

9.1.1 Risk-related Re-assessment

As has been emphasised throughout this book, delivery of the person-focused MIOC framework by the oral healthcare team involves more than just the minimally invasive operative treatment of the consequences of dental disease. It also involves identifying and predicting disease patterns and concerns the control of disease and prevention of lesions by modifying aetiological factors, all in the long term, throughout the life course of the patient. Equally important is the *Re-assessment* of the adherence to changes in patient behaviours, attitudes and responsibility towards the maintenance of their personal oral and dental health, as well as caries risk/susceptibility assessment. *Active surveillance* of the oral cavity and restored dentition ensures that any treatment undertaken, and subsequently improved oral health, are *maintained* and not reversed. This should be accomplished through individualised strategic *recall* regimens. The

tooth-restoration complex (TRC) needs to be *reviewed* regularly and occasionally *refurbished, resealed, repaired* or *replaced* (Section 9.4; the "5Rs"). Therefore, tailored, risk-related, periodic recall/review consultations (inappropriately called 'checkups' by too many!), once an episode of treatment is completed, are just as important as the treatment itself. It is critical that the patient understands the importance of these recall consultations as active surveillance of their ongoing care being offered to help maintain their lifelong oral and dental health.

Three aspects of active surveillance to be carried out in recall consultations include:

- Checking the overall state of the patient's oral and dental health (review) including longitudinal assessment of the patient's caries risk/susceptibility (CRSA) to highlight any changes that have occurred. Thus, appointment frequency ideally should be patient risk-related.
- Reassessing the individual patient's longer-term behavioural response/adherence to previous preventive advice and/or treatment, in moderating any

aetiological factors that could cause future dental disease (re-assessment)

• Status and quality of the restorations/tooth-restoration complexes present (monitor and maintain to ensure the patient remains disease inactive).

The recall consultation follows a pattern similar to the initial assessment detailed in Chapter 2, Section 2.3. The ongoing, updated history will concentrate on what has happened since the clinician and patient last met. For instance, it is important to re-check the medical history carefully, but questions about past dental history need not be dwelt upon except to check that no other dental treatment has been provided in the interim elsewhere. When the clinical examination is carried out, particular attention is paid to areas noted as important or specifically requiring active surveillance, such as caries, restorations and toothwear (see later).

9.1.2 Re-assessment Checklist

• Are existing tooth-restoration complexes stable?
• Is there any clinical evidence for new carious lesions/early surface demineralisation?
• Is there evidence of carious lesion progression on radiographs (Fig. 9.1A–B)?
• Are the risk factors still present? Carry out a new CRSA to allow longitudinal time comparisons.
• Is oral bacterial balance under control?
  ▪ Check oral hygiene (procedures and disclosing solutions).
  ▪ Consider repeating chairside plaque disclosing/saliva tests (see Chapter 2, Section 2.5.4).
• Has preventive home/self care (biofilm control, dietary modifications and use of topical remineralising agents, high-fluoride toothpastes and mouthrinses, etc.) helped? Has the patient adhered to the documented non-operative primary preventive advice offered by the oral healthcare team?

Visual and radiographic examination may be required, with repeated bitewing radiographs every 6 to 12 months for high-risk/caries-active individuals (Fig. 9.1A–B). If the patient has modified the causative factors and reduced their overall risk and susceptibility, becoming caries inactive, then subsequent radiographs may only be required at 18- to 24-month intervals, but these are only guidelines and will be subject to change depending on the patient's ongoing response to treatment and

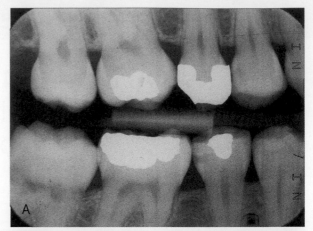

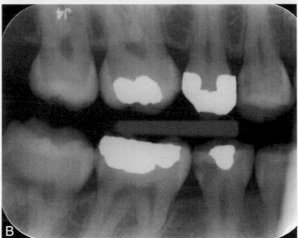

Fig. 9.1 (A) Right bitewing radiograph of a high caries risk patient with early carious lesions evident distal UR4 and distal LR5. (B) Right bitewing radiograph of the same patient 11 months later showing significant progression of the two lesions. The caries control strategies discussed in Chapter 4 (Section 4.2) had not been fully implemented by the patient.

preventive advice. These risk-related intervals should be judged on an individual patient basis, just like the recall consultation frequency (Table 9.1).

9.1.3 Monitoring Toothwear

As toothwear is usually an ongoing problem on first presentation at the dental clinic, it is important to be able to monitor its progress to see if it is getting worse and at what rate, or to see if controlling measures advised are having an effect at reducing the rate or stopping further progress. Active surveillance methods may include:

• *Clinical digital photography*: Standardised digital photography of the patient's teeth as shown in

TABLE 9.1 Average Recall Frequency for Patients With Respect to Lesions Present and Level of Caries Susceptibility

Identify	LESION			NO LESION	
	Cavitated (mICDAS 3, 4; ICCMS moderate/ extensive)	Non-cavitated (mICDAS 1, 2; ICCMS initial)		(mICDAS 0; ICCMS sound)	
	High risk/ susceptibility	*High risk/ susceptibility*	*Low risk/ susceptibility*	*High risk/susceptibility (un-modifiable factors)*	*Low risk/ susceptibility*
Recall frequency	2–6 months	3–6 months	6–12 months	3–6 months	12–24 months

Note: Recall frequencies must be tailored to the individual patient and the figures presented are purely a guide. For more information regarding the mICDAS/ICCMS scores, see Chapter 2, Table 2.3.

figures in this section, with good lighting, can be helpful for comparison over months and years. An overview can be gained from this rather than detailed measurements of any lesion change. Note that in many countries, full written consent from the patient may be required before images can be captured and stored securely (see Chapter 5, Section 5.7.1).

- *Toothwear indices*: These are clinical scoring systems that are available to permit objective numerical scores of the degree of toothwear to be noted, reassessed and compared at a later date. Some indices will also help with the care planning regimen required for the individual patient. Unfortunately, as with many of these indices, they are often complicated and time consuming to use in a busy dental practice. Their use in research and epidemiological studies is recommended, but in general dental practice their use may be limited. However, practitioner-friendly toothwear screening indices do exist to help give an overview of the patient's existing problem. An example includes the Basic Erosive Wear Examination (BEWE; see Table 2.7, Chapter 2).
- *Serial, dated study models* (Fig. 9.2): Casts of the dentition can be made from impressions at 12- to 18-month intervals in patients where active toothwear appears to be progressing, to be able to compare changes and develop future personalised care plans. Again, as with clinical photography, the changes will have to be quite extensive to be noticed with the naked eye. The patient should be given the dated casts to keep safely ensconced in Bubble

Wrap and bring to future appointments. This also may help to better evaluate the attitude and motivation of the individual patient to their toothwear problem. Remember, without the patient appreciating their own responsibility in managing their condition, no form of operative or preventive treatment will be successful in the medium to long term.
- *Profilometry*: Using laboratory-based laser scanners, serial study casts can be scanned to give accurate changes in lesion dimensions over a period of time (Fig. 9.2). This is a useful research tool at present. Intra-oral chairside scanners, initially developed for fixed prosthodontic dental applications, are now being used with specialist software to measure this detailed level of tooth surface morphological change over time and may prove useful in a dental practice setting (Fig. 9.3).

As with all cases of measuring the progression of a relatively slowly developing lesion, disease or condition, the relative impact of the perceived change on the patient's lifestyle plays a significant role in motivating the patient to alter their behaviour to prevent the occurrence of further disease. A patient is less likely to be concerned about a condition that is only developing slowly with little or no detrimental impact to their way of life. However, a rapid obvious deterioration to their health will impact more, spurring them on to change their lifestyle. The screening index that impacts the most on the patient will require the appropriate level of explanation from members of the oral healthcare team in the clinic. The clinical effectiveness of such indices cannot be relied upon without this critical support.

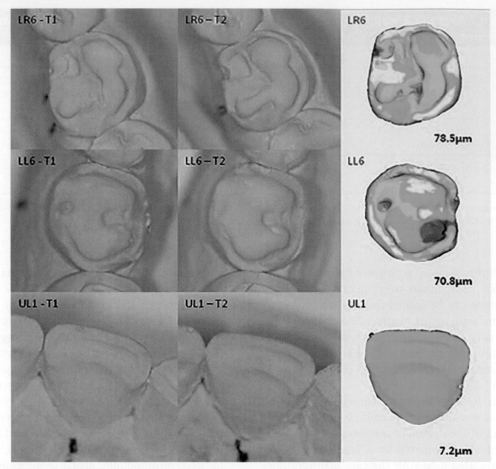

Fig. 9.2 Serial study casts of three different patients, 1 year apart (T1 to T2). From the direct 'naked eye' visual examination of the study casts, there does not appear to be any progressing tooth surface loss, but the non-contact laser profilometry of the casts in a laboratory highlights the actual tissue loss. The colour scale of the profilometry scans indicates green (normal, within the range of natural error of the measuring system, 15 microns), through yellow, to blue regions showing the highest negative surface change between the T1 and T2 images. The figures quoted are the average tooth surface loss measured across the surface of each tooth. Geomagic software was used in these cases for the image superimposition and calculation of the surface change. (Courtesy of Jose Rodriguez.)

9.2 RESTORATION FAILURE

The potential causes of restoration failure have been separated and outlined in Table 9.2. It is important to appreciate that the causes for restoration and tooth failure (Table 9.3) are often multifactorial in nature. Indeed, as the causes for both tooth and restoration failure are inextricably linked, it is wise to consider them together, as a *tooth-restoration complex (TRC)*.

Consider the causes of failure in all the following clinical scenarios. Without appreciating the cause of

failure and addressing this in the first instance, it will be impossible to rectify in the long term.

9.2.1 Aetiology

The multifactorial aetiology of restoration failure is often due to manifestations of inherent long-term weaknesses in the mechanical properties of different restorative materials (e.g., poor edge strength, wear, compressive strength, water absorption) and/or problems in the technical application of the restorative material

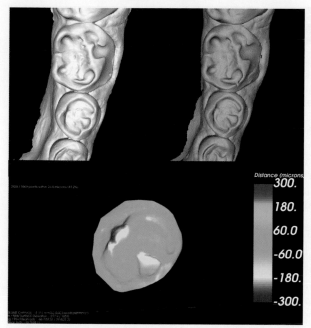

Fig. 9.3 A digital intra-oral scan of a lower-left second premolar and first molar at initial assessment *(left image)* of a patient, and 3 years later *(right image)*. Wear progression can be assessed visually on an intra-oral scan and is visually evident on the first molar buccal and occlusal surfaces. Wear progression is less visually evident on the second premolar. Wear progression can also be digitally assessed. A 3D inspection of the differences between scans on the LL5 reveals areas of wear in red (areas of high wear progression ~300 μm) and yellow (areas of moderate progression ~60–180 μm). Note the areas of blue depicting areas of tissue 'gain'. This demonstrates the systematic error and suggests that values showing loss should be used as a guide and not a precise measure of change. Image analysis done in WearCompare (www.leedsdigitaldentistry.com/Wear-Compare). (Data courtesy the Radboud Tooth Wear Project Monitoring Arm. Saoirse O'Toole and Bas Loomans.)

for the chosen clinical situation (i.e., inappropriate case selection, incorrect choice of material and inadequate placement technique).

9.2.2 Choice of Restorative Material

The chemistries and physical properties of different direct, plastic restorative dental materials at a clinician's disposal have been discussed in Chapter 7. Restorative material longevity will be affected by:

- The differences in physical properties of each material (e.g., bulk dental amalgam has the greatest strength

and resistance to wear; conventional glass-ionomer cement (GIC) has limited long-term wear resistance under high occlusal loads; resin composites exhibit volumetric shrinkage).
- The occlusal loading placed on individual restorations (which might cause some materials to wear, fatigue or fracture more quickly than others).
- The rapid development of dental biomaterial science. As the mechanical properties and placement techniques are continuously being refined, the longevity of new materials will continue to improve.
- The simplicity of the clinical handling characteristics of the material (the easier it is to manipulate by the nurse or clinician and the fewer stages required for its placement, the less chance for iatrogenic weaknesses or errors to be introduced).
- Linked to the preceding point, the clinical skill of the operator. It is these last two points that are most critical in modern minimally invasive conservative dentistry in affecting restoration longevity.

Clinical research studies and statistical meta-analyses of past clinical data have attempted to objectively answer the question of how long restorations should last. However, due to the numerous uncontrollable variables mentioned already (primarily the operator and the patient), obtaining a precise figure is impossible and arguably irrelevant! Often-quoted *average* age ranges of modern restorations at the time of replacement are:

- Amalgam restorations: 10–15 years
- Resin composite restorations: 7–10 years
- GIC restorations: 5-7 years

However, this does not mean, for example, that all GICs will catastrophically fail after 5 years or that all amalgams will last 15 years without any problems. The hotly debated issue regarding the assessment criteria for designating failure (see Section 9.2.3) rears its head when considering the aforementioned longevity figures. It must be appreciated that the weighted clinical importance of some of the criteria for failure assessment (outlined in Table 9.1) will be dependent on the restorative material being assessed. For example, when considering aesthetics as an assessment of restoration failure, a black, tarnished amalgam with ditched, corroded margins on a premolar tooth may be considered functional as replacing it would probably be detrimental to the remaining

TABLE 9.2 **Causes of Restoration Failure and Criteria Used to Assess the Failure With Associated Clinical Comments**

Restoration Failure Criteria	Causes/Comments
Colour match (aesthetics)	• Important to get unbiased patient views especially in the anterior aesthetic zone—they may or may not be concerned. Ability to manage patient expectations is important at the outset of any treatment offered. Care must be taken not to influence or bias the patient views in this regard. • Underlying discolouration from stained dentine. • Superficial discolouration from marginal/surface staining. • Underlying discolouration from corrosion products (e.g., dental amalgam; Fig. 9.4). • Aged tooth-coloured restorative materials become stained and discoloured due to water and/or food stain (tannin) absorption/adsorption onto worn, roughened surfaces, leading to a gradual change in optical properties (Fig. 9.5).
Margin integrity	• Loss of margin integrity (permitting plaque biofilm stagnation and dysbiosis) caused by: 　- Long-term creep/corrosion/ditching of dental amalgams (Fig. 9.6A–F). 　- Margin shrinkage of resin composites/bonding agent (Fig. 9.7). 　- Margin dissolution/shrinkage (on desiccation) of glass-ionomer cements. 　- Margin chipping under occlusal loading due to poor restoration edge strength. Care must be taken when placing such restorations to not leave weak margins in occlusion. 　- Presence of ledges/overhangs, poor contour of margins (Fig. 9.8). • If the patient can keep the failed margin free of plaque and caries and it is not of aesthetic or functional concern, then this partial loss of integrity may not be the sole indicator to repair or replace the restoration.
Margin discolouration	• Micro/macro defects at the tooth–restoration interface will permit exogenous stain (e.g., food stains) to penetrate along the outer perimeter of the restoration as well as towards the pulp. • Poor aesthetics (Fig. 9.9). • An indication of marginal integrity failure? • Not necessarily an indication of secondary/recurrent caries/caries associated with restorations/sealants (CARS).
Loss of bulk integrity	• Restorations may be bulk fractured/partially or completely lost due to: 　- Heavy occlusal loading; inadequate occlusal assessment before restoring the tooth (Fig. 9.10A–B). 　- Poor cavity design leading to weakened, thin-section restorations (especially for amalgams; Fig. 9.11A–B). 　- Poor bonding technique/contamination leading to an adhesive bond failure and lack of retention. 　- Inadequate placement procedures (condensation technique/curing) causing intrinsic material structural weaknesses (e.g., voids, 'soggy bottom' in resin composites). • Patients will often complain of a 'hole in the tooth' where food debris is trapped; ↑ caries risk (Fig. 9.12). • Bulk loss of restoration or occlusal wear may affect the bite/occlusal scheme (Figs. 9.13 and 9.14A–B).

Note: It is vital to appreciate that multiple aetiologies for restoration failure are common and must be considered in conjunction with the causes of tooth failure—that is, the tooth-restoration complex.

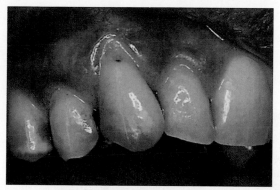

Fig. 9.4 Corrosion products from a distal amalgam in the UR3 causing coronal discolouration which the patient complained about, an example of aesthetic restoration failure.

Q9.4: What restorative material should be used to replace this amalgam restoration?

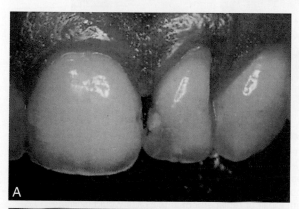

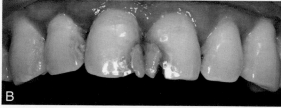

Fig. 9.5 (A) An aged, discoloured mesial resin composite restoration on the UL2. This provided aesthetic concerns for the patient who requested its replacement. (B) Class IV defective resin composite restorations in the maxillary central incisors. Aesthetics, form and function are severely compromised as is plaque biofilm control in the defects, thus warranting restoration replacement (the "5Rs").

Q9.5A: What would be the difficulty faced by the clinician when replacing this Class III restoration?

tooth structure, whereas a mildly partially stained resin composite may be seriously considered for repair or replacement as the repair procedure is perceived to be relatively simple and non-destructive by dentists. So, which restoration has actually 'failed'? The most useful answer to the lead question in this section is one given by an experienced operator who has monitored their own patients over many years and has seen failed restorations they were responsible for placing, appreciated the causes of failure and then repaired or replaced them. This individual can give an honest estimate of the longevity of the restorations placed by their own hand, incorporating the individual patient factors into this.

9.2.3 How May Restorations Be Assessed?

Several clinical indices are available to researchers to help evaluate the causes, extents and timelines for restoration failure made from different dental materials (USPHS, Ryge & Snyder and FDI criteria[1] to name but three). However, interpretation of collected, pooled data depends on what is designated a failure in the first instance. A restoration's success may be judged on:

- Its clinical or radiographic appearance and technical form
- Its clinical function
- Whether the tooth is free of pain and/or disease

The aspects of a restoration to be assessed, either on primary examination or at a recall consultation, are shown in Table 9.1. Each criterion can be given a score on a numerical scale depending on the degree of 'failure'. Restoration failure is mechanical in origin. However, with experience and consideration of the clinical knowledge of the patient and the patient's views, the clinician is able to make a judgment as to the degree of failure and the necessity of operative intervention, in most cases. Note that a 'failed' restoration may require replacement in one patient, but a similar 'failure' in another patient may be accepted without any operative intervention, depending on other factors. Therefore the decision whether to replace or repair the tooth-restoration complex will depend on input from both the experienced dentist and the patient—that is, shared decision-making.

9.2.4 How Long Should Restorations Last?

Numerous factors affect the answer to this important question that many patients will, quite reasonably, ask:

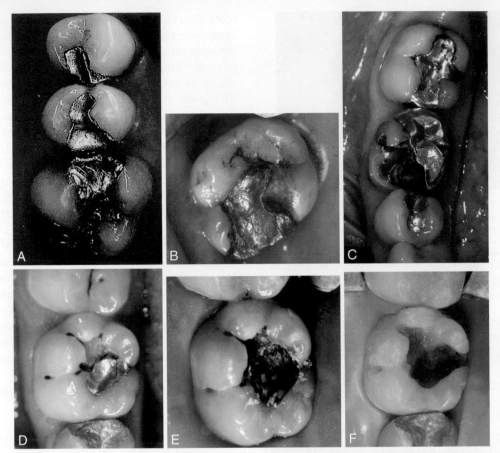

Fig. 9.6 (A) A series of old, ditched and partly corroded amalgam restorations which, when observed on clinical examination, are deemed to be cleansable and are not causing direct problems for the patient. Although the margins and occlusal surfaces are not perfect, should these amalgams be classified as failed restorations? (B) A ditched amalgam UL7 with a marginal defect large enough to accommodate the tip of a periodontal probe, accumulating plaque. A combination of refurbishment with repair or replacement in this case would facilitate plaque control. (C) A complex fracture of the large dental amalgam tooth-restoration complex (TRC), LR6. Either this defect would need to be repaired or the whole TRC would need to be replaced. (From Mackenzie L, Banerjee A. Minimally invasive direct restorations: a practical guide. Brit Dent J. 2017 Aug 11;223(3):163-171. doi:10.1038/sj.bdj.2017.661. (D–F) The LR6 fractured Class I occlusal amalgam restoration with a lost distal portion and associated stained fissures. The fractured restoration was removed, exposing caries associated with restorations and sealants beneath the defective restoration. The final minimally invasive, selective carious dentine cavity preparation using hand excavation, with extension into the undermined lingual enamel. (Courtesy T Viswapurna.)

- The caries risk/susceptibility status of the patient. The higher the caries risk over a prolonged period of time, the less likely it is for restorations, independent of the restorative material used, to last as long without problems due to poor patient adherence to preventive regimens and/or maintenance of oral hygiene.

- The age of the patient. When clinical data from adolescents and adults are compared, restorations last longer in adults. This may reflect the susceptibility to caries of younger people or differences in attitude and abilities towards dental care depending on age.

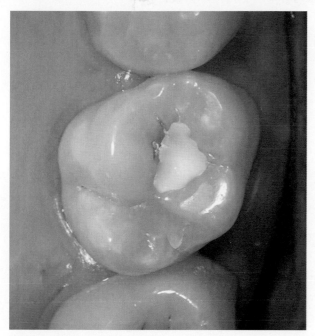

Fig. 9.7 Occlusal resin composites on the UL6. Note the poor aesthetics and margin staining/breakdown. These restorations might be easier clinically to replace rather than repair due to their small size in a high caries risk patient with continuing poor oral hygiene, as plaque stagnation will be a concern at the defective restoration margins.

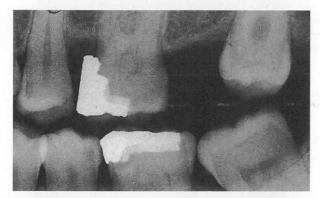

Fig. 9.8 A left bitewing radiograph of an overhanging (positive ledge) radio-opaque dental amalgam restoration on the mesial aspect of the UL6. Due to plaque stagnation, mesial alveolar bone loss has occurred along with radiographic evidence of caries (radiolucency beneath the overhang; care is needed to distinguish this from radiographic cervical burnout).

Q9.8: What has caused this positive ledge to occur in the restoration?

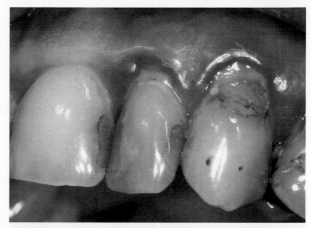

Fig. 9.9 Marginal staining evident on the resin composite restorations on the distal UL1, mesial and distal UL2 and buccal cervical UL3. The patient complained of poor aesthetics. Note the plaque accumulation at the gingival margins of the UL2 and UL3, posing a caries and periodontal disease risk in these areas.

Q9.9: What periodontal condition has been caused by the accumulated plaque and what is its relevance when replacing the restorations?

- The type and size or surface area of restorations. Smaller restorations with a reduced surface area exposed to the oral environment are easier to place and are easier for the patient to clean as their margins will be more easily accessible to effective oral hygiene procedures and thus will last longer than larger ones if maintained.
- The restorative material used in the correct situation (see Section 9.2.3).
- The diagnostic criteria of the clinician. This is particularly important with respect to recurrent and/or secondary caries (CARS), because this is the most common reason dentists give for replacing restorations (see later).
- The age and clinical experience of the operator. Young dentists, with less clinical experience, tend to replace more restorations than older dentists, as they have been less exposed to the deleterious consequences of the destructive operative restorative cycle on the natural life of teeth in their patients.
- Whether the dentist is reviewing their own work or that of another dentist. Changing dentists puts a patient 'at risk' of the diagnosis of failed restorations

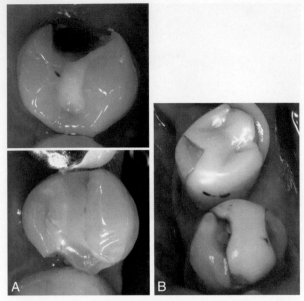

Fig. 9.10 (A) Two clinical examples of fractured resin composite occluso-proximal restorations. A bulk fracture of the distal portion of the restoration, LL5 (top image) and a chipped fracture of the mesial portion of the restoration, LL4 (lower image - both courtesy of Jan Kühnisch, LMU Munich). (B) The 21-year-old resin composite MOD Class II restoration in the LR4 is worn occlusally and has fractured at the margin of the buccal wall. (From Mackenzie L, Banerjee A. Minimally invasive direct restorations: a practical guide. *Brit Dent J.* 2017 Aug 11; 223(3): 163–171. Doi:10.1038/sj.bdj.2017.661.)

> **Q9.10A and B:** What concerns might the patient and/ or clinician have with the clinical situations shown in Fig. 9.10A–B?

and again is dependent on the criteria used to define failure but this time without any prior background clinical information as to how and why the original restoration was placed.

- The care, attitude and motivation of the patient in maintaining their oral and dental health. Restorations are only ever as good as the operator placing them and the patient looking after them.

The actual answer to the question heading this section is 'it doesn't matter'! In the modern era of minimum intervention oral and dental healthcare (MIOC) and minimally invasive operative treatments (MID)

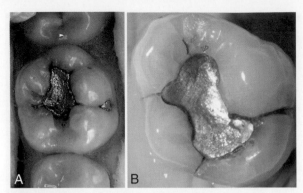

Fig. 9.11 (A) A partially fractured occlusal amalgam restoration in the LL6. (B) Tooth cracks around an ageing dental amalgam Class I occlusal restoration, UR6. Always elicit the cause of the problem before trying to fix it.

> **Q9.11A:** What factors have resulted in this fracture?
> **Q9.11B:** What factors have resulted in these tooth cracks?

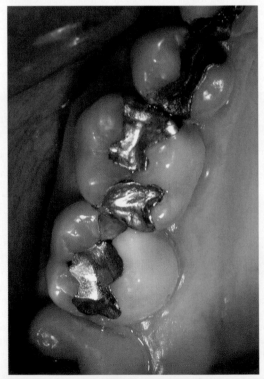

Fig. 9.12 Fractured amalgam restorations on the UR7 mesial and UR4 distal, which need repair due to plaque stagnation and caries associated with restorations and sealants (CARS).

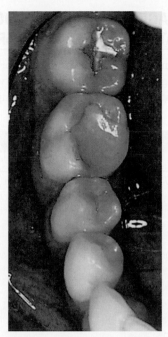

Fig. 9.13 Occlusal wear on resin composite restoration on the LR6.

Q9.13: Does this finding necessitate the replacement of this restoration?

advocated throughout this textbook, the critical question to ask regarding the measure of a successful outcome of dental therapy and treatment is not necessarily just about the technical quality and/or status of restorations placed, but whether natural tooth structure and pulp sensibility have been preserved long term. It is the profession's duty to concern itself, along with the patient, with the maintenance of natural oral and dental health and pulp sensibility as opposed to purely that of the restorations or prostheses placed to repair the consequences of dental disease. It is important to remember that none of the artificial materials used to repair or replace natural teeth come close to replicating the qualities of natural biological tooth structure. These materials will always fail over varying periods of time and will be superceded eventually by newer developments in materials technology, but they are still not as good as biological tissues themselves. Therefore assessment of successful outcomes should no longer be concerned with the simple overall longevity of restorations but with the level of biological response they elicit in the tooth and the ease with which they can be repaired when the time comes without detriment to the remaining viable tooth. Thus perhaps a better title for this section should be 'How long should restored teeth last?'

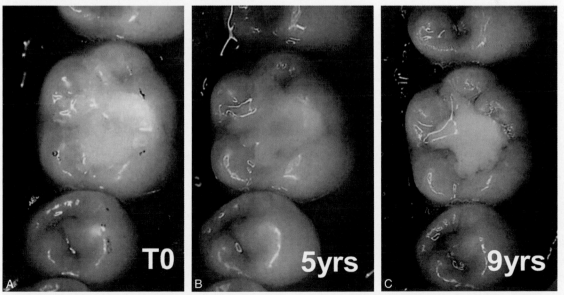

Fig. 9.14 (A) Posterior occlusal restoration on the LL6 at time of placement (blue marks on teeth are made by articulating paper checking the occlusion). (B) The same restoration 5 years after placement showing early signs of occlusal wear. (C) Restoration 9 years after placement, with further loss of occlusal definition. Margins are intact, there were no symptoms from this tooth and aesthetics are a little compromised: this does not constitute a restoration failure and the restoration can continue to be reviewed.

9.3 TOOTH FAILURE

Teeth can fail for *mechanical or structural* reasons and/or *biological* reasons, either together with or independent from restoration failure (consider the *tooth-restoration complex* as a whole) (Table 9.3; Figs. 9.15–9.19).

9.4 MANAGING THE FAILING TOOTH-RESTORATION COMPLEX: THE '5Rs'

As has been stated at the beginning of this chapter, the long-term maintenance and survival of the tooth-restoration complex (TRC) relies upon regular

TABLE 9.3	Causes of Tooth Failure	
Tooth Failure		**Comments**
Mechanical	Enamel margin	• Poor cavity design can leave weak, unsupported or undermined enamel margins which can more easily fracture under occlusal load. • Cavity preparation techniques (burs) cause subsurface micro-cracks within the body of the enamel, thus undermining the surface (see Chapter 5, Fig. 5.35). • Adhesive shrinkage stresses on prisms at the enamel surface can cause them to be pulled apart causing cohesive marginal failure in tooth structure, leading to a microleakage risk (Fig. 9.15).
	Dentine margin	• Adhesive bond to hydrophilic dentine results in a poorer quality bond (compared to that with sound enamel) which hydrolyses over time leading to ↑ risk of microleakage. • Deep proximal cavities often have exposed margins on dentine. Poor moisture control leads to a compromised bonding technique, in turn ↑ risk of microleakage.
	Bulk coronal/cusp fracture	• Large restorations will weaken the coronal strength of remaining hard tissues. • Loss of marginal ridges/peripheral enamel will weaken the tooth crown. • Cusps absorb oblique loading stresses and are prone to leverage/fracture (Fig. 9.16). • Can cause symptoms of food-packing, sensitivity.
	Root fracture	• Often in root-filled, heavily restored teeth (with post-core-crown) under heavy occlusal/lateral loads. • Traumatic injury. • Symptoms variable (pain, mobility, tenderness on biting) but radiographic assessment not always easy to interpret.
Biological	Recurrent/secondary caries/CARS	• New caries at a tooth–restoration gap with plaque biofilm accumulation, stagnation and dysbiosis (Fig. 9.17A and B). • Detected clinically or with radiographs (can be difficult to interpret). • Margin stain is not an indicator of caries associated with restorations and sealants. • Can affect a section of margin and not the whole restoration.
	Pulp status	• Heavily restored teeth are more susceptible to pulp inflammation due to the original disease or the invasive direct operative treatment (Fig. 9.18). • Iatrogenic damage or ongoing disease may cause pulp pathology or necrosis.
	Periodontal disease	• Examination of the periodontium required for loss of attachment, pocket depths, bone levels (Fig. 9.19). • Can be exacerbated by poor margin adaptation of restorations (causing plaque and debris stagnation)/margins encroaching into the periodontal biological width.

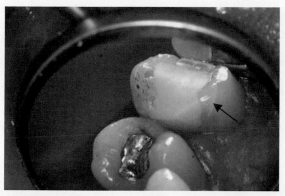

Fig. 9.15 A resin composite restoration in a maxillary premolar with a fine enamel crack evident on the palatal cusp *(white line)* remote to the tooth-restoration interface *(arrow)*.

Q9.15: What has caused this enamel crack?

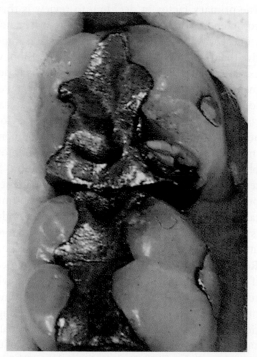

Fig. 9.16 The mesiobuccal cusp of the LR7 has fractured off due to excessive loading of the weakened crown and possible undermining of the cusp when the cavity was originally prepared.

Q9.16: Which coronal structural feature is missing that has contributed to the increased weakness of the remaining tooth structure?

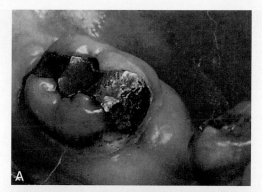

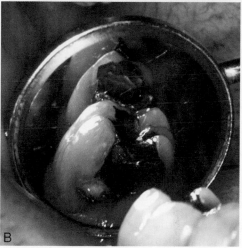

Fig. 9.17 (A) Recurrent/secondary caries (CARS) at the cervical margin gap between the tooth and dental amalgam in a mandibular molar. (B) Active, cavitated CARS adjacent to a dental amalgam restoration with plaque stagnation.

and careful recall consultations (clinical domain 4 of the MIOC delivery framework: active surveillance). At these important appointments, the team is able to review not only the status of existing TRCs, but also the patient's attitude about maintaining them with the appropriate level of well-executed preventive self-care. Nevertheless, all functional tooth-restoration complexes have a finite lifespan, as has been discussed earlier. Modern restorations can be *reviewed, refurbished, re-sealed, repaired* and/or *replaced* (the "5Rs") when deemed necessary by the operator and the patient. The decision to repair or replace a restoration is one that has to be made specifically for the particular situation in the particular patient. When significant portions of the restoration (>50%) have failed or the surrounding tooth structure is structurally and/or functionally

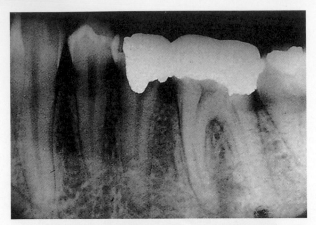

Fig. 9.18 Periapical radiograph of a heavily restored LL5; over time the pulp has become non-vital and there is radiographic evidence of pulp necrosis.

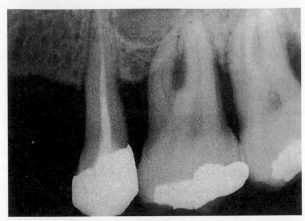

Fig. 9.19 A periapical radiograph of a successful coronally restored UL6. Note the loss of alveolar bone support caused by periodontal disease leading to excessive mobility.

> **Q9.18i:** Can you spot it?
> **Q9.18ii:** What anatomical feature might confuse your diagnosis?
> **Q9.18iii:** The amalgam restoration has not extended into the pulp, so why does it appear as though it has?

compromised, partial or complete replacement of the restoration will often be indicated. In most other cases, especially where the original restoration material type is known, careful minimally invasive repair of the deficient, fractured or weakened sections may be appropriate. When completely removing old adhesive restorations, there is a significant chance of enlarging the cavity with a rotary instrument due to similarities in colour of the restoration and surrounding tooth structure. Therefore other operative technologies may be useful, such as bio-active glass air-abrasion (see Chapter 5, Section 5.8.4). Repairing failing portions of an existing TRC is the more conservative and minimally invasive option available.

The minimally invasive operative and non-operative interventions for managing the tooth-restoration complex that has been diagnosed as failing may be divided into five categories known as the *5Rs*, listed here from least to most invasive:

1. **Review (Fig. 9.14).** If only minor defects are evident such as surface wear roughness or irregularities without concomitant plaque biofilm stagnation, the restoration can be monitored non-operatively.

The primary factor in deciding to review is that by commencing operative treatment there will be no net clinical advantage gained by the patient. It is imperative that the patient is informed of the decision, with explanation as to its rationale, and that this is documented clearly in the notes for both clinical and dento-legal purposes. Assessment of the patient's caries risk/susceptibility and their responsible behavioural adherence to non-operative preventive regimens is imperative. The use of intra-oral clinical photography is recommended to help review restorations long term. Care should be taken to try to standardise the perspective and lighting conditions between images taken as much as possible. Suitable recall periodicity is required and this will be partly dependent upon the attitude the patient has towards their own oral health.

2. **Refurbishment (Fig. 9.20A–C).** This is indicated if there are small defects in the restoration which require intervention, including re-shaping, removal of excess material and/or polishing. If plaque stagnation occurs in such surface defects which the patient cannot remove easily with oral hygiene procedures, or if there is an aesthetic benefit to the finished restoration, refurbishment is indicated. Micro-abrasion techniques to refresh resin composite surfaces especially in the anterior aesthetic zone would be included in this category.

3. **Re-seal (Fig. 9.21A–B).** Re-sealing is defined as the application of sealant into a non-carious, defective margin, gap and/or surface. This is achieved

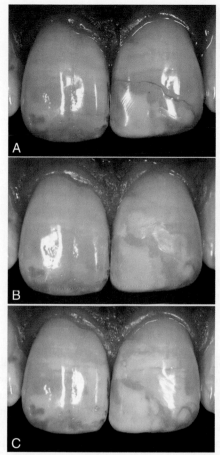

Fig. 9.20 (A) Maxillary upper central incisors with old, stained, roughened Class IV resin composite restorations. (B) Initial refurbishment carried out with mildly abrasive resin composite rotary finishing tips/discs (see Chapter 5, Section 5.8.2). (C) The polished refurbishment has significantly improved the anterior aesthetics of these restorations with no biological cost. (Courtesy *Dental Update*: Green D, Mackenzie L, Banerjee A. Minimally invasive long-term management of direct restorations: the '5Rs'. *Dent Update*. Jun;42(5):413-416, 419-421, 423-426. doi:10.12968/denu.2015.42.5.413.)

through the use of flowable resin-based adhesive systems. Sealing a restoration minimally invasively prevents further ingress, accumulation and stagnation of plaque biofilm and the potential of caries developing.

4. **Repair.** Repair is the addition of a restorative material to an existing restoration. It may involve operative removal of the defective part of the restoration or modification of the existing retained portion to facilitate retention. A minimally invasive approach

endeavours to restore the failing restoration whilst preserving the maximum quantity of tooth structure and maintaining pulp viability.

5. **Replacement.** This is defined as the complete removal of the existing restoration and necessary tooth structure to prevent disease progression or to aid retention and stability and is indicated if there are multiple or severe problems associated with the existing failed tooth-restoration complex in which a segmental repair is not feasible.

It must be appreciated that in the majority of clinical cases, these categories of treatment are not mutually exclusive and should not be considered separately. A more extensive surface refurbishment of a restoration combined with resealing its defective margins might be considered together as a tooth-restoration complex repair. The categories have been defined to allow a better understanding of the minimally invasive approach to biological tooth preservation. Resorting to the 5Rs should not be considered a 'failure' of care, but rather a part of the long-term management of the TRC. These principles should be explained to the patient as part of the overall maintenance regimen when consenting a patient for any restorative treatment and should be documented in the clinical notes accordingly.

In the following sub-sections the 5Rs MI management protocols are applied to different restorative materials.

9.4.1 Dental Amalgam

The most common causes of failure of dental amalgam restorations are secondary caries (CARS; pathological) and TRC fracture (mechanical) (see Tables 9.1 and 9.2).

- *Review.* If only minor deficiencies are present in the restoration, such as a minimal surface defect, reviewing the restoration periodically as per standard recall guidelines is a sensible management option. If there is no clinical advantage to treating the restoration operatively, it should be reviewed. Indeed, operative intervention of old, established amalgams can lead to significant levels of tooth tissue destruction as the corroded alloy offers some 'support' to weakened tooth structure over time. Removing this can accelerate cusp or wall failure, thus complicating the replacement restoration significantly (Fig. 9.6A). Appropriate documentation and informed consent should be gathered from the patient.

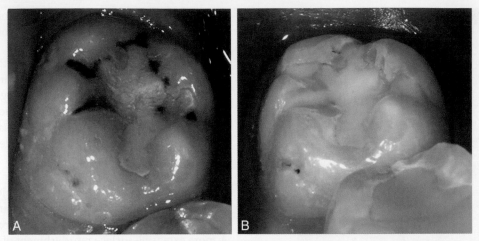

Fig. 9.21 (A) Non-carious, stained and defective margins associated with an occlusal resin composite restoration on a mandibular right second molar. (B) The defective margins were cleaned using air-abrasion with 27 μm alumina particles, acid-etched for 20 seconds, washed and dried. Adhesive was then placed and resealed with a resin-based fissure sealant and photo-cured. (Courtesy *Dental Update*: Green D, Mackenzie L, Banerjee A. Minimally invasive long-term management of direct restorations: the '5Rs'. *Dent Update*. Jun;42(5):413-416, 419-421, 423-426. doi:10.12968/denu.2015.42.5.413.)

- *Refurbish* (or *re-finish*). Existing amalgam restorations may be refurbished or re-finished using brown and green amalgam abrasive rubber polishing points in a slow-speed handpiece; see Chapter 5, Fig. 5.35, and Fig. 9.22A–B. This is a useful treatment for anatomical form defects and refreshing an old tarnished restoration. The refurbishment of anatomical form and surface roughness is a conservative and simple procedure which can enhance the appearance of amalgam restorations and, indirectly, their longevity, as they are less likely to be replaced by clinicians in the future.

- *Re-seal*. The application of a resin composite sealant into a non-carious gap or defect at the margin of an amalgam restoration has been shown to increase the clinical longevity of the amalgam restoration (Fig. 9.22A–B). Prior to application of a flowable resin composite, the amalgam surface and adjacent tooth can be modified using a variety of techniques. Air-abrasion, etching with orthophosphoric acid and application of a dentine bonding agent are all effective protocols cited in the literature.

- *Repair*. It is relatively easy to remove the remaining amalgam restoration or loose fragment. A tungsten carbide (TC) Beaver bur (Chapter 5, Figs. 5.30A and 5.34D) is used to cut through the amalgam restoration from its centre towards the periphery of the portion to be removed (avoiding contact with the tooth cavity margins). Larger fragments are usually easily dislodged or can be flicked away using hand excavators (see Chapter 5, Section 5.8.1).

  - Tooth cavity margins may be 'freshened up' using gentle pressure rotary instrumentation to remove stains or early demineralised hard tissues especially if the restoration is to be repaired or replaced using a tooth-coloured adhesive restorative material.

  - Retention has to be gained macro-mechanically via cavity undercuts, slots or grooves. If replacing the complete restoration, these retentive features will often already feature in the existing cavity design and may only need slight modification. When repairing the damaged portion of the restoration/tooth only, these retentive design features should be cut into the retained portion of the original amalgam restoration to avoid further loss and weakening of the surrounding tooth structure (Fig. 9.23A).

  - Some may advocate the use of chemical retention, using a bonded amalgam technique, in an attempt to conserve remaining tooth structure, but there is limited clinical evidence for long-term success rates of this repair technique (Chapter 7, Section 7.5.3; Chapter 8, Section 8.9).

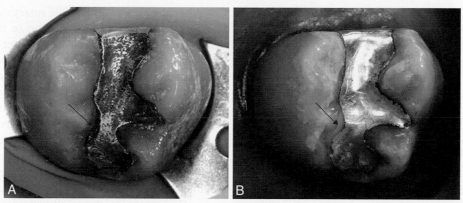

Fig. 9.22 (A) The occlusal surface of an UL7 with a Class II mesio-occlusal amalgam restoration. Note the non-carious defect associated with the palatal margin of the amalgam *(arrow)*. (B) The defect was cleaned and acid-etched, adhesive was applied and re-sealed using flowable resin composite and the remaining amalgam was refurbished using an amalgam finishing bur. (Courtesy *Dental Update*: Green D, Mackenzie L, Banerjee A. Minimally invasive long-term management of direct restorations: the '5Rs'. *Dent Update*. Jun;42(5):413-416, 419-421, 423-426. doi:10.12968/denu.2015.42.5.413.)

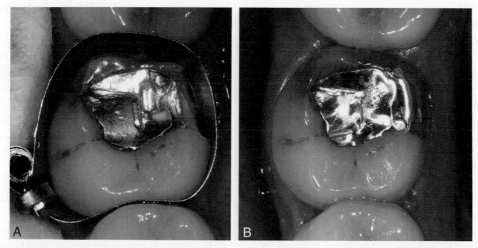

Fig. 9.23 (A) LR6 with an old occlusal amalgam and a recently fractured distolingual cusp. A retentive lock has been cut into what was originally an occlusal amalgam to improve retention for the repair. (B) The repair of the tooth-restoration complex has been successful using amalgam; the image was taken 1 year after the repair was originally carried out. (Courtesy *Dental Update*: Green D, Mackenzie L, Banerjee A. Minimally invasive long-term management of direct restorations: the '5Rs'. *Dent Update*. Jun;42(5):413-416, 419-421, 423-426. doi:10.12968/denu.2015.42.5.413.)

Q9.23A: How else can the amalgam repair bond to the old restoration be enhanced?
Q9.23B: What type of matrix system has been used in this case?

- If these processes can be carried out, then the repair can be completed using dental amalgam (Fig. 9.23B). If not, resin composite (including the use of an etch-and-rinse adhesive [Types 1 and 2]) or chemically adhesive GIC in situations with poor moisture control might be the material of choice. Margins must be contoured appropriately to avoid ledges, overhangs and voids.

9.4.2 Resin Composites/GIC

In contrast to dental amalgam, resin composite restorations present a more complicated chemical substrate for repair. There is variation in the chemical composition of resin composites regarding the type of resin matrix, with additional disparities in inorganic filler quantity and type. The age of the restoration also has a significant deleterious effect on the bond strength between new to old resin composite repairs. Newly placed resin composites, placed incrementally, have cohesion between increments due to the presence of uncured resin monomer after photo-curing (the oxygen-inhibited layer). This degrades rapidly in clinical service and reduces the success of bonding further additions of resin composite for intra-oral repairs.

Dentists have been shown to be more likely to intervene operatively with a defective resin composite restoration in contrast to a defective amalgam restoration. It has been speculated that this difference may be due to the perceived increased longevity of amalgam restorations in general and the lack of correlation between margin breakdown and the presence of caries.

- It is more usual to *refurbish*, *re-seal* or *repair* adhesive restorations rather than *replace* them completely. Polishing, improvement in surface roughness and anatomical form of Class I and II resin composite restorations have been shown to maintain an improvement for 3 years post-intervention (Fig. 9.20A–C). If there is a gross aesthetic or biological concern, old restorations may be veneered or re-surfaced with new material (the old restoration re-surfaced with an up-to-date, shade-matched equivalent rather than replaced completely).

- When *repair* is an option, use rotary instrumentation to remove the defective portion of the restoration. Care must be taken to avoid cavity over-preparation as it can sometimes be difficult to dis-tinguish between the adhesive restoration and cavity margin due to colour similarities. Air-abrasive techniques using alumina or bio-active glass powders might facilitate this process due to their inherent selectivity for resin composites and/or grossly demineralised enamel.
- Fresh cavity margins should expose roughened sound enamel and/or the dentine surface for better micro-mechanical/chemical adhesion.
  - *GIC repair*: Condition all surfaces with 10% polyacrylic acid for 10 seconds, wash thoroughly, blot dry and apply or pack GIC (with suitable matrixing as appropriate).
  - Resin composite repair (Figs. 9.24A–C and 9.25A–C; repairing a fissure sealant):
    - Acid-etch with 37% orthophosphoric acid for 20 seconds (enamel) and 10 to 15 seconds (dentine), wash thoroughly (10 seconds) and dry.
    - A silanating agent may be used to couple a new methacrylate-based resin composite to an old one (painted on the bonding surface of the old restoration and evaporated). This step may be omitted as it can interfere with the adhesive chemistry of the specific dental adhesive used, and it may be clinically difficult to separate these two procedures.
    - The dentine bonding agent is agitated onto the cavity surfaces, gently dried (until no rippling is noticed, indicating solvent evaporation) and light-cured (see Chapter 8, Table 8.12).
    - The resin composite is added in small increments, photo-cured and finished appropriately (see Chapter 5, Fig. 5.33).
- Another factor in the success of resin composite repairs is appreciating the chemistry of the original material and the ability to match new material with old. The use of a dental adhesive also significantly improves outcomes, mainly by increasing the 'wetting' or adaptation of the repairing material.

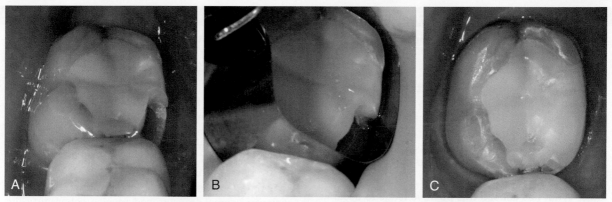

Fig. 9.24 (A) LR7 with an occluso-lingual resin composite restoration and a fractured mesio-lingual cusp. (B) The isolated cavity walls can be freshened with rotary instruments or air-abrasion. The cavity is then silanated to improve the resin composite–composite bond and adhesive is applied and photo-cured. (C) The immediate postoperative image of the resin composite–composite repair. (Courtesy *Dental Update*: Green D, Mackenzie L, Banerjee A. Minimally invasive long-term management of direct restorations: the '5Rs'. *Dent Update*. Jun;42(5):413-416, 419-421, 423-426. doi:10.12968/denu.2015.42.5.413.)

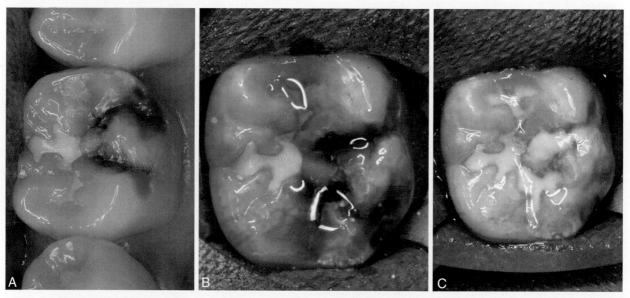

Fig. 9.25 (A) LL6 with hypomineralisation defect (brown discolouration) with remnant of resin-based fissure sealant in the occlusolingual fissure. (B) The LL6 with rubber dam isolation, occlusal surface debrided and 37% orthophosphoric aid etch applied over the remaining exposed occlusal fissures. (C) The acid etch has been washed off and the occlusal surface dried before applying the resin-based fissure sealant using a small ball-ended instrument, teasing the material into the exposed fissures. This is then light-cured, the rubber dam is removed and the occlusion is checked before the patient is discharged. (Courtesy D Raju.)

9.5   ANSWERS TO SELF-TEST QUESTIONS

Q9.4: What restorative material should be used to replace this amalgam restoration?
A: Dental resin composite.

Q9.5A: What would be the difficulty faced by the clinician when replacing this Class III restoration?
A: Aesthetics: matching the natural translucency from the incisal edge through to the mesial aspect of the UL2. An aesthetic layered composite restoration would have to be placed, carefully mimicking the underlying dentine and overlying enamel shades.

Q9.8: What has caused this positive ledge to occur in the restoration?
A: A poorly adapted/wedged matrix band at the cervical margin of the approximal Class II cavity.

Q9.9: What periodontal condition has been caused by the accumulated plaque and what is its relevance when replacing the restorations?
A: Chronic marginal gingivitis. This would need to be remedied with improved oral hygiene techniques prior to any restoration being placed to ensure optimal moisture control during placement of the new composite restorations.

Q9.10A and B: What concerns might the patient and/or clinician have with the clinical situations shown in Fig. 9.10A and B?
A: In Fig. 9.10A, food-packing, gingival trauma, gingival bleeding or gingivitis and ultimately caries due to difficulty for the patient to disrupt the biofilm in the depths of the defect over a period of time. In Fig. 9.10B, aesthetics. As the defect is wide enough and accessible enough for normal effective oral hygiene procedures (toothbrushing), the risk of CARS is low, assuming the patient is using an effective technique.

Q9.11A: What factors have resulted in this fracture?
A: Poor cavity design: the mesial portion of the cavity was too shallow and the amalgam fractured under occlusal load due to its inherent weakness in thin sections and lack of macromechanical retentive features; and inappropriate choice of material: a resin composite may have been a better choice, thus preventing any unnecessary extension of the cavity.

Q9.11B: What factors have resulted in these tooth cracks?
A: Occlusal forces in combination with internal crack propagation from internal cavity line angles over time.

Q9.13: Does this finding necessitate the replacement of this restoration?
A: No. The restoration is fully functional and is not causing any clinical problems.

Q9.15: What has caused this enamel crack?
A: Shrinkage stress from the composite pulling on the prismatic enamel structure and causing cohesive failure in the enamel.

Q9.16: Which coronal structural feature is missing that has contributed to the increased weakness of the remaining tooth structure?
A: A missing mesial marginal ridge.

Q9.18i: Can you spot it?
A: Widening of the periodontal ligament space at the root apex with loss of lamina dura in this area of the LL5.

Q9.18ii: What anatomical feature might confuse your diagnosis?
A: An overlying mental foramen.

Q9.18iii: As the amalgam restoration has not extended into the pulp, why does it appear as though it has?
A: There is an additional buccal cervical amalgam restoration whose radiographic opacity has superimposed itself over the pulp chamber radiolucency.

Q9.23A: How else can the amalgam repair bond to the old restoration be enhanced?
A: Using air-abrasion and/or burs to roughen the surfaces and then using a resin cement in a bonded amalgam technique. However, there is inconclusive evidence as to whether this actually strengthens the adhesive bond between the two amalgams.

Q9.23B: What type of matrix system has been used in this case?
A: A circumferential metal matrix band. This is required as a sectional band would not extend to help contour the mesiolingual aspect of the restoration.

REFERENCE

1. Hickel R, Mesinger S, Opdam N. Revised FDI criteria for evaluating direct and indirect dental restorations-recommendations for its clinical use, interpretation, and reporting. *Clin Oral Investig.* 2023 Jun;27(6):2573–2592. doi:10.1007/s00784-022-04814-1.

MIOC Implementation: Personalised Care Management Pathways

CHAPTER OUTLINE

10.1 MIOC FRAMEWORK: SUMMARY

Fig. 10.1 (see also Chapter 2, Figs 2.1 and 2.2A–E) summarises the MIOC framework to enable oral healthcare teams to deliver person-focused, better long-term oral health, focused on preventive behaviours instilled into and carried out by the patient/caregiver. As has been discussed and explained throughout this textbook, multiple overlapping factors influence the options for delivering care and treatment in each domain. The four clinical domains themselves must not be considered as purely standalone entities, as each will undoubtedly influence the delivery and outcomes of the others. The MIOC framework helps the oral healthcare team work with the patient/caregiver to enable, encourage and facilitate their management of their long-term personal oral and dental health. It provides a logical, simplified structure to a complex process to help create a suitable care management pathway for each individual patient.

10.1.1 Phased Courses of Treatment

The overall care for and management of biofilm-mediated, patient behaviour–related conditions including dental caries and periodontal disease needs to be carried out in a phased approach, often redirecting the patient care regimens back and forth between the clinical domains and team members, until the suitable and pragmatic goals set originally as part of prevention-based behaviour modelling and change are met and maintained (see Chapter 3, Table 3.5). Unfortunately, there are no pre-defined formulae that can be used to calculate the number, length and periodicity of appointments in each of the three care pathway phases: stabilisation, re-assessment/active surveillance and rehabilitation. These will depend upon a host of interlinked factors outlined and discussed in Chapters 2, 3 and 4 as well as the personal characteristics of and dynamic relationship between the patient/caregiver and the clinical team members.

An example of risk/susceptibility-related phased courses of treatment that could be applied to all patients, including those with high clinical needs, vulnerable patient groups and/or those with poor access to care, encompassing the management guidelines for both dental caries and periodontal disease, is shown in Fig. 10.2A–D.

Such phased courses of treatment following the MIOC clinical domains can apply to all age groups and across the restorative disciplines as depicted in Chapter 2, Fig. 2.2A–E. It is by using these risk/susceptibility-based approaches to care that personalised management regimens can be targeted to those most in need with a more appropriate use of resources in terms of workforce deployment, materials and finances. For many healthcare systems around the world, this approach would need a radical shift in professional and public policy as well as to the funding structures that are currently in place.

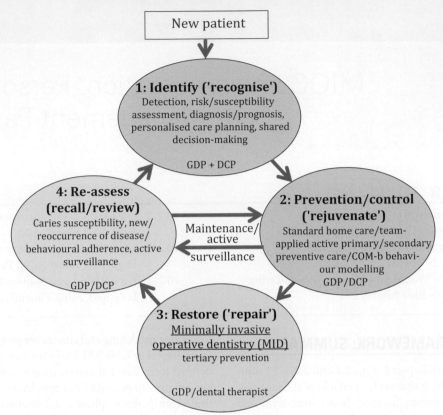

Fig. 10.1 The person-focused MIOC delivery framework showing the four interlinking clinical domains of *identify* (clinical assessment/diagnosis); non-operative, micro-invasive *prevention* of lesions/*control* of disease; *minimally invasive* operative intervention; and *re-assessment* (recall/review/active surveillance). The arrows indicate the direction of the patient pathway through this care delivery framework and within each domain an indication is given of the members of the oral healthcare team who might be involved. *DCP*, Dental care professionals (includes oral health educators, extended duties dental nurses, dental hygienists, dental therapists, practice managers, clinical dental technicians and reception staff); *GDP*, general dental practitioner.

Fig. 10.2 Flowcharts depicting team-delivered phased courses of treatment applied to dental caries management pathways and incorporating periodontal disease management guidelines. These guidelines are related to risk and susceptibility and link to patient-based outcome measures. Definitive oral and dental rehabilitation should only be delivered when targeted prevention goals are achieved and maintained, as per the MIOC domains, to achieve the best possible long-term outcome for the patient. (Acknowledgement to Divyash Patel, Zain Hameed, OCDO England; Jin Vaghela, Kish Patel and Ali Chohan, Smile Dental Academy.)

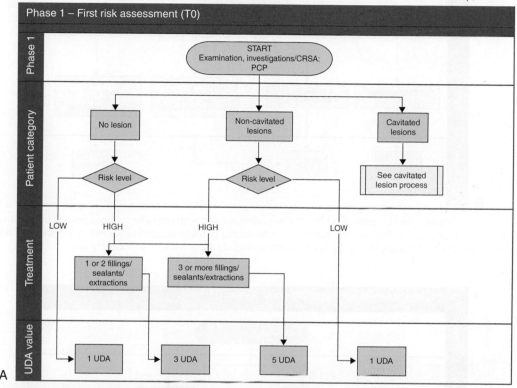

(A) Phase 1: Assessment and stabilisation. After acute pain relief care if required, the patient is assessed as per MIOC Domain 1 and categorised by their caries (and periodontal) risk/susceptibility assessment (CRSA) and presence/absence of carious lesions (cavitated/non-cavitated). A personalised care plan will initially include stabilising primary, secondary and tertiary preventive non-invasive, micro-invasive or minimally invasive care as per MIOC Domains 2 and 3. This can be delivered by the suitably trained workforce. The UK National Health Service reimbursement system is given as a remuneration example for patients with no or early lesions. *PCP*, Personalised care plan; *UDA*, unit of dental activity assigned with a monetary value.

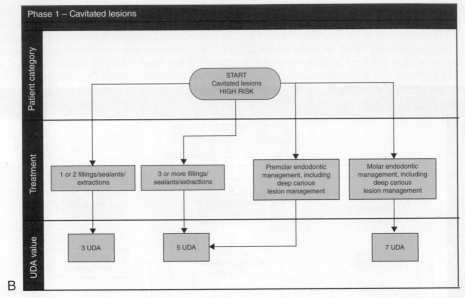

(B) Phase 1: Stabilisation for patients at high risk/susceptibility and with clinically cavitated lesions on presentation (MIOC Domain 3). The number, duration and periodicity of these appointments will vary depending on clinical and practical requirements. *UDA*, Unit of dental activity assigned with a monetary value.

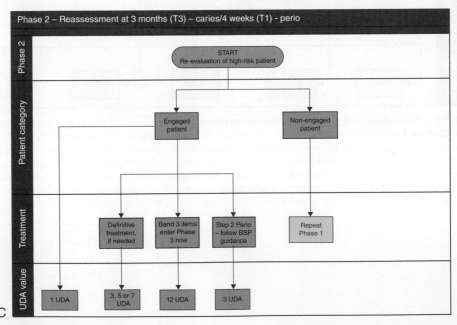

(C) Phase 2: Re-assessment/active surveillance of patients at high risk/susceptibility for caries MIOC Domain 4. This could be carried out between 1 and 3 months after Phase 1 stabilisation is complete. Depending on the level of patient/caregiver engagement and re-evaluation of the CRSA, the patient care pathway may progress to Phase 3, rehabilitation with definitive restorations (MIOC Domain 3), or go back to Phase 1 for further prevention-based stabilisation to try to ensure the pragmatic goals based on the Capability – Opportunity – Motivation – Behaviour change model can be achieved and maintained (MIOC Domain 2). *BSP*, British Society of Periodontology and Implant Dentistry; *UDA*, unit of dental activity assigned with a monetary value.

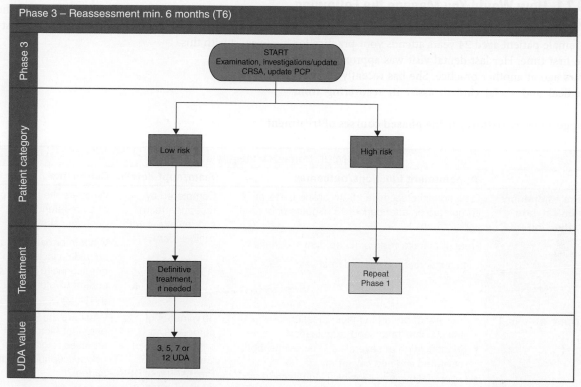

(D) Phase 3: Re-assessment/rehabilitation within approximately 6 months after prevention-based stabilisation has succeeded. If the patient is still at high risk for caries and is non-engaged (MIOC Domain 4) then the care pathway is cycled back again to Phase 1 course of treatment (MIOC Domain 2) for both periodontal disease and dental caries preventive management. *CRSA*, Caries risk/susceptibility assessment; *PCP*, personalised care plan; *UDA*, unit of dental activity assigned with a monetary value.

10.2 CARE MANAGEMENT PATHWAYS: CLINICAL SCENARIOS

This section focuses on four clinical patient scenarios, indicating how a risk/susceptibility-related care management pathway might be configured for a high caries risk adult, a high caries risk child, a high caries risk older adult and low caries risk adult. Using the underpinning basis of the four MIOC clinical domains, each clinical pathway/patient journey indicates how the personalised phased course of treatment might be structured based on appointments (number, frequency and duration), oral healthcare team deployment within their scope of practice and actual preventive care or operative treatment given. These scenarios in no way attempt to standardise this process, but merely provide examples as to how a clinical team might implement all the MIOC principles described in this textbook.

10.2.1 How Would You Manage the Following High-Risk Adult?

A female patient aged 24 years attends your practice for the first time. Her last dental visit was approximately 3 years ago at another practice. She has recently received medical and social care to assist in recovering from substance abuse and pronounces herself "clean". She has been taking a sugar-based medication for the past year to assist with this.

Suggested care pathway using phased courses of treatment

MIOC Domain 1: Identify		
Appointment functions/outcomes	**Team/appt details**	**Comments**
Pre-attendance clinical data collection	Questionnaire accessed from online portal or completed on attendance, 15 minutes prior to appointment 1. Frequent intake of carbonated drinks identified. High sugar diet, no acute dental pain.	Completed by reception team and reviewed with clinical team.	What are the benefits of a pre-attendance questionnaire? What information could/should be included in the questionnaire? https://cgdent.uk/standards-guidance/
Appointment 1	• Review of pre-attendance questionnaire. • Initial consultation and examination. • Identification of several carious lesions, both cavitated and non-cavitated. • Poor oral hygiene – visible plaque seen/documented. • BPE recorded – scores 2 in all sextants. • Photographs and radiographs taken – Radiography in accordance with CGDent guidelines (see https://cgdent.uk/selection-criteria-for-dental-radiography/) – left and right bitewings with apical views as required to confirm apical status/pathology. • Provide diet diary for completion	30 minutes of surgery time and staff time of General Dental Practitioner (GDP)/Dental Therapist (DT) and one dental nurse.	What are the key pertinent factors that are used to glean the risk/susceptibility of the patient?
Initial caries risk/susceptibility assessment (CRSA): High		
	Clinical photographs and radiographs taken by suitably trained member of oral healthcare team on completion of appointment 1 (could use a separate room to avoid surgery usage)	What clinical findings can be seen from this anterior pre-operative intra-oral view? What should the time interval be between appointments 1 and 2 for this patient?

MIOC Domain 2: Disease Control/Lesion Prevention			
	Appointment functions/outcomes	**Team/appt details**	**Comments**
Appointment 2	• Discussion of findings from appointment 1, diagnosis/prognosis. • Findings/significance of CRSA explained. • Primary prevention advice: oral hygiene routines, dietary control, fluoride usage. • Plaque disclosing carried out (*see below*). • Saliva testing (if required). • Discussion of use of fluoride and adjunctive remineralising agents. • Provide diet diary for completion. • Demonstration/observation of oral hygiene procedures. • Suggest goals for improvements in control of disease – COM-B behaviour modelling/goal-setting.	45 minutes of surgery time and staff time of oral health educator/ Dental Hygienist (DH)/DT. With GDP oversight?	The functions/outcomes of appointments 1 and 2 could be merged into one longer appointment, depending on clinical resource and patient logistics.
	CRSA confirmed as HIGH (*see below*).		
Dental plaque disclosing			What do the different three colours of the disclosing agent indicate? What clinical information, in addition to simply the presence/absence of dental plaque, should be recorded in the clinical notes? Consider the importance of patient motivation when planning preventive interventions.

CRSA	Status	High Risk	Low Risk	What should be the interval between appointments 2 and 3?
	Lesions – current or 2 or more new, progressing or restored lesions in the last two years. State of activity.	✓		
	General Factors			
	Diet	✓		
	Fluoride use	✓		
	Health		✓	
	Medications	✓		
	Social	✓		
	Age		✓	
	Oral Factors			
	Oral hygiene	✓		
	Saliva	✓		
	Plaque	✓		
	Bacterial balance in oral biofilm	✓		

Continued

MIOC Domain 2: Disease Control/Lesion Prevention—cont'd			
	Appointment functions/outcomes	Team/appt details	Comments
Appointment 3	• Discuss findings of diet diary. • Explanation of investigations and identification of high caries risk/susceptibility, periodontal risk/susceptibility. • Review outcome of goals set at end of appointment 2. • Advise switch to sugar-free medication (contact medical physician). • Dialogue of options and discussion to include use of caries removal methods as appropriate, e.g. chemo-mechanical, rotary, hand instruments, etc. • Assess COM-B behavioural adherence (good) and finalise phased, personalised care plan with prognosis.	30 minutes of surgery time and staff time of GDP/DT and one dental nurse.	What are the important findings from a diet diary to translate to the patient with regards to her sugar intake and dental caries? Are there other health messages the oral healthcare team can provide? https://www.england.nhs.uk/wp-content/uploads/2016/04/making-every-contact-count.pdf
	Phased, personalised care plan (PCP) *Acute/stabilisation phase:* • Oral hygiene advice, diet recommendation, prescription 5000ppm fluoride toothpaste/other adjunctive remineralisation agents. • Supra- and subgingival professional mechanical plaque removal (PMPR). • Stabilisation of carious lesions – glass-ionomer cements as needed. • Extraction of retained roots/unrestorable teeth. • Re-assess for potential endodontic treatment based on deep carious dentine excavation. *Re-assessment (up to 3 months):* • To help determine if ready to move to restoration phase – plaque scores, improvements to diet and daily self-care routines. • Active surveillance of arrested lesions/tooth-restoration complexes (TRCs). • If CRSA still high/uncontrolled, then cycle phased care back to MIOC Domain 2. *Definitive treatment:* • Definitive direct/indirect restorations as indicated. • Removable partial denture to replace missing teeth. *2-3-month recall consultation:* • Longitudinal CRSA • Review COM-B, goal-setting behavioural adherence to preventive regimens • Active surveillance of lesions/TRCs • If stable, then proceed with possible fixed tooth replacement option as decided with patient, *shared decision-making.*		What are the properties of glass-ionomer cements that make them useful for stabilisation of cavitated carious lesions? What are the differences between temporary, provisional and definitive restorations in terms of the materials used and their clinical indications?

MIOC Domain 3: Minimally Invasive Dentistry (MID)			
	Appointment functions/outcomes	**Team/appt details**	**Comments**
Appointment 4 onwards	• Restore/repair tooth restoration complexes (TRCs) as appropriate ("5Rs"). • Review of plaque score after 6 weeks. • Continue preventive advice and periodontal care. • Reinforcement of preventive strategies to control disease.	Multiple visits of surgery time and staff time of GDP/DT and one dental nurse	
MIOC Domain 4: Recall			
	Appointment functions/outcomes	**Team/appt details**	**Comments**
Recall/ re-assessment appointment(s)	• Longitudinal CRSA • Review COM-B, goal-setting behavioural adherence to preventive regimes • Active surveillance of early/arrested lesions/TRCs If stable, then proceed with possible fixed tooth replacement option as decided with patient, *shared decision-making*.	30 minutes with GDP/DT and dental nurse.	Customised recall interval in accordance with NICE guidelines (https://www.nice.org.uk/guidance/cg19) and local assessment of risk factors. How would you decide on the recall interval for this patient? What goals would you set in preparation for the next recall consultation?

10.2.2 How Would You Manage the Following High-Risk Child?

A female patient, aged 7 years, attends your practice as a new patient. Her last dental visit was approximately 2 years previously at another practice. She attends with her mother, has a history of irregular attendance and has active caries present. Her sister, aged 14 years, also has apparent caries resulting in cavitation of several teeth.

Suggested care pathway using phased courses of treatment

MIOC Domain 1: Identify		
Appointment functions/outcomes	**Team/appt details**	**Comments**
Pre-attendance clinical data collection — Questionnaire accessed from online portal or completed on attendance, 15 minutes prior to appointment 1, by patient and mother regarding presenting medical conditions, dental concerns and expectations.	Completed by reception team and reviewed with clinical team.	What are the benefits of a pre-attendance questionnaire? What information could/should be included in the questionnaire? https://cgdent.uk/standards-guidance/
Appointment 1 — • Review of pre-attendance questionnaire. • Initial consultation and examination. • Identification of carious cavities in ULD, URC. • Early lesions URD, URE, LRE and erupting LL6 and LR6. • Photographs and radiographs taken – radiography in accordance with CGDent guidelines (see https://cgdent.uk/selection-criteria-for-dental-radiography/) – left and right bitewings • Provide diet diary for completion	15–30 minutes of surgery time and staff time of GDP/DT and one dental nurse.	What are the pertinent factors that are used to glean the risk/susceptibility of the patient?
Initial caries risk/susceptibility assessment (CRSA): High		
	Clinical photographs and radiographs taken by suitably trained member of oral healthcare team on completion of appointment 1 (could use a separate room to avoid surgery usage)	What clinical findings can be seen from these images/radiographs? What should the time interval be between appointments 1 and 2 for this patient?

MIOC Domain 2: Disease Control/Lesion Prevention			
	Appointment functions/outcomes	**Team/appt details**	**Comments**
Appointment 2	• Discussion of findings from appointment 1, diagnosis/prognosis. • Findings/significance of CRSA explained. • Primary prevention advice: oral hygiene routines, dietary control, fluoride usage. • Discussion of use of fluoride and adjunctive remineralising agents. • Provide diet diary for completion. • Demonstration/observation of oral hygiene procedures. • Suggest goals for improvements in control of disease – COM-B behaviour modelling/goal-setting including the caregiver.	30 minutes of surgery time and staff time of oral health educator.	The functions/outcomes of appointments 1 and 2 could be merged into one longer appointment, depending on clinical resource and patient logistics. What goals might you consider setting at this time? How would you engage the caregiver?

CRSA confirmed as HIGH *(see below)*.

CRSA				What should be the interval between appointments 2 and 3?

Status	High Risk	Low Risk
Lesions – current or 2 or more new, progressing or restored lesions in the last two years. State of activity.	✓	
General Factors		
Diet	✓	
Fluoride use	✓	
Health		✓
Medications		✓
Social		✓
Age	✓	
Oral Factors		
Oral hygiene	✓	
Saliva	✓	
Plaque	✓	
Bacterial balance in oral biofilm	✓	

| **Appointment 3** | • Discuss findings of diet diary.
• Explanation of investigations and identification of high caries risk/susceptibility, periodontal risk/susceptibility.
• Review outcome of goals set at end of appointment 2.
• Dialogue of options and discussion to include use of caries removal methods as appropriate, e.g. chemo-therapeutic, rotary, hand instruments, etc.
• Assess COM-B behavioural adherence (good) and finalise phased, personalised care plan with prognosis. | 30 minutes of surgery time and staff time of GDP/DT and one dental nurse. | What are the important findings from a diet diary, to translate to the patient with regards to their sugar intake and dental caries?

Are there other health messages the oral healthcare team can provide?

https://www.england.nhs.uk/wp-content/uploads/2016/04/making-every-contact-count.pdf |

Continued

MIOC Domain 2: Disease Control/Lesion Prevention —cont'd			
	Appointment functions/outcomes	**Team/appt details**	**Comments**
	Phased, personalised care plan (PCP) *Acute/stabilisation phase:* • Oral hygiene advice, diet recommendation, fluoride toothpaste/other adjunctive remineralisation agents. • Stabilisation of carious lesions ULD and URC – glass-ionomer cements as needed. Consider lesion stage and risk of symptoms or sepsis before exfoliation. • Topical fluoride application URD, URE, LRE, LR6, LL6. • Use of silver diammine fluoride (SDF)/Hall technique to stabilise/restore. *Review at one month:* • Re-assess risk factors. • Consider further topical fluoride application and preventive fissure sealants to molar teeth as erupt. • Shared decision-making with child and parent(s)		What are the properties of glass-ionomer cements that make them useful for stabilisation of cavitated carious lesions? How can topical fluoride be best applied?
MIOC Domain 3: Minimally Invasive Dentistry (MID)			
	Appointment functions/outcomes	**Team/appt details**	**Comments**
Appointment 4	• Restore ULD and URC – glass-ionomer cement. • Reinforce preventive strategies to control disease. • Topical fluoride application URD, URE, LRE, LR6, LL6. • Preventive fissure sealants for first permanent molars as they erupt.	30 minutes with GDP or DT and dental nurse	
MIOC Domain 4: Recall			
	Appointment functions/outcomes	**Team/appt details**	**Comments**
Recall/ re-assessment appointment(s)	• Longitudinal CRSA • Review COM-B, goal-setting behavioural adherence to preventive regimens (patient and caregiver) • Active surveillance of early/arrested lesions/TRCs	15 minutes with GDP/DT and dental nurse.	Customised recall interval in accordance with NICE guidelines (https://www.nice.org.uk/guidance/cg19) and local assessment of risk factors. How would you decide on the recall interval for this patient? What goals would you set in preparation for the next recall consultation?

785Pathways85

10.2.3 How Would You Manage the Following High-Risk Older Adult Patient?

A male patient, aged 70 years, attends your practice for the second time. He has recently been widowed, and you are aware of a change in his confidence. His last visit had been approximately 18 months previously, and he had been unable to attend sooner because he had been nursing his wife for the past year.

Suggested care pathway using phased courses of treatment

MIOC Domain 1: Identify			
	Appointment functions/outcomes	**Team/appt details**	**Comments**
Pre-attendance clinical data collection	Questionnaire accessed from online portal or completed on attendance, 15 minutes prior to appointment 1, by patient regarding presenting medical conditions, dental concerns and expectations.	Completed by reception team and reviewed with clinical team.	What are the benefits of a pre-attendance questionnaire? What information could/should be included in the questionnaire? https://cgdent.uk/standards-guidance/
Appointment 1	• Review of pre-attendance questionnaire. • Initial consultation and examination. • Identification of carious cavities proximally in LL3, LL4, LL5. • Poor level of oral hygiene – visible plaque seen/documented. • BPE recorded – scores 2/3 in all sextants. • Photographs and radiographs taken-radiography in accordance with CGDent guidelines (see https://cgdent.uk/selection-criteria-for-dental-radiography/). • Provide diet diary for completion.	30 minutes of surgery time and staff time of GDP/DT and one dental nurse.	What are the pertinent factors that are used to glean the risk/susceptibility assessment of the patient? How would you manage this case differently from the other adult cases discussed? It is important to spend personal time with the patient, for social and mental well-being support. https://www.england.nhs.uk/wp-content/uploads/2016/04/making-every-contact-count.pdf
Initial caries risk/susceptibility assessment (CRSA): High			
		Clinical photographs and radiographs taken by suitably trained member of oral healthcare team on completion of appointment 1 (could use a separate room to avoid surgery usage)	What clinical findings can be seen from this anterior clinical pre-operative view? What should the time interval be between appointments 1 and 2 for this patient?

Continued

MIOC Domain 2: Disease Control/Lesion Prevention			
	Appointment functions/outcomes	Team/appt details	Comments
Appointment 2	• Discussion of findings from appointment 1, diagnosis/prognosis. • Findings/significance of CRSA explained. • Primary prevention advice: oral hygiene routines, dietary control, fluoride usage. • Plaque disclosing carried out. • Saliva testing (if required). • Discussion of use of fluoride and adjunctive remineralising agents. • Provide diet diary for completion. • Demonstration/observation of oral hygiene procedures. • Suggest goals for improvements in control of disease – COM-B behaviour modelling/goal-setting.	45 minutes of surgery time and staff time of oral health educator.	The functions/outcomes of appointments 1 and 2 could be merged into one longer appointment, depending on clinical resource and patient logistics. What goals might you consider setting at this stage?
	CRSA confirmed as HIGH *(see below)*.		

CRSA			
Status	High Risk	Low Risk	
Lesions – current or 2 or more new, progressing or restored lesions in the last two years. State of activity.	✓		
General Factors			
Diet	✓		
Fluoride use	✓		
Health	✓		
Medications	✓		
Social	✓		
Age	✓		
Oral Factors			
Oral hygiene	✓		
Saliva	✓		
Plaque	✓		
Bacterial balance in oral biofilm	✓		

Comment alongside CRSA section: What should be the interval between appointments 2 and 3?

Appointment 3	• Discuss findings of diet diary. • Explanation of investigations and identification of high caries risk/susceptibility, periodontal risk/susceptibility. • Review outcome of goals set at end of appointment 2. • Dialogue of options and discussion to include use of caries removal methods as appropriate, e.g. chemotherapeutic, rotary, hand instruments, etc. • Assess COM-B behavioural adherence (good) and finalise phased, personalised care plan with prognosis.	30 minutes of surgery time and staff time of GDP/DT and one dental nurse.	What are the important findings from a diet diary, to translate to the patient with regards to their sugar intake and dental caries? Are there other health messages the oral healthcare team can provide?

MIOC Domain 2: Disease Control/Lesion Prevention—cont'd			
	Appointment functions/outcomes	**Team/appt details**	**Comments**
	Phased, personalised care plan (PCP)		What are the properties of glass-ionomer cements that make them useful for stabilisation of cavitated carious lesions?
	Acute/stabilisation phase:		
	• Oral hygiene advice, diet recommendation, prescription 5000ppm fluoride toothpaste/other adjunctive remineralisation agents.		
	• Stabilisation of carious lesions LL3, LL4, LL5 – glass-ionomer cements as needed.		
	Review at 1 month:		
	• Re-assess risk factors.		
	• Renewal of prescription for 5000ppm fluoride toothpaste.		
	• Consider possible approaches for replacement of missing teeth once CRSA status is low.		
MIOC Domain 3: Minimally Invasive Dentistry (MID)			
	Appointment Functions/Outcomes	**Team/appt details**	**Comments**
Appointment 4	• Restore/repair TRCs as appropriate.	30 minutes with GDP or DT and dental nurse	What would you consider to be an acceptable plaque score?
	• Review of plaque score after 6 weeks.		
	• Continue preventive advice and periodontal care.		
	• Reinforce strategies to control disease.		
MIOC Domain 4: Recall			
	Appointment functions/outcomes	**Team/appt details**	**Comments**
Recall/ re-assessment appointment (s)	• Longitudinal CRSA	20 minutes with GDP/DT and dental nurse.	Customised recall interval in accordance with NICE guidelines (https://www.nice.org.uk/guidance/cg19) and local assessment of risk factors.
	• Review COM-B, goal-setting behavioural adherence to preventive regimens		
	• Active surveillance of early/arrested lesions/TRCs		How would you decide on the recall interval for this patient?
			What goals would you set in preparation for the next recall consultation?

10.2.4 How Would You Manage the Following Low-Risk Adult Patient?

A female patient, aged 29 years, attends your practice for a recall visit. Her last visit was approximately 9 months previously. She has a history of regular attendance.

Suggested care pathway using phased courses of treatment

MIOC Domain 1: Identify			
	Appointment functions/outcomes	**Team/appt details**	**Comments**
Pre-attendance clinical data collection	Questionnaire accessed from online portal or completed on attendance, 15 minutes prior to appointment 1, by patient regarding presenting medical conditions, dental concerns and expectations.	Completed by reception team and reviewed with clinical team.	What are the benefits of a pre-attendance questionnaire? What information could/ should be included in the questionnaire? https:// cgdent.uk/standards-guidance/
Appointment 1	• Review of pre-attendance questionnaire. • Initial consultation and examination. • Identification of stained occlusal fissures on molar teeth. • No obvious changes in appearance for last 2 years. • Periodontal condition – good. BPE recorded (0/1 scores in all sextants). Calculus present lingual lower anteriors. • Photographs and radiographs taken – radiography in accordance with CGDent guidelines (see https://cgdent.uk/selection-criteria-for-dental-radiography/). • Provide diet diary for completion.	15–30 minutes of surgery time and staff time of GDP/ DT and one dental nurse.	What are the pertinent factors that are used to glean the risk/ susceptibility of the patient? How would you manage this case differently from the other cases? Is the diet diary strictly necessary for this patient?
Initial caries risk/susceptibility assessment (CRSA): Low			
		Clinical photographs and radiographs taken by suitably trained member of oral healthcare team on completion of appointment 1 (could use a separate room to avoid surgery usage)	What clinical findings can be seen from this upper occlusal clinical pre-operative view? What should the time interval be between appointments 1 and 2 for this patient?

MIOC Domain 2: Disease Control/Lesion Prevention			
	Appointment functions/outcomes	**Team/appt details**	**Comments**
Appointment 2	• Discussion of findings from appointment 1 and diagnosis/prognosis. • Findings/significance of CRSA explained as well as how to maintain the low level of risk/susceptibility. • Demonstration/observation/reinforcement of oral hygiene procedures. • Suggest goals for improvements in control of disease – COM-B behaviour modelling. • Final personalised care plan made with recall interval of 6 months to review oral hygiene routines and effectiveness, with a view to extending recall interval further if continued stability achieved.	15–30 minutes of surgery time and staff time of oral health educator.	The functions/outcomes of appointments 1 and 2 could be merged into one longer appointment, depending on clinical resource and patient logistics. What goals might you consider setting at this stage?

CRSA

Status	High Risk	Low Risk
Lesions – current or 2 or more new, progressing or restored lesions in the last two years. State of activity.		✓
General Factors		
Diet		✓
Fluoride use		✓
Health		✓
Medications		✓
Social		✓
Age		✓
Oral Factors		
Oral hygiene	✓	
Saliva		
Plaque		
Bacterial balance in oral biofilm		

MIOC Domain 4: Recall			
	Appointment functions/outcomes	**Team/appt details**	**Comments**
Recall/ re-assessment appointment(s)	• Longitudinal CRSA • Review COM-B, goal-setting behavioural adherence to preventive regimens	20 minutes with GDP/DT and dental nurse.	Customised recall interval in accordance with NICE guidelines (https://www.nice.org.uk/guidance/cg19) and local assessment of risk factors. How would you decide on the recall interval for this patient? What goals would you set in preparation for the next recall consultation?

INDEX

Note: Page numbers followed by '*f*' indicate figures, '*t*' indicate tables, and '*b*' indicate boxes.